Vision
and
Reading

Vision and Reading

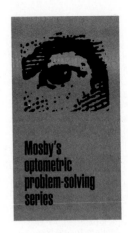

Mosby's Optometric problem-solving series

Edited by

Ralph P. Garzia
OD, FAAO

Associate Professor
School of Optometry
University of Missouri–St. Louis
Chief, Pediatrics/Binocular Vision Service
Director of Optometric Services
Center for Eye Care
St. Louis, Missouri

Series Editor

Richard London
MA, OD, FAAO

Diplomate, Binocular Vision and Perception
Pediatric and Rehabilitative Optometry
Oakland, California

with 54 illustrations

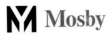 Mosby

St. Louis Baltimore Boston Carlsbad Chicago Naples New York Philadelphia Portland
London Madrid Mexico City Singapore Sydney Tokyo Toronto Wiesbaden

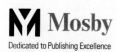
Dedicated to Publishing Excellence

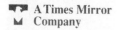
A Times Mirror
Company

Executive Editor: Martha Sasser
Associate Developmental Editor: Kellie F. White
Project Manager: John Rogers
Production Editors: George B. Stericker Jr., Helen Hudlin
Design Coordinator: Renée Duenow
Series Design: Jeanne Wolfgeher
Manufacturing Supervisor: Linda Ierardi
Production and Editing: Carlisle Publishers Services
Cover Photography: John Patrick Phelan

Text in cover photograph modified from Fritz J: *Where do you think you're going Christopher Columbus* (p. 9), New York, 1980, GP Putnam's Sons.

Printed in the United States of America
Composition by Carlisle Communications, Ltd.
Printing/binding by R. R. Donnelley

Mosby–Year Book, Inc.
11830 Westline Industrial Drive
St. Louis, Missouri 63146

International Standard Book Number 0-8151-3438-X

96 97 98 99 00 / 9 8 7 6 5 4 3 2 1

Contributors

John A. Baro, PhD
Instructional Designer
NASA Classroom of the Future
Wheeling Jesuit College
Wheeling, West Virginia

Eric Borsting, OD, MS
Assistant Professor
Southern California College of
   Optometry
Fullerton, California

Michael T. Cron, OD
Professor
Associate Dean
College of Optometry
Ferris State University
Big Rapids, Michigan

Aaron S. Franzel, OD
Assistant Professor
School of Optometry
University of Missouri–St. Louis
St. Louis, Missouri

Ralph P. Garzia, OD
Associate Professor
School of Optometry
University of Missouri–St. Louis
St. Louis, Missouri

Sylvia R. Garzia, RPT
Physical Therapist
City of St. Charles School District
St. Charles, Missouri

Louis G. Hoffman, OD
Professor (retired)
Southern California College of
   Optometry
Fullerton, California

Katie LeCluyse, PhD
Department of Psychology
University of New Orleans
New Orleans, Louisiana

Stephen Lehmkuhle, PhD
Professor
School of Optometry
University of Missouri–St. Louis
St. Louis, Missouri

Richard Littell, PhD
Department of Psychology
University of New Orleans
New Orleans, Louisiana

William F. Long, OD, PhD
Associate Professor
School of Optometry
University of Missouri–St. Louis
Coordinator of Photographic Services
Center for Eye Care
St. Louis, Missouri

William Lovegrove, PhD
Professor
Vice Chancellor's Unit
University of Wollongong
Wollongong, New South Wales
Australia

W. Howard McAlister, OD, MA, MPH

Associate Professor
Director of Residencies
School of Optometry
University of Missouri–St. Louis
St. Louis, Missouri

Steven B. Nicholson, OD

Eyecare Specialties
Hastings, Nebraska

Jack E. Richman, OD

Professor
New England College of Optometry
Director
Pediatric Optometry and Binocular Vision
   Services
The New England Eye Institute
Boston, Massachusetts

Joy Rosner, OD

Associate Professor
College of Optometry
University of Houston
Houston, Texas

Barbara A. Steinman, OD, MS

School of Optometry
University of Missouri–St. Louis
St. Louis, Missouri

Scott B. Steinman, OD, PhD

Associate Professor
Southern College of Optometry
Memphis, Tennessee

Mary C. Williams, PhD

Professor and Chair
Department of Psychology
University of New Orleans
New Orleans, Louisiana

Dale M. Willows, PhD

Department of Instruction and Special
   Education
Ontario Institute for Studies in Education
Toronto, Ontario
Canada

Timothy Wingert, OD

Associate Professor
School of Optometry
University of Missouri–St. Louis
Chief of Primary Care
Center for Eye Care
St. Louis, Missouri

To Sylvia
Nicholas, Camille, Luke
Mom and Dad
Louis and Rose Mastrian

Preface

The National Institute of Child Health and Human Development has spent $30 million over the past 10 years to investigate the nature and causes of learning disabilities. Reading disabilities constitute 80% of learning disabilities. Despite society's efforts, the population of reading disabled is expanding at such an alarming rate that the levels can no longer be considered "special" (i.e., deserving of special pedagogical efforts and placement) but as having a regular place on the landscape of education. Difficulties with reading affect so many individuals that all sources of influence must be considered.

This volume is about vision, visual processing and reading, and anomalies of the visual system that are associated with reading disability. It is obvious even to the most casual observer that normal reading begins with an active visual process. However, this simple association has been lost on many educators, psychologists, and, most disappointingly of all, many eye care practitioners. This was not always the case, however. In decades past, in the era of single-deficit hypotheses of learning disabilities, anomalies of vision and visual development were considered important potential sources of interference with reading acquisition. The fundamental conceptual framework held that the visual processes necessary for reading required extensive and intricate learning.

However, when the causes of learning disabilities were discovered to be multifactorial, the study of the relationship between vision and reading declined, previous lessons were systematically forgotten, and finally regularly ignored. If not for the individual monk and organizational monasteries, the concept that vision is important for reading would have been lost completely.

The explanation for this attitude is not immediately self-evident. One difficulty may be that early vision investigators were probably looking in the wrong place, operating under limited definitional constraints. Vision is intuitively assumed as operating entirely in a spatial domain. Traditional studies of form discrimination, figure-ground perception, and visual closure bear witness to this. However, vision must also be understood as having a temporal component. There must be proper temporal sequence of all visually related processes (perhaps even before integration with language and linguistic processes) for reading to proceed efficiently. Attention must shift, the eyes must move, and the magnocellular and parvocellular visual pathways must have a proper timing differential. It is not just a simple matter of disabled readers having slower visual processing times. If this were the case, the central nervous system would probably adapt to this slower temporal rate. The visual system of a disabled reader is best conceptualized as sputtering, as having inconsistently timed connections between the multiple subcomponents of visual processing.

Through the work of Bill Lovegrove, Mary Williams, Bruno Breitmeyer, and their colleagues, there has been a reviviscence of vision and its relationship to reading. Those interested in vision and reading are indebted to them. However, misology persists. Perhaps this volume will help to reverse this attitude.

The use of the term *dyslexia* to describe children that have difficulty reading has been avoided throughout this volume (except in the Introduction). In its place, the operational description of "reading disability" is used. The use of this nomenclature avoids the incessant confusion surrounding the term *dyslexia*. Originally associated with reading problems caused by brain injury, the term became pejorative and prejudicial and was, therefore, avoided. It has since cascaded into the visual science—and to only a lesser extent—the special education lexicon as a satisfactory synonym for reading disability. Children who make letter reversals or word transpositions when reading, spelling, or writing are often designated as dyslexic, suggesting that this is a special form or subtype of reading disability. Dyslexia has also been described as the particular cause of reading difficulties. For these reasons, it is best to leave "dyslexia" at home.

Acknowledgments

I want to thank Rick London for choosing me to edit a book on vision and reading, Beth Busemeyer for her bibliographic assistance on most of the chapters, and Janice White for creating the jumbled text on the cover. A special thanks also to Kellie White and Amy Dubin of Mosby–Year Book and Cindy Trickel of Carlisle Publishers Services for their patience, cooperation, and hard work.

All of the authors and co-authors of this volume are recognized scholars in their respective disciplines. It is a privilege and honor to have my name associated with theirs.

Ralph P. Garzia
University of Missouri–St. Louis

Contents

Vision
and
Reading

Introduction

Louis G. Hoffman

The relationship between vision and reading continues to be an ambiguous issue for professionals involved in both areas. In the usual reading situation, it appears obvious that reading requires the visual system. In fact, depending on the definition of vision used, even the reading of Braille involves visualization, a facet of visual processing. The complexities of both vision and reading processes make the study of each difficult, and an evaluation of the relationship between the two perplexing.

An important issue in examining this relationship is how vision is defined. A somewhat limited definition will almost certainly reveal a limited relationship, and an expansive definition, a greater relationship. Vision can be defined as a continuous and integrative process that can be divided into three components: (1) visual acuity, including refractive status; (2) visual efficiency, which is composed of oculomotor, accommodative, and binocular vision skills; and (3) visual perceptual- motor skills, which represent the ability to recognize and discriminate visual stimuli and interpret them correctly in the light of previous experiences. These components together constitute the visual information–processing system. Each of them is complex; no single component can be considered a definition of vision, nor can only one test be used for evaluation. Reading is an equally complex process that leads to comparable conclusions—i.e., it is continuous and integrative, defying singular definition and testing.

Attempts at relating vision and reading have tended to focus on simple one-to-one relationships between components. However, it is very difficult to take a complex function, separate it into its constituent elements, and predict the contribution of each to the operation of the entire process. One also must consider that people are quite resilient and can develop compensations for their shortcomings. This can be accomplished naturally, or by the use of artificial devices provided by professionals. The individual with reduced visual acuity may simply hold reading material closer to increase magnification. Surprisingly, reading may continue quite efficiently compared with another individual with normal visual acuity but with other associated problems. A child with visual memory deficits, relying on verbal information, may perform quite well in certain situations under certain conditions (see Chapter 8). However, we also should be aware that tasks requiring the use of a deficient skill are frequently avoided. The child who gets headaches when reading has a simple way of eliminating them!

It is obvious that reading will be impaired by insufficient illumination, low contrast, or veiling glare (see Chapter 5). Nevertheless, many of us can remember reading by a dim hallway light after we were expected to be asleep. The individual who enjoys reading and is proficient can overcome many distractions. This does not mean that illumination, contrast, and glare are not important determinants of reading efficiency but rather that they affect each of us to a different degree.

The ophthalmic and educational literature[1-4] supports the fact that a segment of the reading-disabled population manifests some deficiency in visual information–processing skills (see also Chapters 6 and 7). The impact of this deficiency on reading is dependent on the stage of reading development. For example, visual perceptual-motor skills (directionality, form and figure-ground discrimination, visual closure, visual memory, visual-motor integration) may have a greater effect on a beginning reader than on an established reader, whereas visual efficiency skills (oculomotor, accommodative, binocular vision) may affect both.[1]

Automaticity of visual information processing is necessary for the most efficient reading and learning. Individuals who must devote a portion of their intelligence to the mechanics of seeing will have "less" intelligence left to devote to learning. Therefore, the more intelligent individual may be able to overcome vision problems and continue to read effectively, but not to full potential.

Dyslexia is a term frequently used when discussing *reading disability*. They are different. Dyslexia is a medical term that suggests a specific syndrome of behaviors and etiology (see Chapters 12 and 13). However, there is no generally accepted symptomatology associated with dyslexia, other than reading difficulties. Educators generally consider a child who is below a designated level of reading ability to be dyslexic. The extent of the deficit and the inclusion of other deficits in the description vary depending on the authority quoted. Dyslexia is a language-based reading disability usually in the absence of other specific learning problems. Reading disability is considered a type of learning disability, frequently accompanied by other academic problems. There have been attempts at subtyping dyslexia based on spelling patterns (for example, dysphonesia, dyseidesia, and dyskinesia or a combined form).[5] Reading and spelling are considered, but comprehension is not. Despite many efforts, no unitary definition or system of classification has emerged.

Not all children with learning disabilities have reading difficulties, nor do all children with reading difficulties have learning disabilities.[6] The attention paid to educational problems by the media frequently leads to confusion. At the time of the Soviet Union's launching of the sputnik satellite, the emphasis in the learning disabilities community was on mathematics. Educators subsequently developed the idea of modern math, and the media considered the problem solved. The emphasis then shifted to reading.

Although there are children with reading disability who do not manifest vision problems and children with vision problems who do not manifest reading disability, vision problems can be considered contributory factors.[7] As our understanding of the visual system increases, so will the ability to comprehend its participation and potential interference in the reading process. Recent evidence of magnocellular (M) and parvocellular (P) visual pathway functions is an excellent example. It has been shown[8,9] that a deficient M pathway is associated with reading disabilities (see Chapters 9, 10, and 11). The effect of colored filters on reading performance has been interpreted in the framework of restoring the normal temporal relationship between these pathways (see Chapter 14).

Correction of visual deficiencies with the use of lenses, prisms, and/or vision therapy may result in immediate improvement in reading ability. This scenario is most likely to occur in that individual whose reading skills were well established before the manifestation of the vision problem. The remediation of vision problems cannot ensure an improvement in reading. Often, following remediation, reading deficiencies remain because reading skills are inadequate. The acquisition of appropriate reading skills is within the purview and responsibility of the educator.

This leads to another aspect of reading that must be considered—reading readiness (see Chapters 3 and 4). Educators generally agree that there are prerequisite skills for reading. But the agreement ends there. Children develop at different rates, which means that some do not reach the developmental levels deemed necessary for success in beginning reading. This results in these children having inadequately developed reading-readiness skills when they begin formal reading instruction. Although skills, both acquired and developed, can be enumerated, it cannot be said with certainty that the absence of any particular one will result in reduced reading ability. Reading readiness requires visual and auditory perceptual skills, including auditory-visual and visual-motor integration. The role of the vision care specialist is the screening, evaluation, and remediation of deficits in all components of vision.

There are many disciplines involved with the complex visual processes associated with reading. There are some vision specialists, however, whose approach is simplistic and whose concerns are limited to ocular health and refractive status. Psychologists and educators may be concerned with the visual perceptual-motor development of the child. Speech and language specialists may be concerned with auditory-visual integration. It must be understood that these are all components of vision and that they are interrelated. Frequently, remediation of one aspect of vision will result in improvement in another area.[10] Therefore, it is imperative that vision be evaluated with an understanding of the entire visual information-processing system, so that appropriate relationships with reading can be discerned.

There are two important questions concerning remediation of vision problems: When is it appropriate to recommend remediation? And what constitutes remediation? The remediation of vision problems should be implemented to whatever degree necessary when and if such problems are detected. Children with anomalies in ocular health, refractive status, visual efficiency, and visual perceptual-motor skills should be given appropriate treatment. Treatment is indicated when the existing vision condition is determined to be adversely affecting health, performance, or behavior.

There is a tendency for many vision care and educational specialists to recommend remediation only if there is a high degree of certainty that improved reading performance will result. Such opinions are extremely myopic. The purpose and goal of all forms of remediation is the enhancement of vision performance. It is anticipated that the improvement of vision performance will result in a child better able to benefit from pedagogy. A child with one diopter of myopia may have reading disability, and most clinicians would conclude that this is probably not a significant contributing factor to the reading problem. However, correction of the myopia would be contemplated, probably for its effect on other aspects of vision performance. The same could be said for the treatment of allergies or other conditions that affect comfort and the learning environment. A similar rationale exists for vision problems detected during an evaluation of a reading-disabled child. They can affect many aspects of performance and behavior besides reading and should not be ignored. Sometimes minor deficiencies may have major consequences. This should be explained in as much detail as possible to patients or parents.

Because of the demonstrated relationship of vision to reading, the vision care specialist should perform a comprehensive vision evaluation encompassing all aspects of vision for any patient having reading problems. The educator should be provided with information relative to the patient's visual strengths and weaknesses and, if possible, how these might affect reading performance. This information would be crucial for the selection of the appropriate teaching methodology for the individual. Finally, the eye care specialist should provide remediation to whatever degree necessary for detected vision problems. This might include lenses, prisms, vision therapy, or any combination of these.

The goal of all professionals involved in vision and reading should be to provide a well-developed and efficiently functioning visual system, with the best environmental conditions for learning. Continued research and the development of more sophisticated and precise testing methods will certainly enhance our understanding of the role of vision in reading.

References

1. Flax N: The contribution of visual problems to learning disability, *J Am Optom Assoc* 41:841-845, 1970.
2. Solan HA, Mozlin R: The correlations of perceptual-motor maturation to readiness and reading in kindergarten and the primary grades, *J Am Optom Assoc* 57:28-35, 1986.
3. Solan HA: A comparison of the influence of verbal-successive and spatial-simultaneous factors on achieving readers in fourth and fifth grade, *J Learn Disabil* 20:237-242, 1987.
4. Grisham JD, Simons HD: Refractive error and the reading process: a literature analysis, *J Am Optom Assoc* 63:411-417, 1992.
5. Boder E: Developmental dyslexia: a diagnostic approach based on three typical reading-spelling patterns, *Dev Med Child Neurol* 15:663-687, 1973.
6. Solan HA: Overview of learning disabilities. In Scheiman MM, Rouse MW (eds): *Optometric management of learning related vision disorders*, St Louis, 1994, Mosby.
7. Garzia RP: The relationship between visual efficiency problems and learning. In Scheiman MM, Rouse MW (eds): *Optometric management of learning related vision disorders*, St Louis, 1994, Mosby.
8. Garzia RP, Nicholson SB: Visual function and reading disability: an optometric viewpoint, *J Am Optom Assoc* 61:88-97, 1990.
9. Lovegrove WJ, Martin F, Slaghuis W: A theoretical and experimental case for a visual deficit in specific reading disability, *Cogn Neuropsychol* 3:225-267, 1986.
10. Hoffman LG: The effect of accommodative deficiencies on the developmental level of perceptual skills, *Am J Optom Physiol Opt* 59:254-262, 1982.

Public Health Issues and Reading Disability

W. Howard McAlister
Ralph P. Garzia
Steven B. Nicholson

Key Terms

epidemiology	readability	sex differences
public health	readability formulae	stability
literacy	distribution	

Literacy

Health has traditionally been defined as merely the absence of disease or disability. This definition has evolved over the years to a more positive meaning. In the Constitution of the World Health Organization health is defined as a state of complete physical, mental, and social well-being and not merely the absence of disease and infirmity. This has been expanded also to include the ability to lead a socially and economically productive life. Given the current definition, illiteracy could easily be classified as a health anomaly. Illiteracy decreases the quality of life for the afflicted individual as well as society as a whole. This makes illiteracy of vital public health importance.

Literacy should be considered more than those skills that are taught in school and reported as reading or writing levels attained in achievement test scores. What is important for most individuals is the functional aspects of literacy. Functional literacy is those literacy skills practiced in the extra-scholastic environment, the reading and writing skills, that are necessary to understand and utilize the printed materials to which one is exposed in the environment for work, leisure, and personal survival[1]—in other words, reading for daily living.

CLINICAL PEARL

Literacy should be considered more than those skills taught in school and reported as reading or writing levels attained in achievement test scores. What is important for most individuals are the functional aspects of literacy.

As the definition of health has changed over time, so has that of literacy. There are no codified and universally accepted standards for defining literacy. A standard used just a century ago was a person's ability to sign his or her name. Today nearly all young adults can do that. Functional literacy was first defined by a government agency in the 1930s as 3 or more years of formal schooling.[2] The level of education necessary for functional literacy has increased steadily since then. During World War II, the United States Army used a fourth grade educational level.[3] In 1947 the Census Bureau designated fifth grade, and raised the level to the sixth grade by 1952.[4] The U.S. Office of Education placed the standard at the eighth grade in 1960.[5] From the 1970s, high school completion is a frequently used criterion level of educational attainment for functional literacy.[6] The mean educational level for the nation is now near twelfth grade. In 1930, 88% of the adult population had at least a third grade education. In 1950 nearly 90% had completed at least fifth grade. However, in 1960 only 78% of the adult population had at least an eighth grade educational level. By 1980 only 68.7% had completed high school.[2] If one uses high school graduation as the criterion for literacy, then 45 million adult Americans in the 1980s were illiterate.

Several studies have attempted to quantify the reading level of young adults. The National Center for Health Statistics[7] issued a report in 1973 indicating that in the 12-to-17-year-old group, 4.8% did not attain a literacy level of beginning fourth grade reading performance. Fisher[8] reported that of adults 14 years of age or older 7% read below a fifth grade level, with 30% below the eighth grade. The U.S. Department of Defense statistics indicate that 18-to-23-year-olds have a median reading level of 9.6, with 18% below seventh grade level.[9] The Young Adult Literacy Study found that 6% of young adults read below fourth grade level and one in four below eighth grade.[10]

The ability to read is crucial to function effectively to any degree in our society. All demographic groups—whether broken down by occupation, race, educational level, or sex—read for information, political awareness, social development, and entertainment to varying degrees.[11] Street and traffic signs, billboards, and printed directions also account for a substantial amount of daily reading activity. Studies on what and when adults read have shown that newspapers are the most commonly read material. In the Adult Functional Reading Study, 7 of 10 adults read or looked at a newspaper daily for an average of 35 minutes.[10] There was an average of 61 minutes of reading at work, and on average 47 minutes/day reading books. The most commonly read book was, not surprisingly, the Bible, which is read about 29 minutes/ day. In a survey sponsored by the book-publishing industry,[12] 33% of adults 16 years and older read at least one book a month and 55% read at least one book in the last month. However, nearly 40% never read books, and 6% don't read anything! Approximately 3 in 10 said they don't like reading.

CLINICAL PEARL

All demographic groups—whether broken down by occupation, race, educational level, or sex—read for information, political awareness, social development, and entertainment to varying degrees.

Different reading materials can have significantly different demands on reading skill level. This is considered their "readability." The lead articles in prominent magazines (e.g., *Reader's Digest, Saturday Evening Post, Popular Mechanics*) are written at the twelfth to thirteenth grade level. This has remained largely unchanged over the past 40 years.[13] See Table 2-1 for a few more examples.[14-16]

Based on these estimates of readability, best sellers are written at the level of the bottom 30% of the population, with 18% having a reading skill level below that required for the average best seller. The only activity listed that falls within the reading level of the bottom 30% of the population is a driver's license manual.

This has important implications for clinical practitioners. The readability of instructional materials given to patients can have enormous impact on their effectiveness. If materials are written above the reading level of the patient, then their educational potential will be lost. There is fairly strong evidence[17-19] that such disparity exists for a wide range of health materials and the reading skills of their target populations.

TABLE 2-1

Readability Levels

Reading materials	Grade level
Leading magazine articles (*Reader's Digest, Popular Mechanics,* etc.)	12 to 13
Newspaper articles	9 to 12
Best sellers	>6 to 9
Apartment leases	>12
Food stamp notices	>12
Insurance policies	12
Aspirin bottle label	10
Tax forms and directions	8
Cooking instructions	8
Driver's license manual	6

Based on information from Monteith M: *J Read* 23:460-464, 1980; Kozol J: *Illiterate America,* New York, 1985, Anchor/Doubleday; and Wellborn SM: *U.S. News & World Report,* pp. 53-57, May 17, 1982.

CLINICAL PEARL

The readability of instructional materials given a patient can have enormous impact on their effectiveness. If materials are written above the reading level of the individual, then their educational potential will be lost.

There are several formula constructed to determine the reading difficulty of written materials. Readability formulas use, for example, the number of words per sentence and the number and percentage of polysyllabic words in the passage to establish readability. The SMOG, Fry, Gunning-FOG, Flesch, and Cloze are the more commonly used formulas. They do not always produce the same readability index, but they are usually within close range.

The following is an example of an informational/instructional sheet describing insurance for visual training patients.[20]

Following the first month of visual training, the claim form will be filled out and returned to the patient to be submitted; if the insured wishes the office to submit the form directly to the insurance company, include an addressed and stamped envelope. . . . If the claim is honored, thereafter, each month, included in the monthly statement, will be an insurance receipt covering the past month's visual training that is to be submitted to the insurance company; there will be no need for us to fill out an additional company form.

When readability formulas are applied to this selection, the results indicate a rather sophisticated level of required reading skill for the patient. The SMOG formula estimates this passage at a fifteenth grade level, Fry thirteenth grade, Gunning-FOG 12.8, and Flesch 13.1. Although this information sheet was probably appropriate for the patients in the practice for which it was developed, this is not the case for all practices, and it would have been difficult for many adults to fully understand.

What are the reading level demands of functional tasks that most adults 16 years and older can manage? The results of several literacy studies[21-23] can be found in the box below. They indicate that 3 to 7 million adults would have problems with the simplest tasks. Filling out job applications would pose difficulty for 5% to 8% of the adult population. The estimates are that 20% of the adult population, or 35 million people, have serious difficulties with common, everyday reading tasks. Another 10% have only marginal functional literacy.

CLINICAL PEARL

Estimates are that 20% of the adult population, or 35 million people, have serious difficulties with common everyday reading tasks, and another 10% have only marginal functional literacy.

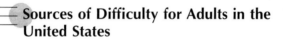

Sources of Difficulty for Adults in the United States

0.1% had difficulty recognizing the word "milk" on a bottle

2.0% made more than 1 error in understanding telephone dialing instructions

5.0% had difficulty reading housing advertisements

7.0% were unable to mark the place where their name needed to be entered on an application

8.0% scored <90% when asked simple information like height, weight, name

14% could not perform map reading, address an envelope, or write out a check

21% could not follow instructions on medicine bottles

33% failed on airline and train schedules

40% could not read 2 short paragraphs describing a blood donation program or identify the person they needed to contact

>50% had trouble completing tax forms (W-4) and calculating miles per gallon

Compiled from Murphy RT: Assessment of adult reading competence. In Nielsen DM, Hjelm HF (eds): *Reading and career education*, Newark, Del, 1975, International Reading Association; Murphy RT: *Adult functional reading study*, Princeton NJ, 1973, Educational Testing Service; and Harris L et al: *The 1971 national reading difficulty index*, Washington, DC, 1971, National Reading Center.

In 1980 only 68.7% of students completed high school. This is not a problem for a labor intensive industrial economy requiring no sophisticated communication or computational skills. However, three fourths of all jobs today require some form of information-handling capabilities, such as preparing reports, filling out forms, filing and retrieving some form of information, and following or learning from written procedures or instructions. By the year 2000, work force analysts forecast that up to 98% of all U.S. jobs will require such skills.[24]

Nearly all new employees today must possess at least basic reasoning and learning skills. In order to fully realize the productive potential of the new electronic information systems, a workplace literacy gap cannot be allowed to develop. Between now and the year 2000, for the first time in history, a majority of new jobs will require postsecondary education.[24] The jobs that are losing employment are those requiring lower skill levels; those jobs requiring little verbal aptitude will continue to decline.[25] All U.S. workers, from the bottom to the top, will need to be equipped with more sophisticated communication skills, reasoning skills, and computational and analytical skills than have ever been required. By 2000, 24% of jobs will require 4 or more years of college education, and jobs requiring the lowest skill levels will drop from 9% to 4%. In the same time period, jobs requiring the highest skill levels will increase from 24% to 41%.[24] It is clear that the quality as well as quantity of potential employees is of ever increasing importance to employers. As the next century will require increased abilities to communicate in order to empower the learner, society as a whole will pay the cost of illiteracy.[25]

It has been long established that individuals have different learning styles, for which different teaching methods are most appropriate. As long as America's employers only needed 30% to 50% of the workforce to possess a mastery of higher-order reasoning and problem-solving skills, public education could get by with a single uniform pedagogy from which only a majority of students could learn effectively.[26] It is now apparent that more attention should be given to individualized instruction in reading.

Numerous factors contribute to illiteracy. Health disorders, physical trauma, lack of educational opportunity, emotional disturbance, economic disadvantages, sensory or motor deficits, mental retardation, lack of family support and reinforcement, and inadequate medical and vision care all can hamper an individual's ability to learn to read.

CLINICAL PEARL

Health disorders, physical trauma, lack of educational opportunity, emotional disturbance, economic disadvantage, sensory or motor deficits, mental retardation, lack of family support and reinforcement, and inadequate medical and vision care all can hamper an individual's ability to learn to read.

Illiteracy can have profound and lasting impact on family functioning and the life chances of the affected individual. Not only does it interfere with academic success, but self-esteem and peer relationships also are negatively influenced. Strains are placed on parental resources and equanimity. Illiteracy is costly and burdensome to society, requiring special services in schools, institutions, and industries.

African-Americans, other minorities, Southerners, and the foreign born have been less literate on average than native-born middle class whites.[1] Poverty and unemployment also are associated with lower rates of literacy. One fifth of all children today live below the poverty level. Often associated with poverty is poor nutrition, lack of encouragement, poor medical and vision care, and decreased exposure to reading and reading materials. Illiterate adults employed in Missouri today, for example, make 42% less than those with a high school education.[25] The education of employees with illiteracy is a considerable expense to employers. Unfortunately, a too frequent destination for those who do not graduate from high school is poverty or imprisonment.[25]

With any health care anomaly, the method of management that minimizes human suffering and financial expenditure is primary prevention. With many infectious diseases this is accomplished through immunizations. To reduce the prevalence of illiteracy, we need to ensure good health and social well-being. This begins with proper prenatal care, followed by proper medical care, nutrition, and nurturing into the early adult years. Good nutrition is essential for proper development of the central nervous system. Once developed, a proper diet is required for the body's ability to use its innate capacity to learn. If primary prevention is unsuccessful, then a secondary prevention (i.e., early detection, diagnosis, and treatment) must be provided.[27] Home support in the learning process is imperative, as the education of one generation determines the economic success of the next generation.

CLINICAL PEARL

With any health care anomaly, the method of management that minimizes human suffering and financial expenditure is primary prevention. With many infectious diseases this is accomplished through immunizations. To reduce the prevalence of illiteracy, we need to ensure good health and social well-being.

Optometrists can play a key role in the prevention and treatment of reading problems by alleviating potential visual obstacles that could interfere with the patient's educational and learning opportunities. The ability to read standard print depends on a number of basic visual skills. Reduced visual acuity, double vision, and faulty visual perception are several of the visual deficits that can hinder reading ability. A child with bilateral deprivation or refractive amblyopia, or reduced acuity from ocular disease, may never be able to read standard print without timely and appropriate vision care. A presbyopic adult with illiteracy may not be able to progress in a reading program without the appropriate near point correction. School-age children with visual perceptual or processing problems may experience significant delays in acquiring reading skills, while others learn the reading basics but fail to develop fluency.

Visual anomalies such as hyperopia, binocular dysfunction, poor saccadic eye movements, and inefficient visual perceptual processing (among other dysfunctions) have been implicated[28-30] as creating adverse effects on reading performance and sustainability. Refractive errors can easily be managed by ophthalmic lens correction. Dysfunctions of binocular vision and visual perceptual delays may respond to orthoptics and vision therapy.

Third-party reimbursement has a sizable impact on the consumption of given health care services. A large segment of health care insurance plans have either not covered the treatment of reading disability or resisted compensating for such services when provided by doctors of optometry. Thus many in need of these services must either pay for the services themselves or do without such care. While many middle-class white children have received appropriate treatment, many poor African-American and Hispanic children have not.

Reading Disability

Adult illiteracy begins in childhood as reading disability. To determine that a child is a low achiever is relatively straightforward. To determine what is contributing to the reading problem and to design an effective intervention program is extremely complex and has puzzled researchers and educators for decades. Approximately 2 million children in 1989 received special education services for a learning disability. This represents just under 5% of the school-age population, and it is estimated that 75% of the identified learning-disabled students have a primary deficit in reading.[31] While these figures were compiled nationally, there are significant variations in how individual states define and identify children who are learning disabled.

CLINICAL PEARL

Approximately 2 million children in 1989 received special education services for a learning disability. This represented just under 5% of the school-age population, and it is estimated that 75% of the identified learning-disabled students had a primary deficit in reading.

The number of children identified as reading disabled has increased significantly since the enactment of the Education of All Handicapped Children Act in 1975.[32] Hallahan[33] proposed several reasons for this increase following the initial issuance of the federal regulations in the mid-1970s. One reason is that parents and educators now have a better understanding of the condition, enabling them to be more adept at identifying children with difficulties learning to read. A second responsible factor could be the impact of social/cultural changes. Increasing pollution, a rise in drug-exposed births, deficient prenatal care, broken homes, and an increase in poverty not only place the development of the central nervous system at risk, they also increase the degree of psychological stress on the families. Families are less able to provide the emotional and practical nurturing that can help a child learn. Hallahan[33] also pointed out that stress and a disruption of the family support system are a potential problem for families at all income levels. All families are faced with many demands on their time and resources, which can interfere with maintaining the optimum learning environment.

CLINICAL PEARL

The number of children identified as reading disabled has increased significantly since the enactment of the Education of All Handicapped Children Act in 1975.

In 1975 Rutter and Yule[34] provided evidence that reading ability has a bimodal distribution. This means that disabled readers are represented by a lower-end "hump" in the distribution of reading performance, which was interpreted to mean that reading disability is a discrete entity, perhaps with a specific causal mechanism(s). Later studies have not found this hump but rather a normal distribution of reading abilities. Most recently Shaywitz et al.[35] used data from the Connecticut Longitudinal Study and found that reading performance was continuous and normally distributed. They were unable to locate a group of readers who were not predicted by a normal distribution. The study followed 414 elementary-age children for 6 years. Intelligence tests were obtained for grades 1, 3, and 4, and achievement scores were administered yearly. Intelligence scores were used to determine aptitude, and standard discrepancy calculation methods were used to identify the reading-disabled students. Shaywitz et al.[35] found no distinct cutoff point delineating the reading-disabled population; instead, they found their performance to represent simply the lower end of a normally distributed reading continuum.

In addition to finding a normal distribution of reading performance, Shaywitz et al.[35] found that the diagnosis of reading disabilities was not consistent over time. Using a criterion of discrepancy of 1.5 SD between the observed achievement level and the predicted achievement level based on IQ, they found a prevalence of 6% to 7% in each grade. But, only 28% of the children classified as disabled in first grade were also classified as disabled in third grade. Only 17% of the children classified as reading disabled in first grade were still identified in sixth grade. Yet the overall prevalence in each grade was similar. While the findings may indicate that many of the students made progress and no longer met the criteria for identification, it also points out that the testing was not sensitive in the early grades to those students who would later encounter severe academic difficulty. These findings run counter to the belief that a specific reading disability is stable over time. The findings may provide further evidence of the inadequacy of the current methods of identifying those children. As Shaywitz et al.[35] discussed, these results greatly confound attempts to identify early predictors of, or a screening battery for, reading disability.

Reading-disabled populations are usually thought to comprise significantly more males than females.[36,37] In some instances males outnumber females by 3:1. Shaywitz et al.,[38] however, found no significant difference in the prevalence of reading disabilities between second and third grade boys and girls in the Connecticut Longitudinal Study. The study included a comparison of identification methods. The prevalence of reading disabilities determined by strict research criteria was compared with the prevalence of children identified and placed in special education programs by the schools. The research criteria consisted of using a regression equation to determine the discrepancy between a child's actual reading achievement and his or her predicted achievement based on the results on the WISC-R Full Scale IQ. A discrepancy of 1.5 SDs or more classified them as research-identified, reading-disabled children. School-identified children qualified for the study if they were designated as reading disabled by the school and were receiving special education services. The results revealed no significant difference between the percentage of boys and girls in the research-identified classification. But, significantly more boys were present in the school-identified group. For example, in second grade 8.7% of the 196 boys and 6.9% of the 216 girls were research-identified as having a reading disability, while 13.6% of the boys and 3.2% of the girls were identified by the school.

To better understand these differences, teachers' ratings of the children's behavior and activity were obtained with the Multigrade Inventory for Teachers. Boys received significantly poorer ratings than girls in assessments of activity, behavior, attention, fine-motor skills, and academic performance. No gender differences were found when overall ability and achievement were compared. In third grade only 45% of the school-identified children met the research-identification criteria. Shaywitz et al.[38] concluded that school-identified samples are

subject to referral bias toward boys and recommended caution when relying solely on school classifications when researching these children.[38]

Recommendations

Parents, teachers, school administrators, and society in general must
promote reading development in young children. The Report of the
Commission on Reading[39] developed the following recommendations
for producing citizens who can read with skill, with frequency, and
with satisfaction.
1. Parents should read to preschool children and informally teach
   them about reading and writing.
2. Parents should support school-aged children's continued
   growth as readers.
3. Preschool and kindergarten reading readiness programs should
   focus on reading, writing, and oral language.
4. Teachers should maintain classrooms that are both stimulating
   and disciplined.
5. Teachers of beginning reading should present well-designed
   phonics instruction.
6. Reading primers should be interesting and comprehensible,
   and should give children the opportunity to apply phonics.
7. Teachers should devote more time to comprehension instruction.
8. Children should spend less time completing workbooks and
   skill sheets.
9. Children should spend more time reading independently.
10. Children should spend more time writing.
11. Textbooks should contain adequate explanations of important
    concepts.
12. Schools should cultivate an ethos that supports reading.
13. Schools should maintain well-stocked and well-managed
    libraries.
14. Schools should introduce more comprehensive assessments of
    reading and writing.
15. Schools should attract and hold more able teachers.

It is important for all health care providers to be aware of these
recommendations and to educate individuals in the community regarding the importance of literacy development for all its citizens.

References

1. Stedman LC, Kaestle CF: Literacy and reading performance in the United States,
   from 1880 to the present, *Read Res Q* 22:8-46, 1987.
2. Floger JK, Nam CB: *Education of the American population*, Washington, DC, 1967,
   Government Printing Office.
3. Ginzberg E, Bray DW: *The uneducated*, New York, 1953, Columbia University Press.

4. U.S. Bureau of the Census: School enrollment, educational attainment, and illiteracy. In *Current population reports,* series P-20, no. 45, Washington, DC, 1953, Government Printing Office.
5. Fisher DL: *Functional literacy and the schools,* Washington, DC, 1978, National Institute of Education.
6. Carroll JB, Chall JS: *Toward a literate society,* New York, 1975, McGraw-Hill.
7. Vogt DK: *Literacy among youths 12–17 years in the United States,* Rockville, Md, 1973, National Center for Health Statistics.
8. Fisher DL: Functional literacy tests: a model of question-answering and an analysis of errors, *Read Res Q* 16:418-448, 1981.
9. Kirsch IS: *NAEP profiles of literacy: an assessment of young adults' development plan,* Princeton NJ, 1985, Educational Testing Service.
10. Kirsch IS, Jungeblut A: *Literacy: profiles of America's young adults,* Princeton NJ, 1986, National Assessment of Educational Progress.
11. Costa M: *Adult literacy/illiteracy in the United States: a handbook for reference and research,* Santa Barbara, Calif, 1988, ABC-CLIO.
12. Yankelovich, Skelly & White, Inc: *The 1978 consumer research study on reading and book purchasing,* Report no. 6, 1978, Book Industry Study Group.
13. Sticht TG: *Reading for working: a functional literacy anthology,* Alexandria, Va, 1975, Human Resources Research Organization.
14. Monteith M: How well does the average American read? Some facts, figures, and opinions, *J Read* 23:460-464, 1980.
15. Kozol J: *Illiterate America,* New York, 1985, Anchor/Doubleday.
16. Wellborn SM: Ahead: a nation of illiterates? *U.S. News & World Report,* May 17, 1982, pp. 53-57.
17. Taylor AG, Skelton JA, Czajkowski RW: Do patients understand patient education brochures? *Nurs Health Care* 13:305-310, 1982.
18. Vivian AS, Robertson EJ: Readability of patient education materials, *Clin Ther* 3:129-136, 1980.
19. Patient literacy and the readability of smoking education literature, *Am J Pub Health* 79:204-206, 1989.
20. Classé JG: *Legal aspects of optometry,* Boston, 1990, Butterworths.
21. Murphy RT: Assessment of adult reading competence. In Nielsen DM, Hjelm HF (eds): *Reading and career education,* Newark, Del, 1975, International Reading Association.
22. Murphy RT: *Adult functional reading study,* Princeton, NJ, 1973, Educational Testing Service.
23. Harris L, et al: *The 1971 national reading difficulty index: a study of functional reading ability in the United States,* Washington, DC, 1971, National Reading Center.
24. Johnstone WB: *Workforce 2000: work and workers for the 21st century,* Indianapolis, 1987, Hudson Institute.
25. Ashcroft J, Blunt R, Bartman R: *Jobs without people: the coming crises for Missouri's workforce,* Jefferson City, Mo, 1989, Governor's Council on Literacy.
26. Martin EW: Developing public policy concerning "regular" or "special" education for children with learning disabilities, *Learn Disabil Focus* 3:11-16, 1987.
27. Mausner JS, Kramer S: *Epidemiology: an introductory text,* Philadelphia, 1985, WB Saunders.
28. Flax N: Visual function in dyslexia, *Am J Optom Arch Am Acad Optom* 45:574-587, 1968.
29. Flax N: The eye and learning disabilities, *J Am Optom Assoc* 43:612-617, 1972.
30. Simons HD, Gassler PA: Vision anomalies and reading skill: a meta-analysis of the literature, *Am J Optom Assoc* 65:893-904, 1988.
31. McCormick S: *Remedial and clinical reading instruction,* Columbus, Ohio, 1987, Merrill Publishing.
32. Frankenberger W, Fronzaglio K: A review of states's criteria and procedures for identifying children with learning disabilities, *J Learn Disabil* 24:495-500, 1991.

33. Hallahan D: Some thoughts on why the prevalence of learning disabilities has increased, *J Learn Disabil* 25:523-528, 1992.

34. Rutter M, Yule W: The concept of specific reading disabilities, *J Child Psychol Psychiatry* 16:181-197, 1975.

35. Shaywitz SE, Escobar MD, Shaywitz BA, et al: Evidence that dyslexia may represent the lower tail of a normal distribution of reading ability, *N Engl J Med* 326:145-150, 1992.

36. Critchley M: *The dyslexic child,* ed 2, Springfield, Ill, 1970, Charles Thomas.

37. Finucci JM, Childs B: Are there really more dyslexic boys than girls? In Ansara A, et al (eds): *Gender differences in dyslexia,* Towson, Md, 1981, Orton Dyslexia Society.

38. Shaywitz SE, Shaywitz BA, Fletcher JM, Escobar MD: Prevalence of reading disabilities in boys and girls, *JAMA* 264:998-1002, 1990.

3

Risk Factors for Reading Disability

Michael T. Cron

Key Terms

risk factors	prenatal factors	risk modification
case history	postnatal factors	predictions
perinatal factors		

The visual system and its processing of information are extremely complex. When viewed in the context of its contributions to reading, it becomes nearly impossible to attribute causality of reading problems to one specific exposure or the existence of any one condition. Only devastating events can have such predictable effects. What we are left to deal with, in the main, are people with mild to moderate learning delays without obvious causation.

In spite of this, there is good reason to want to have an idea of how many known or suspected risk factors are present. If you are seeing a child early in the educational process, this information could help you determine how likely a future problem might be. Details about potential risks also help in formulating conclusions about the prognosis for recovery or improvement following treatment or therapy. Awareness of the potential impact of risk factors can lead to prevention of problems for future patients. Thus the case history will ultimately affect case management in the areas of prognosis, points to be addressed in case summation, potential recommendations for such things as genetic counseling, and assistance in choosing the best treatment course.

CLINICAL PEARL

Awareness of the potential impact of risk factors can lead to prevention of problems for future individuals. Thus the case history will ultimately affect case management in the areas of prognosis, points to be addressed in case summation, potential recommendations for such things as genetic counseling, and assistance in choosing the best treatment course.

This chapter will provide a discussion of history taking relevant to the multidimensional act of learning to read from the standpoint of noting the type, severity, and number of past occurrences that are potentially contributory to visual and learning difficulties. Although they might not be known to be causative, many past events are at least coincidental with learning difficulties. This is the concept of risk—that a child has a better than average chance of having a condition (e.g., reading disability) based on some historical event or medical condition. It is best thought of in epidemiological terms such as odds ratio or relative risk. If a child has a positive history of an exposure, then he or she is statistically more likely to have an unfavorable outcome. For example, if the odds ratio of a child having severe learning disabilities when the mother was on antidiabetic medications was 1.99, that would mean the child was twice as likely to have the disability as a child of a nondiabetic mother (all else being equal). In addition to the importance of singular events, there is evidence that cumulative and interactive effects of multiple exposures may be even more significant.

It is important that a careful and knowledgeable history be obtained. This cannot be overstated. Initially, a professional seeing a child with reading problems should query the parent and patient about the chief complaint or reason for presentation. Careful attention must be paid to the nature of the symptoms or problems, when they occur, and whether they are getting better or worse. It is also helpful to find out what, if any, treatments or therapies have been pursued and their results.

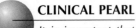

CLINICAL PEARL

It is important that a careful and knowledgeable history be obtained. This cannot be overstated. Initially, a professional seeing a child with reading problems should query the parent and patient about the chief complaint or reason for presentation.

A good history review must ultimately move beyond this stage, however, in two pursuits: The first should be history information from whatever additional sources are available and pertinent. These could include teacher, principal, school psychologist, teacher consultant or remedial teacher, physician or pediatrician, audiologist, occupational therapist, physical therapist, or additional caregivers (e.g., baby-sitter or grandparent). The second pursuit should be a systematic survey of other potential problems or sources of difficulty. These could include the patient's health history, academic history, and developmental history beginning with prenatal events. Also to be included would be family health and academic histories, including sibling and parental information. Many practitioners accomplish this portion of the history with a detailed checklist form to be filled out by the parent or guardian. Often this is mailed to the household before the appointment. This method has the advantage of allowing the parent time to recall events and to consult with others or with additional resources such as doctor's reports or baby books.

A case history should not be viewed as a fishing expedition, but as a strategy to satisfy your interest and need to address the most possible problems with all relevant background data at your disposal.

CLINICAL PEARL

A case history should not be viewed as a fishing expedition, but as a strategy to satisfy your interest and need to address the most possible problems with all relevant background data at your disposal.

It is generally a good idea before proceeding with an evaluation to review with parent and child your summary of the reason they are seeing you and what it is they want you to do for them. In this way, all parties will have a clear understanding of the situation.

What follows is a fairly complete, but not exhaustive, listing of conditions reported to be risk factors for physical, physiological, or behavioral disorders that might eventually result in visual and reading problems. As will become evident, most of these factors have not been studied in sufficient depth to determine whether they cause reading or other learning delays. Some have been investigated only for their effects in the immediate postnatal period, or during infancy. Many have concentrated only on physical changes and have not looked at behavioral or learning outcomes at all. There continues to be a large volume of research generated on this topic, and longitudinal studies with learning outcomes are beginning to emerge. More are needed, as you will see.

The potential risk factors will be presented in categories loosely defined by when the event was likely to occur—prenatally, perinatally, or postnatally.

Prenatal Factors

Prenatal factors encompass both the genetic material the father and mother donate to the embryo and the environment the parents provide for the developing child from conception to birth.

Maternal Age

The age of the mother is typically discussed in terms of increased risk for having a child with Down syndrome (usually trisomy 21). While the frequency of Down syndrome in the general population is 1:700, the risk in women under the age of 30 is 1:1000. And the rate rises slowly with increasing age—being 1:750 in women between 30 and 34, 1:300 in women 35 to 39, 1:100 in women 40 to 44, and between 3:100 and 6:100 in women 45 years of age and older.[1] The cause of this particular anomaly is abnormal cell development, either improper chromosomal separation during mitosis or translocation of chromosomal material during cell division. These types of cell division abnormalities can occur with many other chromosomes as well. The risk for these also increases with maternal age—the rate of all chromosomal anomalies being 1.5% in mothers aged 35 to 40, 3.4% over age 40, and as high as 10% over age 45.[2]

CLINICAL PEARL

While the frequency of Down syndrome in the general population is 1:700, the risk in women under the age of 30 is 1:1000. And the rate rises slowly with increasing age—being 1:750 in women between 30 and 34, 1:300 in women 35 to 39, 1:100 in women 40 to 44, and between 3:100 and 6:100 in women 45 years of age and older.[1]

Consideration of risk to the child also needs to be given the other end of the age spectrum. When biological factors may not be highly significant, environmental concerns can contribute to poor outcomes.[3] The environment of the infant born to a teenager and raised by one parent (who is often an unemployed high school dropout) is not conducive to helping the child achieve its full potential. The resultant lower achievement may be the equivalent of a learning disability.

Obstetrical History of the Mother

Two important concepts influence the significance of the mother's obstetrical history—maternal insufficiency and parity effects. Maternal insufficiency (also referred to as maternal inadequacy, uterine inadequacy, or reduced optimality) is the tendency among some mothers for a higher than normal frequency of such prenatal and perinatal complications as bleeding, toxemia, prematurity, and miscarriage.[4] It has been described[5] as an important risk factor in many conditions, including minimal brain dysfunction. This tendency for some mothers to have bad pregnancies has been shown to be familial.[6] For example, aunts and sisters of mentally retarded children have more mental retardation, miscarriages, and stillbirths in their families than do the uncles and brothers of mentally retarded children.[7] Thus, because of the familial nature of uterine inadequacy, the outcome of one pregnancy may predict the outcome of the next, especially regarding such factors as birth weight, prematurity, and neonatal death.

Parity effects are the systematic changes in some measurable parameter of children with increasing pregnancy order. The incidence of most forms of complications during labor and delivery increases with birth order, the later-born being at greater risk.[8] These parity effects are observed in minimal brain dysfunction.[9] A retarded, hyperactive, or learning-disabled child is more likely to have been later in the birth order.

Malnutrition

The significance and form of detrimental effects of intrauterine malnutrition will depend on the period of pregnancy when they occurred. The brain develops first by proliferating cell numbers at a rapid rate (as many as 250,000 new cells per minute,[10]) and then enlarging these cells and developing glial cells. In the human brain, malnutrition during the first 26 weeks of gestation will affect only the number of neurons; if it occurs late in the pregnancy, it will selectively affect glial cell number. The latter case will have much less impact on intelligence than the former.[11]

Infections

In general, infectious processes can cause different types of damage to the developing fetus and the newborn. Multiple systems may be involved depending on the type of infection and the period of gestation in which it occurs. Some infectious agents can damage the central nervous system and produce varying amounts of brain damage with manifestations such as mental retardation, seizures, and cerebral palsy. Learning and reading disabilities are certainly also potential complications of these infections. In general, however, multiple handicaps are noted.[12]

CLINICAL PEARL

In general, infectious processes can cause a variety of types of damage to a developing fetus and the newborn. Multiple systems may be involved depending on the type of infection and the period of gestation in which it occurs.

There are a number of conditions that will increase the likelihood of any of these infections[13]—premature or prolonged rupture of membranes, maternal fever, prematurity, low birth weight, low socio-economic status, or maternal drug use.

Rubella

The effects of congenital rubella have been well documented. Commonly seen damage to the child includes deafness, mental retardation, microcephaly, cataracts, salt-and-pepper retinopathy, and heart defects. Learning disabilities also appear to occur in some children.[14]

Toxoplasmosis

Congenital toxoplasmosis is a serious condition with an often fatal outcome from generalized infection. Chorioretinitis, seizures, microcephaly, and significant mental retardation are consequences. Only 8% to 16% of affected children are normal at 4 years of age.[15] There is as yet little evidence of the number of less severely affected who might have learning disabilities.

Syphilis

Despite awareness of the damaging effects on children of congenital syphilis, early congenital syphilis continues to occur in the United States. The risk to the child exists throughout pregnancy since the spirochete can cross the placenta at any time and invade the tissues of the fetus. If the central nervous system is affected, paresis and permanent mental impairment can result.[12] Other common signs include rash, chorioretinitis, iritis, Hutchinson's teeth, and deafness. Learning disabilities also may appear, but have not been studied as such.

Cytomegalovirus

Cytomegaloviruses are a frequent cause of congenital infection in the United States. Fetal infection results from hematogenous spread from the mother, or less commonly from ascending infection via the birth canal. Although some newborns will have severe cytomegalic inclusion disease, this is relatively rare. High-tone hearing loss is a common consequence, along with mild to moderate mental retardation, microcephaly, and hydrocephaly. Chorioretinitis is often observed. Learning disabilities also can be a result of cytomegalic infection.[16] It appears that children with symptomatic cytomegalovirus infection become bimodally distributed with respect to overall development and intelligence: One group is severely affected; the other has more subtle problems, including hyperactivity, speech difficulties, and learning problems.[17]

Drugs

Heroin, methadone, cocaine

The possible associations between exposure to street drugs in utero and subsequent learning or reading problems have yet to be established. A multitude of studies have investigated neonatal and infant effects with a variety of study designs. However, few if any well-designed studies have gone beyond the 4- or 5-year-old level. At this age, exposure to drugs does not seem to seriously affect IQ or neurological development, but subtle effects that might show up as more sophisticated learning is undertaken have not been studied. [18-20]

Antiepileptics

The neurotoxic effects of phenytoin have been described for some time. Phenytoin is known to be associated with fetal hydantoin syndrome (FHS). Exposure prenatally to phenytoin, either alone or with other anticonvulsants, results in neurotoxic consequences. Of particular significance among the problems noted in FHS are visual-motor problems and difficulties with performance subtests on the WISC.[21] Learning disabilities are a common consequence.

Phenobarbital

A discussion of prenatal exposure to drugs must include phenobarbital. Although its use in pregnant women has declined, it is still commonly taken—in maybe as high as 10% of pregnancies.[22] Phenobarbital exposure has been correlated significantly[23] with learning disabilities at age 7 years. The mechanism of the drug's effects has been investigated in animals.[24] The physiology and morphology of cells in the central nervous system were shown to change because of early phenobarbital exposure, as were hormone levels. As a result, learning and behavior of exposed animals can be affected.

Alcohol (fetal alcohol syndrome)

Prenatal exposure to alcohol has received considerable investigation. It is well known from this literature that maternal alcohol consumption during pregnancy results in reduced neonatal weight, length, and head circumference. However, the role of size measures alone may be over-rated. One recent longitudinal study[25] found that the observed alcohol effects on weight, length, and head circumference at birth were not sustained at 18 months or at 4, 7, or 14 years of age. This is not to say that neurobehavioral effects are not observed, for they were reported in the same cohort of children; rather, it implies that birth size reduction apparently does not predict neurobehavioral deficits later.

The deficits that do persist can be manifest into adulthood. Although puberty may mask some of the dysmorphic facial features so characteristic of fetal alcohol syndrome (FAS), cognitive, behavioral, communicative, and socialization difficulties may well persist.[26] Memory problems and attentional difficulties are commonplace in school-age FAS children and need to be addressed with environmental and interventional strategies.[27]

Smoking

Smoking by the pregnant mother throughout her pregnancy has been associated with a 28% increase in late fetal and neonatal mortality rates and with an average reduction of 170 g in birth weight when controlled for other factors.[28] Followed over time, these children show significant reading retardation at ages 7 and 11 years.[29]

Exposure to nicotine does not have to come directly from the mother's smoking to affect the infant. In a study of newborns of nonsmoking mothers whose fathers smoked more than 20 cigarettes/day,[30] the average birth weight deficit was 88 g. Cotinine levels were measured in the cord serum to ensure that the mothers were nonsmokers. The effect of birth weight reduction indeed related to passive exposure to tobacco smoke by the mother and consequently also the fetus.

Anesthesia

The potentially adverse effects of general anesthesia exposure in utero are little known. In a large case-control study,[31] however, striking associations were seen between first-trimester anesthesia exposure and hydrocephalus with other defects, the most common being eye defects such as cataracts. It remains to be determined if more subtle neurological deficits, including learning problems, become evident in first trimester–exposed children without major CNS defects or in children exposed to anesthesia in utero some time during the last two trimesters.

Other pharmaceuticals

Our society faces the problem of inadequate knowledge of potential neurotoxicity of many drugs that are currently available. The surface has barely been scratched.[32] One recent example is isotretinoin, marketed as Accutane for severe cystic acne, which has been widely used for the treatment of regular acne. Unfortunately, although approved by the FDA as a category X drug (contraindicated during pregnancy) this agent was used by childbearing women. The results have been many mentally retarded and learning-disabled children born to women who exposed their fetuses to isotretinoin.[33]

Chronic Maternal Health Problems

Diabetes

Pregnancy in an insulin-dependent diabetic who is not well controlled may result in a macrosomic infant with multiple congenital anomalies.

The risk of fatality and of central nervous system anomalies can be as much as 28 times higher in infants born of diabetic mothers compared with those of nondiabetic mothers.[34] The risk increases with the length of time the mother has had diabetes. If metabolic control is to be effective in reducing the incidence of malformation, the diabetic woman must control her disease meticulously from before conception until delivery, with particular emphasis on the first 2 months.[35]

CLINICAL PEARL

Pregnancy in an insulin-dependent diabetic who is not well controlled may result in a macrosomic infant with multiple congential anomalies. The risk of fatality and of central nervous system anomalies can be as much as 28 times higher in infants born of diabetic mothers compared with those of nondiabetic mothers.

Hypertension

Chronic hypertension in the pregnant woman can exert a hazardous influence on the fetus. Adequate blood supply and, consequently, sufficient oxygen and nutrients can be prevented from reaching the fetus because of an improperly developed placenta or placental degeneration. Both of these are possible consequences of maternal hypertension.[36] As such, any of the consequences of malnutrition or hypoxia are possible.

Allergies

A common complaint of parents of learning-disabled children is their proneness to allergies. Clinicians also have observed an apparent increase in the frequency of allergies among children with learning problems. In fact, research to investigate such associations has begun,[37] and abnormal immunoresponses have been shown in autistic children. A theory called the immunoreactive theory is being put forward to explain many of the trends seen in childbirth.[38] The major premise of this theory is that pregnancy is an immunological phenomenon of maternal tolerance. The immunoprotection of the fetus can break down, resulting in maternal-fetal immunoreactivity similar to Rh or ABO incompatibilities but attributable to other antigens. The theory strongly suggests that in further investigations (of such things as parity effects, prenatal and perinatal complications, maternal insufficiency, and intellectual development) the familial proclivity to autoimmune and allergic disorders be considered. A maternal history of allergies may be a very significant factor.

CLINICAL PEARL

A common complaint of parents with learning-disabled children is their proneness to allergies. Clinicians also have observed an apparent increase in the frequency of allergic patients among children with learning problems.

Irradiation

The teratogenic effects of radiation in pregnant women or women before pregnancy have been noted and are usually substantial. These effects include increased risk of microcephaly or mental retardation,[39] leukemia and other cancers,[40] and spontaneous abortion due to chromosomal abnormalities.[41] Studies of the more subtle effects of lesser doses of radiation have not yet been noted.

Hypothyroidism

Thyroid hormones are extremely important to the normal development of the human brain. Among their contributions are control of neuronal proliferation and differentiation, stimulation of development of axons and dendrites, and progress of myelinization. Maternal hypothyroidism can result in children with a higher-than-normal prevalence of neurological and behavioral problems,[42] particularly hyperactivity. Congenital hypothyroidism is seen in 1:5000 U.S. newborns[43] and if untreated can result in significant problems, including mental retardation. Long-term studies of children treated with replacement hormone[44] still show a number of residual behavioral problems, including visual-motor discrimination and eye movement control.

Polychlorinated biphenyls (PCBs) and dioxins in low doses can block the actions of thyroid hormones and, in higher doses, potentiate these actions. Permanent brain damage, with subsequent functional and behavioral abnormalities, may result if thyroid function in the mother or fetus are altered during critical periods of neurological development of the child.[45] It is conceivable that PCB or dioxin exposure of the mother or child in the prenatal and perinatal period could result in harmful effects through action on the thyroid hormones.

Genetics

A conscientious practitioner needs to be aware of the potential influences of genetic conditions. The prevalence of associated physical problems that must be dealt with, the problems the child might encounter in adapting to the world, and the risks for future generations all emphasize the significance of understanding heritable problems.

Gender

Because there is so much information detailing gender differences in many capacities and functions, it is easy to identify the risk group according to gender. What is perplexing to many is the explanation for these differences. Males are selectively afflicted with most neurological, psychological, and developmental disorders of childhood. The sex ratio is used to express the occurrence of conditions relative to gender and is calculated by dividing the number of males by the number of females and multiplying by 1000. The sex ratios of important neurodevelopmental disorders range from 120 for seizure disorders and 130 for severe mental retardation to 219 for learning difficulties, 300 for hyperkinesis, 400 for stuttering, and 430 for dyslexia.[38]

CLINICAL PEARL

Males are selectively afflicted with most every neurological, psychological, and developmental disorders of childhood.

These sex differences in neurodevelopmental disorders of childhood follow four distinct trends[38]—males are more commonly affected; when females are affected, the manifestation is more severe; in females, genotype is the likely cause of the condition and thus the manifestations are more specific; in males, manifestations are more diverse owing to a stronger interaction between genotype and environmental factors (including many of the prenatal risks mentioned here).

Another factor relating to risk and being male merits mention, the antecedent brother effect. Males born immediately following a previous male sibling are at increased risk of many problems, from pregnancy complications to learning difficulties.

The immunoreactive theory, mentioned previously, is one possible explanation for these gender differences. Some investigators also believe that hormonal influences play a contributory role. The exact nature of the causation remains unknown, but the fact of greater male risk remains.

Handedness

An increased occurrence of left-handedness, along with immune disease among the learning disabled, has been reported.[46] The explanation for this association is unclear, but it may be the manifestation of a genetic predisposition toward autoimmune disorder and the impact of negative environmental factors. Further study of the relationships of handedness, learning disorders, and allergic responses is needed.

Family academic history/dyslexia

Two aspects of this topic should be of concern in history taking, one environmental and the other genetic. It is useful as part of the assessment of a child's environment to ascertain the highest level of education of the parents or caregivers. This information will contribute to an evaluation of the opportunity for the child to overcome possible mild problems with an enriching environment and the level of sophistication that the recommended management or treatment involving the parents might reach.

The second aspect is that of problems either parent might have had with learning, particularly learning to read. It has become evident that certain types of reading problems, particularly the dyseidetic form of dyslexia, are hereditary. Dyseidetic dyslexia appears to be transmitted in an autosomal dominant fashion.[47] An awareness of this condition in the family would alter the approach to treatment and recommendations for further supplemental testing.

Metabolic disorders

Both progressive and nonprogressive metabolic disorders of a hereditary nature have been cited as producing learning problems. For example, boys aged 4 through 8 with adrenoleukodystrophy might initially be diagnosed as learning disabled because of the manifestations of hyperactivity and school failure.[48] This progressive neurodegenerative disorder is a sex-linked, genetically determined, condition. Children with nonprogressive but genetically determined metabolic disorders of amino acid metabolism (e.g., histidinemia) may present with concomitant learning disabilities as well. Even individuals who are heterozygous for these conditions may demonstrate subtle cognitive disturbances. Individuals heterozygous for genetic disorders of the urea cycle have shown depressed verbal IQ compared with performance IQ.[49]

Fragile X syndrome

Fragile X syndrome is the most common form of hereditary mental retardation.[50] It is associated with levels of academic difficulty ranging from mild learning disability to significant mental retardation. In general, males are more severely affected than females. It is the result of the repetition of a DNA sequence on the X chromosome with gaps or breaks in the chromosome. From a counseling standpoint it is important to note that the repeating sequence gets longer with succeeding generations and the longer the sequence the more severe the manifestations.[51] Visually, high refractive errors are noted and as many as half of the affected people are strabismic.[52] As a result, vision specialists may be consulted and may be the first to suspect the presence of fragile X syndrome in an affected individual. It has been recommended[53] that any child with significant learning problems or mental retardation and strabismus be screened for fragile X syndrome.

Perinatal Factors

Infections

Herpes

Passage through an infected birth canal is the principal cause of herpes simplex virus (HSV) infection. HSV type 2 is the causative factor in most genital, and thus neonatal, infections. It is a serious condition, with a 60% fatality rate and major neurological and ocular sequelae in half of the survivors.[54] Central nervous system disease is common and in milder forms may eventuate in various forms of learning disorders.

Low Birth Weight

One of the best-studied risk factors of infancy is low birth weight. This is true because (1) it has been classically thought of as increasing a child's risk, (2) those at risk are very easily identified, and (3) there are increasing numbers of survivors because of modern technological and medical advancements. A classification system for children below normal weight has been developed. Those with birth weights less than 2500 g are called low birth weight (LBW), below 1500 g very low birth weight (VLBW), and below 1000 g extremely low birth weight (ELBW).

CLINICAL PEARL

One of the most well-studied risk factors of infancy is low birth weight. This is true because (1) it has been classically thought of as increasing a child's risk, (2) those at risk are easily identified, and (3) there are increasing numbers of survivors due to modern technological and medical advancements.

Some VLBW children are the result of pregnancies in mothers with a treatable medical condition. The risk of VLBW deliveries in black women is significantly increased if they have essential hypertension or a urinary tract infection. The risk is higher in white women who have essential hypertension, a urinary tract infection, pregnancy-induced hypertension, or diabetes mellitus.[55] These are treatable medical conditions that may appear in the maternal history. Low–birth weight rates also are higher among women who receive inadequate prenatal care.[56]

The future need for additional educational services in children with reduced weight at birth, particularly those with ELBW, has been demonstrated.[57] Even when IQ was normal, ELBW children achieved lower math scores than normal-birth weight children did. As might be expected, ELBW children also scored lower than the other reduced–birth weight groups in both mathematics and reading achievement. When controlled for maternal education and neonatal stay, lowered birth weight increases the prevalence of grade failure, placement in special classes, and classification as handicapped. Other investigators have found significant learning disabilities, defective language comprehension, and visual-motor integration problems in VLBW children with normal or borderline intelligence.[58]

One confounding factor in any investigation of exposure risk factors is the environment. This consideration must be kept in mind for all of the items detailed in this chapter, but it has been researched in few. One area where socioeconomic status (SES) has been considered in research is with low birth weights. In an evaluation of children at double risk for reduced cognitive abilities because of VLBW and low SES, it was found[59] that the SES factor was more significant than the birth weight alone and that the medical main-effect model was not necessarily the best for detecting developmental delay.

Additionally, psychosocial stress in the environment also influences the developmental outcome of VLBW children, at least during the first 2 years.[60] As reflected by a maternal appraisal of daily stress, psychosocial risk accounted for a significant reduction in cognitive outcome over and above biological risk from the birth weight.

Prematurity

Undesirable consequences of prematurity as they relate to later learning capabilities are not necessarily directly related to the prematurity itself, but to associated causes of the prematurity or related conditions. An overview of children initially treated in a neonatal ICU would show that such things as mean intellectual function were normal. The conclusion might be that infants with abnormal or transiently abnormal neurological examinations had few academically related sequelae. Careful assessment, however, would suggest that risk truly exists for special class placement, hyperactivity (in males), and learning and motor problems.[61]

Obstetrical Medications

Although the immediate effects on infants of pharmaceuticals used during labor and delivery are of some interest, we are more concerned with the long-term effects. The physical and behavioral outcomes immediately after birth have been studied in significant detail. Fewer studies have looked at outcomes in school-related performance. Although there is some disagreement, poorer performance on intelligence tests and reading have been seen at age 7 among children exposed to oxytocin induction and inhalation anesthetics.[62] A fourfold increase in the use of inhalation anesthetics has been reported[63] among mothers who had children with minimal brain dysfunction in Israel. The use of inhalation anesthetics was a significant predictor of educational difficulties at age 7 among 994 low achievers in the Collaborative Perinatal Project as well.[64]

Birth Trauma

There are a number of indicators of difficulty with labor and delivery that are overrepresented in the case histories of children with reading and learning problems.

Prolonged labor

In a study of children classified with minimal brain dysfunction,[63] complications of labor and delivery (including prolonged labor and use of forceps) were highly associated with this group of children. Other investigators[65] have documented the same pattern of increased prevalence of minimal brain dysfunction among children with histories of labor complications.[65]

Hemorrhages

Intracranial vascular injury with resultant hemorrhage can have fatal consequences. These are, fortunately, rare. However, with premature or difficult deliveries, small intracerebral hemorrhages can occur and lead to eventual motor abnormalities, seizures, learning difficulties, or mental retardation.[66]

Asphyxia/hypoxia/anoxia

Interference with the circulation and oxygenation of the blood is termed *asphyxia*. Prolonged perinatal asphyxia can have significant consequences. Some of the more common causes[66] include premature placental separation, cord prolapse, difficult labor, obstruction of the airway, and depression of the respiratory center secondary to excessive anesthesia.

Because of the delicate nature of the blood vessels surrounding the ventricles of the brain, and their susceptibility to hypoxia, intraventricular hemorrhage is a possible manifestation of asphyxia. During the period of recovery from asphyxia by resuscitation, many changes may occur in the newborn. Acidosis, hypoglycemia, and serious loss of potassium or calcium may result. Other potential sequelae[67] of asphyxia include congestive heart failure, renal disorders, cerebral edema, and poor gastrointestinal motility.

One study of asphyxiated infants[68] found that half died in the neonatal period, and the other half were normal. The survivors had a normal distribution of IQ scores, with many in the above-average range. Of the survivors, 72.3% had no abnormalities.

Respiratory distress syndrome

One of the most common risk factors occurring in premature infants is respiratory distress syndrome. This occurs in about 20% of preterm infants, and the risk increases with increasing prematurity.[69] The lungs are the last organ to develop, and the surfactant that coats the alveoli is not adequately produced until 34 to 36 weeks of gestation. If delivered before this time, the infant is at risk of having collapsed lungs. Supplemental oxygen or artificial respiration could be required. Periods of reduced blood oxygenation may occur at various times for these infants. The premature infant also is prone to periods of irregular respiration or apnea due to central nervous system damage. Lowered blood oxygen levels and slowed heart rate are a part of the apnea picture.[70]

Cerebral vascular accidents

Prenatal and perinatal stroke can have significant consequences on later learning potential. In a study of 17 children with ischemic or hemorrhagic infarct or intraparenchymal cerebral hemorrhage,[71] full scale, verbal, and performance IQs were all significantly below those of a well-matched control group. This occurred despite the fact that the subjects ranged in age from 4 to 20 years, and were equally mixed with left hemisphere or right hemisphere damage. Still, all subjects had IQ scores within the normal range and evidence of partial compensation and reorganization despite the global deficits.

Breech presentation

In a comprehensive study of the effects of prematurity and breech presentation on almost 1100 children, two interesting findings were noted. Among the premature children, 20% were hyperkinetic and/or learning disabled, and the percentage was the same for breech or vertex presentation. However, among the full-term children, hyperkinesis or learning disability was present in 19% of the breech and only 4% of the vertex presentations. Interestingly, if cesarean section was performed, the percentage of breech babies who were hyperkinetic or learning disabled dropped from 20% to 1%.[72]

Postnatal Factors

Kernicterus (hyperbilirubinemia)

It is well established that unconjugated bilirubin is toxic to the central nervous system.[67] The mechanism of excess bilirubin-produced damage is not clear, but bilirubin staining of the brain (known as kernicterus) is found. Both immediate and long-term effects are noted. Long-term sequelae include sensorineural hearing loss and other consequences (e.g., motor abnormalities, intellectual impairment) that may manifest as learning difficulties.[73] However, in a study of 240 children at ages 4 and 7 who had previously had jaundice,[74] no significant differences in IQ or school readiness were noted.

Rh and ABO Blood Incompatibilities

Although the incompatibility actually occurs during the prenatal period, maternal-fetal blood incompatibilities are discussed here because they result in hyperbilirubinemia in the newborn. Rh disease and ABO blood group incompatibility are allergic reactions of the mother to the baby's blood. Once sensitized to the blood, the mother's antibodies will destroy the fetal red blood cells. Red blood cell destruction results in the release of bilirubin, which the newborn's liver cannot conjugate sufficiently. The resultant hyperbilirubinemia can have the effects noted above. In general, the potential damage from Rh disease is far more serious than from ABO incompatibility.[36]

Malnutrition

Cellular development occurs in the normal brain until about 6 years of age, at which time adultlike levels are reached (with the exception of the cerebellum, where adultlike levels are reached by age 2). Postnatal malnutrition during this period can therefore affect brain development. Timing is of the essence in brain development, and interference with one segment of the developmental chain will negatively affect all subsequent events. Malnourished children have been shown[75] to have much reduced numbers of brain cells. Most pediatricians, in assessing a child's progress, will measure head circumference. Unfortunately, these head circumference values do not correlate well with brain cell numbers.[76] Thus, studies showing that undernourished children catch up in head circumference do not address the entire problem. The real question is whether poor nutrition in early life has long-term effects on intellectual abilities. The answer is not yet clear, because some studies show an effect, but others do not.[77] However, in one well-designed study of children malnourished for differing lengths of time and to varying degrees,[78] significant differences were noted after 6 years of optimum environmental surroundings. IQ and achievement scores were lower for the children who were more severely malnourished and for those who were malnourished for a longer time before age 6.

CLINICAL PEARL

Cellular development occurs in the normal brain until about 6 years of age, at which time adultlike levels are reached (with the exception of the cerebellum, where adultlike levels are reached by age 2). Postnatal malnutrition during this period can therefore affect brain development.

While many of the risk factors detailed here involve exposures to potentially harmful events, humans can experience learning or processing problems as a result of the lack of essential exposures as well. One specific deficiency shown to be detrimental is zinc. Zinc is necessary for normal brain development and function, and essential for neurotransmission. Lower levels of zinc in the diet can lead to decreases in sensory-motor skills, attention span, memory, and spatial skills.[79] Neurological abnormalities do not typically occur in persons exposed to higher than normal levels of zinc.[80]

Hypoglycemia

Persistent hyperinsulinemic hypoglycemia of infancy (PHHI) is a condition of elevated insulin levels with nonketotic hypoglycemia. The diagnosis must be made early, and intervention initiated promptly. Mental retardation and other serious complications have become less common because of early recognition. However, when of school age, these children display both learning disabilities and motor control difficulties.[81]

Phenylketonuria

Phenylketonuria (PKU) is an inborn error of metabolism that is inherited in an autosomal recessive fashion. The inability to hydroxylate phenylalanine to tyrosine that these individuals possess results in depressed levels of dopamine. Because of good neonatal screening and prompt treatment by eliminating phenylalanine from the diet, normal IQ scores can be achieved by these early-treated PKU children. Despite dietary control, some cognitive deficits (particularly executive function deficiencies) have been reported in preschoolers with PKU.[82] However, it appears that by school age these reported executive function deficits are no longer evident.[83] This suggests that a developmental delay, possibly related to availability of dopamine and norepinephrine, rather than a developmental deficit is acting. Visual-motor integrative (VMI) scores did remain lower in the school-aged PKU children than in the control group.

Infections

Encephalitis

Inflammation of the brain, (encephalitis) leads to neuronal injury. It may be either primary or secondary in nature. Primary encephalitis is caused by such viruses as mumps and herpes simplex. Measles is the most common of the secondary encephalitides. Fortunately, there has been a dramatic reduction in the number of deaths from acute measles encephalitis since the introduction of the measles vaccine in 1963.[84]

Meningitis

Meningitis is an infection of the meninges (lining the brain) with resultant inflammation and increases in intracranial pressure. Antibiotics have been very effective in reducing the mortality from bacterial meningitis, but survivors in early infancy display effects that include neuromuscular problems, vision and hearing losses, seizures, and cognitive deficits.[85]

Otitis media

Recurrent ear infections (otitis media) in young children have been thought to impair hearing and result in auditory processing skill deficits that may persist into the school years. However, in 151 children who had prolonged otitis in their preschool years, serious lasting consequences at age 7 were not noted.[86] Spelling ability was somewhat reduced, but reading ability was not. Investigators also found no effects on spelling or reading from treatment with ventilation tubes.

Toxins

High-level exposures to known toxins can have immediate and irreversible consequences. What might go undetected, however, are more subtle changes, which may not be manifest until after some delay. Longitudinal and behavioral studies may begin to demonstrate these subclinical neurotoxic effects,[87] such as reduced intelligence, impaired reasoning skills, and poor attention.

CLINICAL PEARL

High-level exposures to known toxins can have immediate and irreversible consequences. What might go undetected, however, are more subtle changes, which may not be manifest until after some delay.

Lead

Serious consequences of exposure to lead have been documented for centuries. A number of learning difficulties have been associated with excessive but lesser levels of lead exposure. Children with elevated lead levels have shown deficits in IQ, speech processing, and attention, and have had problems in classroom behavior.[88] Subsequently, a fourfold increase in the occurrence of verbal IQ scores below 80 was observed in children with high lead exposure.[89] In another study,[90] lead exposure showed an inverse relationship to IQ scores in young children. However, when evaluated 5 years later, the same children with now lowered lead levels showed no significant correlation between lead level and IQ scores when other significant factors such as maternal IQ and home environment were controlled.[90] In a study of children 8 to 12 years of age,[91] those with higher lead concentrations did have significantly slower simple reaction times and less flexibility in shifting attention.

Methylmercury

Serious effects of excessive exposure to methylmercury have been documented in a few tragic epidemics of significant proportion. Profound cortical atrophy and thinning of cerebellar gray matter have been seen.[92] Whether smaller doses will have similar results on a lesser scale, leading to more subtle behavioral or learning dysfunctions, has not been adequately investigated.

Organophosphates

The long-term effects of organophosphate poisoning have been shown on neurobehavioral tests. One recent study of these effects in adults[93] showed significantly worse performance of the exposed group in sustained visual attention tasks (continuous performance). There is every reason to believe that the same types of effects will be seen when children are exposed to organophosphate pesticides.

Medications

The side effects of medications prescribed for children to treat medical conditions may result in impairments of behavior or learning. These concerns have been addressed for only a few prescription drugs.

Anticonvulsants/phenobarbital

Behavioral disturbances have been reported with the use of anticonvulsant medications. Commonly reported with barbiturates, they include hyperactivity, erratic sleep patterns, and irritability. Additionally, subtle behavioral disturbances may adversely affect academic performance and learning.[94] In an evaluation of the effects of phenobarbital on preschoolers,[95] IQ levels were found to be unaffected. However, memory was reduced as a function of the blood serum level, and comprehension impaired, related to the length of time the drug had been taken. A more recent investigation of children aged 3 months to 15 years[96] concluded that anticonvulsant medications, particularly phenobarbital, can cause behavioral disturbances, most frequently hyperactivity.

Theophylline

A bronchodilator often prescribed for childhood asthma, theophylline has been implicated in behavioral and learning problems of children who use it for asthma. However, there continues to be controversy in the literature on this issue. In a double-blind placebo-controlled trial,[97] parental reports of children's behaviors did not support any conclusion of behavioral side effects involving attention, impulsivity, memory, activity level, or mood. In another large study with a matched control group of siblings,[98] academic achievement was unaffected by asthma or its medical management. There were no differences between children with or without asthma, or between those taking theophylline and those taking other asthma medications. Although individual susceptibilities can vary, in general it appears that theophylline is safe and effective for managing chronic childhood asthma.[99] Recent studies have alleviated concerns over side effects such as cognitive impairment.

Accidents

Near drowning

Although not as serious as periods of asphyxia during the birth process, if prolonged oxygen deprivation occurs later in life significant neurological consequences will result. Near drownings can lead to anything from subclinical deficits, if the anoxic period is brief, to permanent coma or death. Most drownings or near drownings occur among poorly supervised children who cannot swim.[100]

Closed head trauma

Traumatic head injury is the result of a definite blow or wound to the head, causing an alteration in consciousness, even if brief, and associated neurological or behavioral dysfunction.[101] There is little question that victims of traumatic head injury experience specific learning problems.

Falls

Most of the head injuries that occur in children under the age of 2 years come from falls. The majority of these household falls were found to be neurologically benign.[102] Translational forces to the head did not result in acute clinical consequences or retinal hemorrhages. Behavioral sequelae were not reported.

Motor vehicle accidents

In the infant and toddler group aged less than 2 years, subdural hematoma and retinal hemorrhage are observed secondary to motor vehicle accidents.[102] Owing to the severity of the trauma in a few cases, some brain damage with subsequent learning impairment may occur.

Child abuse

The majority of cases of retinal hemorrhage seen in young children suffering trauma come from inflicted injuries.[102] The rotational forces induced by shaking and battering can lead to retinal trauma and an increase in subdural hemorrhages and diffuse axonal injury. Child abuse is a common cause of head trauma; 24% of the cases reported by Duhaime et al.[102] were presumed to be inflicted (i.e., nonaccidental) and another 32% were suspicious for the same.

Moderation and Modification of Risk

As has been noted in the discussion of low birth weight, environmental factors play a significant role in the level to which neurological impairments manifest themselves. Encouraging, nurturing, and stimulating surroundings can reduce the impact of risk factors on learning, performance, and life skills. Similarly, an environment of deprivation and isolation with poor nutrition and nurturing can exacerbate the problem. Research studies have investigated some of these effects. Higher measures of anxiety are associated with poor perinatal outcomes—including premature births, longer labors, more use of analgesia, and low birth weights. Depression has many of the same effects as anxiety. Stressful life events are related to similar pregnancy complications. These negative effects can be mitigated, however, by other variables. Beneficial effects can be seen from positive attitudes toward the pregnancy, a feeling of control over oneself, and a readily available social support network.[103]

CLINICAL PEARL

Environmental factors play a significant role in the level to which neurological impairments manifest themselves. Encouraging, nurturing, and stimulating surroundings can reduce the impact of risk factors on learning, performance, and life skills.

Predictions

It would seem that, with an awareness of all the aforementioned risk factors, a scale or scoring device could be constructed that would predict the likely outcome for any given child. Several attempts have been made at such scales. They consist of differing numbers of items, with different weightings, and are used for different purposes—for medical predictions of morbidity and mortality rates and for estimates of developmental outcomes. Included are the University of Colorado Neonatal Morbidity Risk Scale, the High Risk Pregnancy Screening System, the Obstetrical Complications Scale, the Maternal-Child Health Care Index, the Scale of Optimal Obstetric Conditions, and the

Rochester Research Obstetrical Scale. The validity of these scales is not universal for perinatal outcomes and is even less for predicting later childhood behaviors.[103] Other screening instruments designed specifically to identify children at risk for impaired learning potential have been proposed.[104] The factors included as significant were prematurity, prolonged labor, difficult delivery, cyanosis, blood incompatibility, adoption, late walking, prolonged tiptoe walking, late or abnormal speech, and ambidexterity after age 7. Subsequently, problems during pregnancy and low birth weight have been added. However, these systems remain no better than a screening without proving cause. At this point it would appear that a careful history with an ear toward the types of events described here and a careful noting of the number, type, and severity of problems encountered would be the most practical approach to an assessment of risk.

References

1. Donnell GN et al: Chromosomal abnormalities. In Koch R, delaCruz F (eds): *Down's syndrome (mongolism): research, prevention, and management,* New York, 1975, Brunner Mazel.
2. Sells CJ, Bennett FC: Prevention of mental retardation: the role of medicine, *Am J Ment Defic* 82:117-129, 1977.
3. Geronimus AT: The effects of race, residence, and perinatal care on the relationship of maternal age to neonatal mortality, *Am J Public Health* 76:1416-1421, 1986.
4. Costeff H et al: Pathogenic factors in idiopathic mental retardation, *Dev Med Child Neurol* 23:484-493, 1981.
5. Gillberg C, Rasmussen P: Perceptual, motor, and attentional deficits in seven-year-old children: background factors, *Dev Med Child Neurol* 24:752-770, 1982.
6. Keller CA: Epidemiological characteristics of preterm births. In Friedman SL, Sigman M (eds): *Preterm birth and psychological development,* New York, 1976, Academic Press.
7. Ahern FM, Johnson RC: Inherited uterine inadequacy: an alternative explanation for a portion of cases of defect, *Behav Genet* 3:1-12, 1973.
8. Niswander KR, Gordon M: *The women and their pregnancies,* Philadelphia, 1972, WB Saunders.
9. Badian N: Reading disability in an epidemiologic context: incidence and environmental correlates, *J Learn Disabil* 17:129-136, 1984.
10. Dobbing J: The later development of the brain and its vulnerability. In Davis JA, Dobbing J (eds): *Scientific foundations in pediatrics,* London, 1974, Heinemann.
11. Chase HP: Undernutrition and growth and development of the human brain. In Lloyd-Still JD (ed): *Malnutrition and intellectual development,* Lancaster, England, 1976, MTP Press.
12. Sever JL: Perinatal infections and damage to the central nervous system. In Lewis M (ed): *Learning disabilities and prenatal risk,* Urbana, 1986, University of Illinois Press.
13. Klein JO, Marcy SM: Bacterial sepsis and meningitis. In Remington JS, Klein JO (eds): *Infectious diseases of the fetus and newborn infant,* Philadelphia, 1990, WB Saunders.
14. Desmond MM et al: The longitudinal course of congenital rubella encephalitis in nonretarded children, *J Pediatr* 93:584-591, 1978.
15. Eichenwald HF: Congenital toxoplasmosis: a study of one hundred and fifty cases, *J Dis Child* 94:411-415, 1957.

16. Williamson WD et al: Symptomatic congenital cytomegalovirus: disorders of language learning and hearing, *J Dis Child* 15:902-905, 1982.

17. Conboy TJ: Early clinical manifestations and intellectual outcome in children with symptomatic congenital cytomegalovirus infection, *J Pediatr* 111:343-348, 1987.

18. Robins LN, Mills JL: Effects of in utero exposure to street drugs, *Am J Public Health (Suppl)* 83:19, 1993.

19. Carta JJ, et al: Behavioral outcomes of young children prenatally exposed to illicit drugs: review and analysis of experimental literature, *Top Early Child Spec Educ* 14:184-216, 1994.

20. Shriver MD, Piersel W: The long-term effects of intrauterine drug exposure: review of recent research and implications for early childhood special educators, *Top Early Child Spec Educ* 14:161-183, 1994.

21. VanOverloop D et al: The effects of prenatal exposure to phenytoin and other anticonvulsants on intellectual function at 4 to 8 years of age, *Neurotoxicol Teratol* 14:329-335, 1992.

22. Reinisch JM, Sanders SA: Early barbiturate exposure: the brain, sexually dimorphic behavior and learning, *Neurosci Biobehav Rev* 6:311-319, 1982.

23. Nichols PC, Chen PC: *Minimal brain dysfunction: a prospective study,* Hillsdale, NJ, 1981, Lawrence Erlbaum.

24. Gray DB, Yaffe SJ: Prenatal drugs and learning disabilities. In Lewis M (ed): *Learning disabilities and prenatal risk,* Urbana, 1986, University of Illinois Press.

25. Sampson PD et al: Prenatal alcohol exposure, birthweight, and measures of child size from birth to age 14 years, *Am J Public Health* 84:1421-1428, 1994.

26. LaDue RA et al: Clinical considerations pertaining to adolescents and adults with fetal alcohol syndrome. In Sonderegger TB (ed): *Perinatal substance abuse: research findings and clinical implications,* Baltimore, 1992, Johns Hopkins University Press.

27. Olson HC: The effects of prenatal alcohol exposure on child development, *Infant Young Child* 6:10-25, 1994.

28. Butler NR et al: Cigarette smoking in pregnancy: its influence on birth weight and perinatal mortality, *Br Med J* 2:127-130, 1972.

29. Butler NR, Goldstein H: Smoking in pregnancy and subsequent child development, *Br Med J* 4:573-575, 1973.

30. Martinez FD et al: The effect of paternal smoking on the birthweight of newborns whose mothers did not smoke, *Am J Public Health* 84:1489-1491, 1994.

31. Sylvester GC et al: First-trimester anesthesia exposure and the risk of central nervous system defects: a population-based case-control study, *Am J Public Health* 84:1757-1760, 1994.

32. Vorhees CV: Developmental neurotoxicity induced by therapeutic and illicit drugs, *Environ Health Perspect (Suppl)* 102:145-153, 1994.

33. Adams J, Lammer EJ: Relationship between dysmorphology and neuropsychological function in children exposed to isotretinoin "in utero." In Fujii T, Boer GJ (eds): *Functional neuroteratology of short-term exposure to drugs,* Tokyo, 1991, Teikyo University Press.

34. Pederson J: *The pregnant diabetic and her newborn,* Copenhagen, 1977, Munsgaard.

35. Menutti MT: Teratology and genetic counseling of the diabetic mother, *Clin Obstet Gynecol* 28:486-495, 1985.

36. Baroff GS: *Mental retardation: nature, cause and management,* New York, 1986, Hemisphere Publishing.

37. Stubbs FG, Crawford ML: Depressed lymphocyte responsiveness in autistic children *J Autism Child Schizophr* 7:49-55, 1977.

38. Gualtieri CT: Fetal antigenicity and maternal immunoreactivity: factors in mental retardation. In Schroeder SR (ed): *Toxic substance and mental retardation: neurobehavioral toxicology and teratology,* Washington, DC, 1987, American Association on Mental Deficiency.

39. Rugh R: X-irradiation effects on the human fetus, *J Pediatr* 52:531-538, 1958.

40. National Research Council, National Academy of Sciences: *The effects on population of exposure to low levels of ionizing radiation,* Washington, DC, 1972, Government Printing Office.

41. Alberman E et al: Parental x-irradiation and chromosome constitution in their spontaneously aborted fetuses, *Ann Hum Genet* 36:185-194, 1972.

42. Man EB et al: Thyroid function in human pregnancy. VII. Development and retardation of 4-year-old progeny of euthyroid and hypothyroxinemic women, *Am J Obstet Gynecol* 109:12-18, 1971.

43. Dussault JH et al: Modification of a screening program for neonatal hypothyroidism, *J Pediatr* 92:274-277, 1978.

44. Rovet JF: Congenital hypothyroidism: intellectual and neuropsychological functioning. In Holmes CS (ed): *Psychoneuroendocrinology: brain, behavior, and hormonal interactions,* New York, 1990, Springer-Verlag.

45. Porterfield SP: Vulnerability of the developing brain to thyroid abnormalities: environmental insults to the thyroid system, *Environ Health Perspect (Suppl)* 102:125-130, 1994.

46. Geschwind N, Behan P: Left-handedness: association with immune disease, migraine, and developmental learning disorder, *Proc Natl Acad Sci USA* 79:5097-5100, 1982.

47. Fatt HV, Griffin JR: *Genetics for primary eye care providers,* Chicago, 1983, Professional Press.

48. Moser HW et al: Adrenoleukodystrophy: studies of the phenotype, genetics and biochemistry, *Johns Hopkins Med J* 147:217-224, 1980.

49. Batshaw ML et al: Cerebral dysfunction in asymptomatic carriers or ornithine transcarbamylase deficiency, *N Engl J Med* 302:482-485, 1980.

50. Sutherland G, Richards R: Fragile X syndrome: the most common cause of familial mental retardation, *Acta Paediatr Scand* 35:94-101, 1994.

51. Maino DM et al: Ocular health anomalies in patients with developmental disabilities. In Maino DM (ed): *Diagnosis and management of special populations,* St Louis, 1995, Mosby.

52. Maino DM et al: Optometric findings in the fragile X syndrome, *Optom Vis Sci* 68:634-640, 1991.

53. Maino DM, King R: Oculo-visual dysfunction in the fragile X syndrome. In Hagerman R, McKenzie P (eds): *1992 International fragile X conference proceedings,* Dillon, Col, 1992, Spectra.

54. Committee on the Fetus and Newborn, Committee on Infectious Diseases, American Academy of Pediatrics: Perinatal herpes simplex virus infections, *Pediatrics* 66:147-148, 1980.

55. DeBaun M et al: Selected antepartum medical complications and very low-birthweight infants among black and white women, *Am J Public Health* 84:1495-1497, 1994.

56. Kotelchuck M: The adequacy of prenatal care utilization index: its US distribution and association with low birthweight, *Am J Public Health* 84:1486-1489, 1994.

57. Klebanov PK et al: School achievement and failure in very low birth weight children, *Dev Behav Pediatr* 15:248-256, 1994.

58. Hunt JV et al: Learning disabilities in children with birth weights <1500 g, *Semin Perinatol* 6:280-287, 1982.

59. Smith L et al: Very low birth weight infants (<1501 g) at double risk, *Dev Behav Pediatr* 15:7-13, 1994.

60. Thompson RJ et al: Developmental outcome of very low birth weight infants as a function of biological risk and psychosocial risk, *Dev Behav Pediatr* 15:232-238, 1994.

61. Ellison P et al: The outcome of neurological abnormality in infancy. In Harel S, Anastasion NJ (eds): *The at-risk infant: psycho/socio/medical aspects,* Baltimore, 1985, Paul H Brookes.

62. Broman SH: The collaborative perinatal project: an overview. In Mednick SA et al (eds): *Handbook of longitudinal research,* New York, 1984, Praeger Publishers.

63. Kaffman M et al: Obstetric history of kibbutz children with minimal brain dysfunction, *Isr J Psychiatry Relat Sci* 18:69-84, 1981.

64. Broman SH et al: *Low achieving children: the first seven years,* Hillsdale NJ, 1985, Lawrence Erlbaum.

65. Colletti L: Relationship between pregnancy and birth complications and the later development of learning disabilities, *J Learn Disabil* 12:25-29, 1979.

66. Chamberlin HR: Mental retardation. In Farmer TW (ed): *Pediatric neurology,* New York, 1975, Harper & Row.

67. Ensher GL, Clark DA: *Newborns at risk: medical care and psychoeducational intervention,* Gaithersburg, Md, 1994, Aspen Publishers.

68. Mulligan JC et al: Neonatal asphyxia. II, Neonatal mortality and long-term sequelae, *J Pediatr* 96:903-907, 1980.

69. Batshaw ML, Perret YM: *Born too soon, born too small: children with handicaps, a medical primer,* Baltimore, 1986, Paul H Brookes.

70. Winderstrom AH et al: *At-risk and handicapped newborns and infants: development, assessment, and intervention,* Englewood Cliffs, NJ, 1991, Prentice-Hall.

71. Ballantyne AO, Scarvie KM, Trauner DA: Verbal and performance IQ patterns in children after perinatal stroke, *Dev Neuropsychol* 10:39-50, 1994.

72. Fianu S, Joelsson I: Minimal brain dysfunction in children born in breech presentation, *Acta Obstet Gynecol Scand* 58:295-299, 1979.

73. deVries LS et al: Relationship of serum bilirubin levels to ototoxicity and deafness in high risk low birth weight infants, *Pediatrics* 76:351-354, 1985.

74. Rubin RA et al: Neonatal serum bilirubin levels related to cognitive development at ages 4 through 7 years, *J Pediatr* 94:601-604, 1979.

75. Winick M et al: Cellular growth of cerebrum, cerebellum, and brain stem in normal and marasmic children, *Exp Neurol* 26:393-400, 1970.

76. Winick M, Rosso P: Head circumference and cellular growth of the brain in normal and marasmic children, *J Pediatr* 74:774-778, 1969.

77. Morgan BLG: Nutrition and brain development. In Pueschel SM, Mulick JA (eds): *Prevention of developmental disabilities,* Baltimore, 1990, Paul H Brookes.

78. Lien NM et al: Early malnutrition and late adoption: a study of their effects on the development of Korean orphans adopted into American families, *Am J Clin Nutr* 30:1734, 1977.

79. Penland JG: Cognitive performance effects of low zinc (Zn) intakes in healthy adult men, *FASEB J* 5:A938, 1991.

80. Walsh CT et al: Zinc: health effects and research priorities for the 1990s, *Environ Health Perspect (Suppl)* 102:5-46, 1994.

81. Gross-Tsur V et al: Neurobehavioral profile of children with persistent hyperinsulinemic hypoglycemia of infancy, *Dev Neuropsychol* 10:153-163, 1994.

82. Welsh MC et al: Neuropsychology of early treated phenylketonuria: specific executive function deficits, *Child Dev* 61:1697-1713, 1990.

83. Mazzocco MM et al: Cognitive development among children with early-treated phenylketonuria, *Dev Neuropsychol* 10:133-151, 1994.

84. Centers for Disease Control: Childhood immunization initiative: United States, 5 year follow-up, *MMWR* 31:232, 1982.

85. Sell SH et al: Long-term sequelae of hemophilus influenzae meningitis, *Pediatrics* 49:206-211, 1972.

86. Peters SAF et al: The effects of early bilateral otitis media with effusion on educational attainment: a prospective cohort study, *J Learn Disabil* 27:111-121, 1994.

87. Landrigan PJ et al: Environmental neurotoxic illness: research for prevention, *Environ Health Perspect (Suppl)* 102:117-120, 1994.

88. Needleman HL et al: Deficits in psychologic and classroom performance of children with elevated dentine lead levels, *N Engl J Med* 300:689-695, 1979.

89. Needleman HL et al: Does lead at low dose affect intelligence in children? *Pediatrics* 68:894-896, 1981.
90. Schroeder SR, Hawk B: Psycho-social factors, lead exposure, and IQ. In Schroeder SR (ed): *Toxic substances and mental retardation,* Washington, DC, 1987, American Association on Mental Deficiency.
91. Minder B et al: Exposure to lead and specific attention problems in schoolchildren, *J Learn Disabil* 27:393-399, 1994.
92. Needleman HL: Prenatal exposure to pollutants and neural development. In Lewis M (ed): *Learning disabilities and prenatal risk,* Urbana, 1986, University of Illinois Press.
93. Steenland K et al: Chronic neurological sequelae to organophosphate pesticide poisoning, *Am J Public Health* 84:731-736, 1994.
94. American Academy of Pediatrics: Behavioral and cognitive effects of anticonvulsant therapy, *Pediatrics* 76:644-647, 1985.
95. Camfield CS et al: Side effects of phenobarbital in toddlers: behavioral and cognitive aspects, *J Pediatr* 95:361-365, 1979.
96. Domizio S et al: Anti-epileptic therapy and behavior disturbances in children, *Child Nerv Syst* 9:272-274, 1993.
97. Bender B, Milgrom H: Theophylline-induced behavior change in children: an objective evaluation of parents' perceptions, *JAMA* 267:2621-2624, 1992.
98. Lindgren S et al: Does asthma or treatment with theophylline limit children's academic performance? *N Engl J Med* 327:926-930, 1992.
99. Milgrom H, Bender B: Current issues in the use of theophylline, *Am Rev Respir Dis* 147:33-39, 1993.
100. O'Carroll PW et al: Drowning mortality in Los Angeles County, 1976-1984, *JAMA* 260:380-383, 1988.
101. Begali V: *Head injury in children and adolescents: a resources and review for school and allied professionals,* Brandon, Manitoba, 1992, Clinical Psychology Publishing.
102. Duhaime AC et al: Head injury in very young children: mechanisms, injury types, and ophthalmological findings in 100 hospitalized patients younger than 2 years of age, *Pediatrics* 90:179-185, 1992.
103. Molfese VJ: *Perinatal risk and infant development: assessment and prediction,* New York, 1989, Guilford Press.
104. Hoffman MS: Early indications of learning problems, *Acad Ther* 7:23-45, 1971.

C H A P T E R

4

Reading Readiness

Joy Rosner

Key Terms

reading readiness	perceptual skills	auditory analysis
prerequisites	visual analysis	remediation
visual factors		

The concept of reading readiness as an indicator of a child's ability to make satisfactory progress in a formal reading instruction program is well established, albeit not well defined. It dates from the 1920s, reflecting the views of developmental psychologists who documented the behavioral changes of preschool children displayed as a function of maturation[1] and who then attempted to identify among those behaviors the ones that would be predictive of subsequent school performance.

Concurrent and supportive of this was the hypothesis[2] that the main cause of school learning problems was immaturity. This had been spawned by a body of research that showed first-grade children with mental ages of 6½ to 7 years to be more successful in reading than those with mental ages below 6½. These findings were applauded by many early childhood investigators.[3-6]

Over the years a number of skills and abilities that contribute to a child's reading readiness have been identified. This has led to the development of a number of tests designed to evaluate reading readiness (e.g., the *Metropolitan Readiness Test*).[7,8]

Prereading instruction programs designed to foster reading readiness also have been developed, and many have been adopted by schools in the United States. A chief goal of virtually every kindergarten teacher in the United States is to ensure that his or her pupils will be ready for the academic demands of first grade, especially when it comes to learning to read.

This chapter is based on the proposition that the primary care optometrist has a role to play in monitoring and, to some degree, guiding a child's acquisition of reading readiness. To accomplish this, it will

1. Identify the skills, knowledge, and experiences that have been defined by various educators as representative of reading readiness
2. From these, identify the skills, knowledge, and experiences that are especially relevant to the optometrist, and explain why
3. Identify the visual factors that influence reading readiness—factors that school-based, standardized tests ignore, but the optometrist addresses
4. Describe how the optometrist can serve children whose reading readiness skills are lagging by collecting relevant data and, on the basis of this, communicating effectively with parents and teachers regarding appropriate treatment options
5. Describe how the optometrist can facilitate children's reading readiness by identifying and monitoring the implementation of appropriately designed remedial programs

Reading

Reading is a multicomponent and highly complex behavior involving many cognitive processes that defy exact description. We can do it, but we cannot explain it. A glance at the dictionary will corroborate this statement. Most dictionaries offer at least 10 definitions, each sounding more or less correct, yet none completely correct.

Rather than attempt to unravel the mystery of what happens in our brain when we read (an impossible mission, given our limited knowledge of complex cognitive processes), we will apply a very simple yet empirically accurate definition.

For the purposes of this chapter, it is sufficient to define reading as *the mapping of meaningful language onto symbols;* or, said differently, *the reconstituting of language from its symbolic form into its original state.*[9]

This definition applies not only to normal individuals (who read by converting standard graphic symbols into spoken language), but also to blind persons (who read by mapping language onto tactile symbols) and to deaf persons (who map the unique language of the profoundly deaf onto standard orthography) and even to Morse code operators, who translate acoustical signals into words. Hence, reading per se is not exclusively a "visual" or an "auditory" behavior but, rather, is a blending of the two in a way that enables one to convert a visual, a tactile, or an acoustical code into meaningful information.

A Global Analysis of the Steps in Learning to Read

Before we can address the behaviors that are considered to be evidence of a child's readiness for learning to read, and the optometrist's role in this regard, we should identify the learning objectives a child must master to become a reader—i.e., what it is that the so-called readiness skills subserve. We also must describe the circumstances under which learning to read is expected to take place (the standard public school, primary grade classroom). We will start with the latter.

The standard primary grade classroom can be described as having three components: (1) an "average" teacher (2) using mass-produced instructional programs and materials designed specifically for the "average" student and (3) in a classroom containing about 25 children whose cognitive abilities range from below to above average.[*] As such, the standard primary grade classroom requires children to do a considerable amount of independent learning—self-instruction, learning from example, remembering by association. The teacher in the standard classroom has very little opportunity for individualized instruction, regardless of how dedicated he or she may be.

CLINICAL PEARL

The standard primary grade classroom requires children to do a considerable amount of independent learning—self-instruction, learning from example, remembering by association. The teacher in the standard classroom has little opportunity for individualized instruction, regardless of how dedicated he or she may be.

Objectives to be Mastered in Learning to Read

In analyzing the process of learning to read, four separate yet interrelated sets of basic abilities can be identified. These are described below, in sequence. However, the fact that they are in sequence should not be interpreted as suggesting that the first must be fully mastered before the second or the second before the third, etc. A beginning reader will be able to start to learn some of the second set after making headway with the first. In other words, progress through the sets is

---

[*]The word *average* here is not meant to be pejorative but should be interpreted literally, as meaning midway between the two extremes of distribution.

reiterative: the child learns in synchronous fashion; the first set leads the second somewhat, and the second, the third, etc., while being overlapped by the third, and so on.[10]

The first ability: Knowing the language

It should be no surprise that the principal behavior in learning to read is knowing the language that is to be read or mapped onto symbols. It is not enough to be able to transform the printed words into their oral form. Certainly this is an important step along the way, but it is not enough. For example, if you have an understanding of the letter-sound conventions of Latin (a very "regular" system in which letter-sound relationships are completely consistent), it is easy to convert printed Latin text into its acoustical counterpart. But if you lack an understanding of Latin, then this cannot be called reading; it is decoding. Hence, the primary behavior in learning to read is being able to understand the language that is represented by the printed words.

CLINICAL PEARL

The principal behavior in learning to read is knowing the language that is to be read or mapped onto symbols.

The second ability: Identifying the letters of the manuscript alphabet and the conventions that govern their use in reading

Limiting this discussion to the child with normal sight and hearing, we must realize that it is not enough merely to discriminate the subtle similarities and differences between certain manuscript letters (the *b* and the *d* for example). Even the beginning reader must know and remember which is which. Similarly, the reader must be securely aware of the spatial organization rules that govern the management of printed symbols in English (i.e., that letters are sequenced from left to right, that the spaces separating words are larger than those separating the letters in a given word, that the lines of print are organized from the top to the bottom of the page, that sentences begin with a capital letter and end with a period).

CLINICAL PEARL

It is not enough that a child is able to discriminate the subtle similarities and differences between certain manuscript letters (the b *and the* d, *for example). Even the beginning reader must know and remember which is which.*

The third ability: Decoding

Hearkening back to our definition of reading (and, once again, limiting this discussion to children with normal sight and hearing), it becomes evident that another pivotal behavior in the process of learning to read is decoding: transforming the printed symbols that constitute words into their oral form. Reading specialists sometimes refer to this as word attack, or word recognition, or word analysis skills.

CLINICAL PEARL

Another pivotal behavior in the process of learning to read is decoding: transforming the printed symbols that constitute words into their oral form.

The competent reader is a fluent decoder. The child who decodes slowly and/or ineptly will not be able to obtain meaningful information from the printed page easily. Fluent decoding, in turn, depends at least in part upon how far the child has progressed in learning the letters of the printed manuscript alphabet. (Other skills are also required, as will be discussed). Children who have to pause before determining if a given letter is a *b* or a *d* or a *p* will have inept decoding skills and, as such, will suffer the consequences when it comes to the desired terminal behavior: understanding the language they are generating as they decode.

The Ultimate Behavior: Comprehension

Indisputably, the true goal of learning to read—and the true proof that one can read—is being able to access information from the printed page. Comprehension, therefore, is the highest-order ability of the four.

CLINICAL PEARL

The true goal of learning to read—and the true proof that one can read—is being able to access information from the printed page. Comprehension, therefore, is the highest-order ability.

Competent reading comprehension obviously depends on the three subordinate skills described above, plus one more: a knowledge of the subject matter being read. In other words, even though a child may be fully familiar with the spoken form of the language he or she is learning to read, and with the graphic symbols on the page, and even though he or she is a competent decoder, the child will still not fully comprehend the text he or she is decoding if the subject matter of the text is beyond his or her understanding. An example: consider how much (or how little) a 6-year-old child will comprehend as he or she decodes, albeit fluently, a description of the solar system or how to tell time. The words may be kept short and simple, but the concepts expressed by those words will be beyond a 6-year-old child's comprehension.

Reading Readiness

Having defined the act of reading and identified the four basic abilities a child must have to be able to read, defining reading readiness is not so challenging. Following the rule of pragmatics, reading readiness can be defined as being prepared—as having acquired and/or developed the basic abilities and knowledge that are prerequisite to learning to read under standard instructional conditions.

But, in fact, it is not all that clear cut. Although reading experts may disagree on a precise definition of the act of reading, they disagree little on identifying it when it is performed. They recognize competent reading when they see it.

The same is not true of reading readiness. All educators generally agree that there are prerequisites to learning to read and that, in the aggregate, these constitute a state called reading readiness. There is much debate, however, about just what those prerequisites are. Some reading specialists favor a behavioral approach that emphasizes specific skills and knowledge; others lean toward a more global approach that avoids identifying and teaching specific behaviors and, instead, stresses the importance of prereading environments and experiences.

CLINICAL PEARL

There are prerequisites to learning to read and these, in the aggregate, constitute a state called reading readiness. There is much debate as to just what those prerequisites are.

The Knowledge-Skills Approach to Reading Readiness

The following lists a number of behaviors representative of the knowledge-skills approach.[11] They are organized into two subgroups: *knowledge* that is acquired (experience dependent, learned from birth on) and *skills* that are developed (biologically dependent, emerging as a function of age rather than of specific experiences).

Both these lists could be extended, the first much more than the second, but what is offered is sufficient to illustrate the broad array of items that show up on reading readiness inventories.

Acquired knowledge

1. Identify and name the primary colors
2. Identify and name major body parts
3. Respond correctly to requests of "your last name," "age," "birthday," etc.
4. Repeat short meaningful sentences verbatim
5. Count up to 50 by rote and count up to 10 objects accurately
6. Recite the alphabet in correct sequence
7. Detect an out-of-sequence printed number, up to 10
8. Print first and last names accurately and legibly
9. Print the numerals 1 to 10 accurately and in correct sequence
10. Detect an out-of-sequence printed letter
11. Print lower and upper case letters dictated out of sequence
12. Understand and use words in a manner typical of the average kindergarten child
13. Respond accurately to questions about a short story that has just been read aloud
14. State the sound representative of a given letter (e.g., what sound does the letter *m* make?)
15. State a word that rhymes with a given word
16. Use correctly such phrases as "more than," "less than," "the same as"
17. Position objects in accord with such stated words as "under," "over," "up," "down"

Developed skills

1. Detect similarities and differences between line drawings and between spoken words
2. Copy uncomplicated geometric designs that may, but need not, be identifiable by name (e.g., circle, square, plus sign, cross, triangle)
3. Identify a picture on the basis of its beginning sound
4. Carry out visually directed gross and fine motor actions (e.g., walk on a plank of wood, draw designated pencil marks in a row of circles, cut with scissors along a drawn line, build a cube tower)
5. Group objects according to one or more physical characteristics (e.g., sort painted cubes according to their color and/or size, identify rhyming words)

The Global Approach to Reading Readiness

As mentioned, not all educators approve of the behavioral approach but support, instead, a more global and humanistic approach that stresses the prereading experiences a child should have rather than specifically what should be learned. The following, excerpted from a recent publication,[12] is representative:

1. Surround children with many forms of print and a variety of devices for creating it (e.g., magazines, workbooks that involve coloring letters, painting, chalkboards, typewriters, etc.). Children must want to find out about the pictures and the messages contained within books.
2. Use good literature and encourage thinking (e.g., after reading a story, ask the child "What would you have done?" "Why do you think . . . ?).
3. Provide real experiences to enhance children's experiences with print (e.g., visit the zoo, the post office, etc.).
4. Develop oral language ability (e.g., by using films, tape recorders, etc.).
5. Establish the relationship between spoken and written language. Show that spoken words can be written down.
6. Stimulate thinking (engage the children in problem-solving activities; encourage the use of predictions).
7. Provide opportunities to gain a sense of story structure (e.g., point out how a geographical setting, a time of day, a time of year, contributes to a story).
8. Provide essential support and feedback. Be patient and tolerant when answering endless questions and nurture positive feelings about reading and books.

The author of this list concludes her thesis[12] (p. 25) as follows:

It is vital to remember that reading is a complex and enjoyable thinking process. Structured readiness programs, workbook pages, and drills do not provide an adequate basis for beginning reading instruction. The experiences, knowledge, and environmental factors cited above will provide prereaders with a foundation for an understanding of the process and for later success in reading.

On the surface, it is difficult to argue against this proposition. Indeed, it is probably correct that all some children need is the right kind of environment. But it also is evident that depending exclusively on environment and inspiring, enriching experiences and ignoring specific prereading skills and knowledge is not sufficient for other children.

CLINICAL PEARL

It is probably correct that all some children need is the right kind of environment. But it also is evident that depending exclusively upon environment and inspiring, enriching experiences and ignoring specific prereading skills and knowledge is not going to be sufficient for other children.

This chapter is written for that latter group: those children whose reading readiness skills will not emerge as the result of enriching experiences alone. Many of these can be aided by your intervention.

The Optometrist's Role

Visual Factors That Do and Do Not Influence Reading Readiness

Typically, a comprehensive vision evaluation of preschool children comprises an assessment of visual acuity, refractive status, oculomotor integrity, binocular status, and ocular health. Some of these, if impaired, may have a significant negative influence on a child's reading readiness. (A more extensive discussion of this topic is presented in Chapter 6.)

Recently many optometrists, acknowledging their obligations as primary care practitioners, have added to this list of clinical concerns a developmental screening battery that includes evaluation of visual and, in some cases, auditory perceptual skills. Because these skills are very closely related to reading readiness, we will include them in this discussion of visual factors.

Visual acuity

The importance of adequate near and far visual acuity in the standard classroom is self-evident; no elaboration is needed here.

Refractive status

This topic cannot be covered so quickly; there are unresolved questions. Although no optometrist would hesitate to prescribe compensatory lenses for the preschool child whose visual acuity improves significantly and/or whose ocular discomfort symptoms are alleviated by the appropriate lenses, there are many who would hesitate to prescribe lenses for the asymptomatic child with moderate hyperopia.

This dilemma is understandable. The child with moderate hyperopia (e.g., somewhat in excess of 1.00 D) typically enjoys excellent visual acuity and rarely manifests signs or symptoms that would link school-related difficulties with a vision problem. The rationale generally applied in considering treatment for such cases is that the moderately hyperopic preschool child has ample accommodation and, provided he or she has no associated binocular problem, can cope easily with the ametropia; thus, compensatory lenses would be superfluous.

However, a series of recently reported, interrelated studies tends to support a contrary view.

1. Hyperopic children, even those with moderate hyperopia, are much more susceptible to delays in visual perceptual skills

development than emmetropic children (the relevance of this will be explained later) and the latter, in turn, are more susceptible than myopic children. In one study involving 710 6- to 12-year-old children (all eye clinic patients),[13] only 24 of 177 myopes displayed substandard visual analysis skills as compared with 181 of 479 emmetropes and 46 of 61 hyperopes (p < 0.001).

A second study,[14] involving 378 randomly selected first to fifth graders (who were not eye clinic patients), yielded similar results, with hyperopic children again displaying significantly poorer visual analysis skills than their myopic classmates.

2. Early application of compensatory lenses appears to facilitate visual perceptual skills development. A follow-up study of the eye clinic patients mentioned previously,[15] involving only the hyperopic group, showed that of the 15 children in that group who did have satisfactory visual analysis skills 13 had started to wear corrective lenses before the age of 4; it also showed that, conversely, only 5 of the 33 hyperopic children with substandard visual perceptual skills obtained their first glasses before their fourth birthday.

3. Hyperopic children not only are more prone to delayed development of visual analysis skills, they also seem to make slower progress in the classroom than their emmetropic and myopic classmates do. A recently conducted study of the relationship between ametropia and classroom performance (as measured by standardized achievement tests) of second through fifth grade randomly selected children[16] showed that hyperopes trailed significantly.

All of this should sensitize you to the potential importance of prescribing compensatory lenses for the preschool (and, for that matter, school-aged) moderately hyperopic patient, even in the absence of reduced visual acuity and asthenopia. True, a critical level of hyperopia has yet to be established, and it ultimately may be discovered that anything less than some substantial amount (2.00 or 3.00 D) can be safely ignored. But, for the present, the evidence is too incriminating to simply ignore. You should adopt the position that, until demonstrated to the contrary, hyperopia (even moderate hyperopia) might warrant lens application, at least for near work.

CLINICAL PEARL

All of this should sensitize you to the potential importance of prescribing compensatory lenses for the preschool (and, for that matter, school-aged) moderately hyperopic patient, even in the absence of reduced visual acuity and asthenopia.

Oculomotor integrity

Oculomotor integrity refers to the child's ability to demonstrate unhampered and efficiently controlled/coordinated eye movements in all positions of gaze. Unfortunately, the topic is moot. True (and justifiably), very few optometrists would consider the manifestation of limited and/or poorly controlled and coordinated eye movements to be inconsequential, but the available research regarding a connection between these manifestations and reading readiness is equivocal. Some investigators[17] assert that inadequate oculomotor processes have a direct and negative effect on a child's reading ability; others[18] take the opposing position.

The solution: You need to exercise judgment regarding the management of oculomotor dysfunction based on the standard criteria rather than on a documented connection between it and school performance. In other words, oculomotor dysfunction is worthy of treatment in its own right, regardless of how it may or may not influence classroom performance.

Binocular status

This aspect of visual behavior overlaps to some degree with oculomotor integrity, but it goes beyond that—it also encompasses the ability to maintain clear, single, binocular vision at all viewing distances, in all positions of gaze, and under dynamic conditions. As with oculomotor functions, there is disagreement among optometrists (and among members of other disciplines as well) about the effects of binocular disorders on school achievement. There are studies that show a link between certain binocular functions and school performance;[19] there are others that fail to substantiate that link.[20]

The solution is the same as that stated previously for oculomotor integrity. You should exercise clinical judgment regarding the management of binocular disorders based on the standard criteria of the profession rather than on a documented connection between binocular function and school performance. In other words, binocular dysfunction is worthy of treatment for its own sake, regardless of whether or not it influences classroom performance.

Ocular health

Clearly, no discussion of this subject is required.

Perceptual skills

Although this topic has already been introduced, the required skills have not yet been adequately defined. The perceptual skills that contribute to reading readiness and that are of interest to you will be the naturally developed learning aptitudes that have been labeled visual and auditory analysis skills.

The former skill is the extent to which a child has developed the ability to analyze spatially organized patterns into the concrete features of quantity, magnitude, and fixed relationships[21] (i.e., to recognize that, although it may vary in appearance, spatially organized information consists of a finite number of structural components that interrelate in specific and definable ways). If this ability is present, the child can recognize (or be taught) that subsets of spatially organized patterns (e.g., manuscript letters, sets of numbers) share certain characteristics that facilitate their recall even though they also give them a unique identity. (For example, consider *b*, *d*, *p*, and *q*; these are uniquely different, yet they share characteristics that when correctly identified will help the child remember which is which.) Note that the behaviors identified here as visual analysis skills are the same as one of the basic abilities on the developed readiness skills list discussed earlier. Visual analysis skills tests are usually based on assessing a child's ability to copy geometric designs (e.g., the *Test of Visual Analysis Skills*, the *Developmental Test of Visual Motor Integration*).

The latter skill—auditory analysis—also refers to the child's ability to analyze patterns in terms of their concrete features but, in this modality, the patterns are spoken words and the features are the phonological elements of those words. Stated in the same manner as for visual analysis skills, it is the ability to recognize that, although they may vary as to how they sound, spoken words (i.e., acoustically organized information) all consist of a finite number of structural (concrete sensory) components that interrelate in specific ways. Once this is established, the child can then recognize (or be taught) that subsets of acoustical information share characteristics that give them unique identity yet facilitate their recall. (For example, consider "big," "fig," and "jig.") Auditory analysis skills tests relevant in this context are based on assessing the child's ability to identify specific sounds within words (e.g., the *Wepman Auditory Discrimination Test*, the *Test of Auditory Analysis Skills*).

The Relationship Between Visual and Auditory Analysis Skills and Learning to Read

Both visual and auditory perceptual skills subserve learning to read in very important ways. Recall the four sets of abilities defined previously. Visual analysis skills influence strongly how easily a child learns to identify the letters of the manuscript alphabet with consistent accuracy; auditory analysis skills, in turn, have a powerful effect on how readily the child recognizes the letter-sound relationships that govern decoding. Visual analysis skills also provide the basis for organizational strategies that the reader can exercise when attempting to remember and comprehend the information gained from decoding. Hence, it is predictable that the child with substandard visual perceptual skills will display inept handwriting, persistent letter reversal tendencies, a disorganized approach to the execution of activities that require step-by-step interrelated actions, and difficulty remembering information (regardless of whether it is heard or read).[22] (Although this chapter is devoted to reading, it is essential to mention that visual perceptual skills also have a very significant effect on how well a child masters the concepts of mathematics.)

CLINICAL PEARL

Visual analysis skills influence strongly how easily a child learns to identify the letters of the manuscript alphabet with consistent accuracy; auditory analysis skills, in turn, have a powerful effect on how readily the child recognizes the letter-sound relationships that govern decoding.

CLINICAL PEARL

The child with substandard visual perceptual skills will display inept hand-writing, persistent letter reversal tendencies, a disorganized approach to the execution of activities that require step-by-step interrelated actions, and difficulty remembering information.

The child who has age-appropriate visual and auditory analysis skills upon entering a standard first grade reading class will recognize the system (the rules) on which reading is based—a system wherein letters represent sounds and the spatial arrangement of those letters represents the temporal sequence of those sounds, therefore making unfamiliar words less difficult to read if they can be associated with a word that is familiar. For example, the word "took" will be easier to read on its first exposure if the child already recognizes the word "look" and has the visual and auditory analysis skills expected of a first grader. (True, this is not always the case in English, where unusual spellings occur, but it is the system despite those variations.) Understanding the system makes learning to read (and spell) accomplishable. Attempting to learn to read (and spell) without recognizing an underlying set of rules reduces learning to rote memorization, a process that cannot possibly work when learning how to read.

The Optometrist as a Monitor of Readiness

The readiness abilities listed at the beginning of this chapter were organized into two major categories, knowledge that the child has acquired since birth and skills that the child has developed during this time. The former depend upon experiences—formal and informal—and reflect the child's cultural background; the latter depend upon development and therefore reflect the child's prenatal, perinatal, and postnatal neurological status. (Remember: We are not considering the holistic approach discussed earlier, because it fails to meet the needs of those children who will not acquire/develop readiness abilities "on their own" despite the motivational power of the experiences they are provided.)

The former category, acquired knowledge, is extensive because it encompasses the broad array of information that the typical child is expected to learn during the first 5 years of life. The list provided in this chapter consists of representative "samples" of that category, which if valid allows one to extrapolate the extent of the child's general knowledge base and, as such, gain insight into his knowledge of the language he or she is about to be asked to learn to read. (After all, there is no reason to believe that knowing the location and/or name of a specific body part—or, for that matter, a birthday, family name, or the sequence of the letters in the alphabet—before commencing reading instruction is that critical in and of itself.)

The latter category, developed skills, is relatively limited, and properly so. It comprises seminal behaviors that are expected to evolve at a predictable rate in all children by virtue of their genetic heritage and neurological status, behaviors that reflect the child's inherent ability to recognize order—to "induce systems"—in the environment.[23]

How Do You, the Optometrist, Fit into All of This?

First, you are the individual best trained to assess and, if needed, treat the various basic visual functions that influence school performance.

Second, you can monitor the child's visual (and auditory) analysis skills—skills that have long been recognized by educational psychologists as critical to reading readiness and (in respect to visual analysis) skills that recently have been shown to be closely associated with a very prevalent refractive condition: hyperopia. (Optometrists have only recently become interested in auditory analysis skills, not because of a desire to expand their scope of activity but, rather, because of the recognition that some reading problems stem from a deficit in that area in addition to, or instead of, a visual deficit and therefore should not be ignored.)

Third, you are a facilitator of perceptual skills development, not solely by identifying a need for and prescribing compensatory lenses for ametropia, but also by designing and supervising the implementation of treatment programs that will improve the child's deficient perceptual skills.

And finally, you are a consultant to parents and teachers when it becomes apparent that, because of some underlying neurophysiological condition or some other relevant circumstance, the only acceptable treatment option is not remediation but, rather, modification of the child's instructional program in ways that effectively accommodate existing deficits. (The principles of this treatment approach [i.e., modification of the teaching program] are very familiar to optometrists; it is the one we employ when we recommend [nonstandard] large-print books for young patients with acuity impairments that are not eliminated by compensatory lenses.[24])

The first and second of these roles do not require any elaboration. The latter two might.

Fostering perceptual skills development

A number of optometrists agree that appropriately designed intervention can facilitate perceptual skills development. However, many disagree about what constitutes "appropriately designed intervention."

Some accept the credo that, because perceptual skills are but one facet of an exquisitely complex multidimensional process called "development," the only effective way to treat a lag in the process is to search for any lower level (underlying) developmental deficits that may exist, treat those first, and delay treating the higher-order perceptual skills until a firm foundation of underlying skills has been established.[25] Others believe that there is no need (and, in fact, that it wastes too much time) to search for and treat the so-called lower-level skills before attempting to remediate the child's perceptual skills deficits.[26]

Both groups have their "proof," evidence of successful outcomes from their respective treatment approaches. Given that their evidence is valid, a reasonable explanation emerges: It is not essential to treat "underlying" deficits in order to foster perceptual skills development. True, in a perfect world it might be desirable to do this, but we have to be practical and counterbalance desirability with available resources, such as patient energy, motivation, and time.

How can (visual and auditory) perceptual skills be fostered? The best way is to engage the child in a program of sequentially organized activities that teach how to look at and/or listen to sensory patterns analytically and how to identify the concrete features in those patterns, especially features that relate to the symbolic codes of the classroom. There are a number of such programs available. (See Appendix.)

CLINICAL PEARL

Visual and auditory preceptual skills can be fostered by engaging the child in a program of sequentially organized activities that teach how to look at and/or listen to sensory patterns analytically.

You may elect to assume responsibility for implementing the program or simply play the role of advisor to school-based individuals (or to parents) who assume the responsibility for implementation. It matters little who implements, as long as the prognostic indicators are favorable. If they are not favorable, then an alternative treatment option—classroom accommodation—should be considered.

Determining the prognosis for perceptual skills remediation in the child who is not "ready"

Perceptual skills remediation is not always desirable. Certain prognostic factors should be examined and respected before a treatment decision is made. The following are favorable prognostic indicators: (1) there is no evidence of a neurological deficit; the developmental (perceptual-skills) lag seems to be attributable to individual differences rather than to a physiological circumstance, such as an at-risk birth or a history of seizures; (2) there is a minimal educational deficit; in other words, the child is not yet significantly behind in school—for example, a first or second grader who lags 4 to 6 months in achievement as contrasted to a sixth grader who is 2 years behind his classmates; (3) there is sufficient time, energy, motivation, and personnel to engage successfully in a sustained remedial effort.

If all of these conditions are satisfied, perceptual skills remediation should be implemented; if not, then it is much more prudent to seek an alternative approach to helping the child. (Obviously, the second factor can usually be ignored with children who have not yet entered into reading instruction. They have not had a chance to fall that far behind their classmates in school achievement.)

Alternative Approaches

There are two alternatives to remediation: (1) delay entry into formal instruction or (2) modify the instructional conditions to accommodate the existing deficits.

When should the first be selected? There is no simple way to answer this; it is a complex question. It involves more than testing a set of skills. Delayed entry into school is perceived by some as tantamount to failure, to being cognitively inadequate. As such, it affects family dynamics, emotions, and the child's own self-esteem.

Consider the circumstances. Most schools in the United States enroll children into first grade (and formal reading instruction) in the September following their sixth birthday. Thus, an entering first grade class will comprise children who range from just past their sixth birthday to just short of their seventh birthday. The differences between the just-6-year-old child and the about-to-be-7-year-old child is great, not only physically but also in the basic cognitive processes, which in this context means the child's visual and auditory analysis skills. The child whose readiness status is below what it should be (for first grade) will probably be served best by being retained in a pre-first grade setting for an additional year.

CLINICAL PEARL

The child whose readiness status is below what it should be (for first grade) will probably be served best by being retained in a pre-first grade setting for an additional year.

However, this solution ignores the other factors mentioned previously. How will the child's family (immediate and beyond) and, for that matter, his neighbors and his parents' friends perceive this delaying action? Will they react (in actions and/or words) in ways that disturb the child's parents, who in turn will respond to the child in a resentful manner? Is there a sibling who is just 1 year behind and exhibits no signs of a similar problem? Do the child's school authorities view delayed entry sympathetically, or will the decision color their perceptions of the child in a way that lowers their expectations for him or her when the child does enter first grade? There are other questions as well, but these will serve to illustrate the complexity of the question.

How, then, should you counsel the parent of the 6-year-old child whose reading readiness skills are not up to an appropriate level? Dispassionately. You are neither obliged nor trained to act as an educational counselor but are obliged to apply professional judgment (and that does not preclude feelings) when advising a patient. All else being equal, the child who is not "ready" should not enter a first grade standard instructional setting. This does not preclude remedial efforts during that year, however. Indeed, the 1-year delay provides an excellent opportunity to provide the experiences that will ensure the child's "readiness" 1 year later.

Principles for Accommodating the Child with Deficient Reading Readiness Abilities

Clearly, some children will be entered into first grade despite their "unready" state. If they are to succeed, their deficits will have to be accommodated. (Admittedly, some of these children will succeed; either they will have a spontaneous "spurt" in development or they will be fortunate enough to have a teacher who knows how to teach them despite their condition and is willing and has the opportunity to do it. But one should not depend on this.)

The key to successful classroom accommodation for the child whose reading readiness skills are substandard is to recognize what should be altered and why. Earlier in this chapter, we identified the three components of a standard classroom—(1) an average teacher, (2) instructional materials and programs designed for the average child, and (3) such physical factors as a 1:25 teacher/student ratio, a heterogeneous group of children, and so forth. One or more of these components will have to be changed for successful accommodation.

CLINICAL PEARL

The key to successful classroom accomodation for the child whose reading readiness skills are substandard is to recognize what needs to be altered and why.

The teacher

The child we are discussing needs a teacher who understands the links between readiness skills and learning to read, a teacher who knows how to teach reading rather than depends upon the manual that accompanies the instructional program. (Remember, the manual was written with the "average" child in mind; the child with substandard readiness abilities is not average.)

The instructional program

The instructional program must be designed so it makes apparent, in an unambiguous fashion, specifically what the child must pay attention to if he or she is to learn from the lesson—in a way that reveals clearly the underlying "system" and thereby makes it possible for the child to learn by association (relating what has been learned before with what is being learned now) rather than by rote memorization.

Physical conditions of the classroom

The size of the group must be reduced, and its makeup must be reasonably homogeneous—all children being at more or less the same instructional level—so the teacher has the opportunity to provide direct on-target instruction to the group, along with individual attention when it is required.

Will this work? Can children who enter first grade unready succeed? Yes. But it requires special circumstances—circumstances that many schools cannot (or will not) provide. The outcome in those cases: the child "fails," a cruel and inaccurate term, considering that the decision to enroll in first grade was not made by him, nor was it his fault that an inadequate instructional approach was used.

Conclusion

Optometrists have a long history of professional interest in vision as it pertains to learning, commencing with Gesell's work on the development of vision.[27] It is not difficult to understand this connection. First, vision is important to the optometrist. Second, many children are referred to the optometrist because of classroom difficulties that appear to be linked with vision (e.g., difficulty copying from the chalkboard, disorganized paper work, printing and reading letter/word reversals). Third, the optometrist is trained to understand the connections between visual development and the other facets of development. And fourth, there are now recognized links between hyperopia, visual perceptual skills, and classroom achievement.

The results of all this: Optometrists are highly capable of providing competent guidance to educators and parents in regard to the topic of reading readiness in general, and in regard to the various (and best) ways for managing children who approach (or enter) first grade unready.

References

1. Hughes S: Metropolitan Readiness Test. In Keyser DJ, Sweetland RC (eds): *Test critique,* Kansas City, Mo, 1986, Test Corporation of America, vol 6.
2. Ames L: Learning disabilities: the developmental point of view. In Myklebust H (ed): *Progress in learning disabilities,* New York, 1968, Grune & Stratton.
3. Morphett M, Washburn C: When should children begin to read? *Element School J* 31:496-503, 1931.
4. Gesell A: *The first five years of life,* New York, 1940, Harper & Row.
5. Olson W: *Child development,* Boston, 1949, DC Heath.
6. Kirk S: Amelioration of mental abilities through psychodiagnostic and remedial procedures. In Gervis G (ed): *Mental retardation,* Springfield, Ill, 1967, Charles C Thomas.
7. *Metropolitan Achievement Test,* New York, 1978, Harcourt, Brace, Jovanovich.
8. Barrett TC: Predicting reading achievement through readiness tests. In Farr R (ed): *Measurement and evaluation in reading,* New York, 1970, Harcourt, Brace & World.
9. Rosner J: *Helping children overcome learning difficulties,* ed 2, New York, 1979, Walker Publishing.
10. Rosner J, Rosner J: *Vision therapy in a primary care practice,* New York, 1988, Professional Press.
11. Gordon RR: Increasing efficiency and effectiveness in predicting second-grade achievement using a kindergarten screening battery, *J Educ Res* 81:238-244, 1988.
12. Carver NK: Reading readiness, *Child Educ* 62:256-259, 1986.
13. Rosner J, Gruber J: Differences in the perceptual skills development of young myopes and hyperopes, *Am J Optom Physiol Opt* 62:501-504, 1985.
14. Rosner J, Rosner J: The relationship between ametropia and visual perceptual skills. Abstract, AAO meeting 1992, Orlando, Fla.
15. Rosner J, Rosner J: Some observations of the relationship between the visual perceptual skills development of young hyperopes and the age of first lens correction, *Clin Exp Optom* 69:166-168, 1986.
16. Rosner J, Rosner J: The relationship between ametropia and school achievement, *Optom Vis Sci* (suppl) 69:104, 1992.
17. Pavlidis GT: Eye movement differences between dyslexics, normal, and retarded readers while sequentially fixating digits, *Am J Optom Physiol Opt* 62:820-832, 1985.
18. Brown B, Haegerstrom-Portnoy G, Yingling CD, et al: Tracking eye movements are normal in dyslexic children, *Am J Optom Physiol Opt* 60:376-383, 1983.
19. Hoffman LG: Incidence of vision difficulties in children with learning disabilities, *J Am Optom Assoc* 51:447-451, 1980.

20. Rosner J, Rosner J: Comparison of the visual characteristics of children with and without learning difficulties, *Am J Optom Physiol Opt* 64:531-533, 1987.
21. Rosner J, Rosner J: *Pediatric optometry,* ed 2, Boston, 1990, Butterworths.
22. Rosner J: *Learning disabilities can be overcome,* New York, 1995, Walker Publishing.
23. Simon H: *Science of the artificial,* Cambridge, Mass, 1969, MIT Press.
24. Rosner J, Rosner J, Mazow M: Including perceptual skills testing in an ophthalmic examination. Why? How? *Am Orthopt J* 38:186-194, 1988.
25. Ayres AJ: Learning disabilities and the vestibular system, *J Learn Disabil* 11:18-29, 1978.
26. Rosner J: *Perceptual skills curriculum,* New York, 1973, Walker Educational Book Corporation.
27. Gesell A et al: *Vision–its development in infant and child,* New York, 1949, Paul B Hoeber.

Appendix

Bernell Corporation, 750 Lincolnway East, PO Box 4637, South Bend, IN 46634.

DLM Teaching Resources, PO Box 4000, Allen, TX 75002.

OEP Foundation, 1921 E. Carnegie Ave, Suite 3-L, Santa Ana, CA 92705-5510.

5

The Ergonomics of Reading

William F. Long
Ralph P. Garzia
Timothy Wingert
Sylvia R. Garzia

Key Terms

ergonomics	illuminance	video display
lighting	typography	terminal (VDT)
photometry	legibility	posture
luminance		positioning

Ergonomics is the study of the relationship between human beings and their environment, with special reference to anatomical, physiological, and psychological factors. This topic has gained considerable attention in recent years from industry, education, and individuals. The reason for this interest in ergonomics is its effect on employment productivity, performance efficiency, and injury creation in the workplace or in personal endeavors. The study of ergonomics also includes a preventive component—lowering the relative risk of injury and reducing the prevalence and severity of injury, including discomfort.

This chapter explores several aspects of the ergonomics of reading tasks. Beginning with the traditional component of lighting, it follows with discussions of the legibility of print and the special problems associated with video display terminal use. The concluding section discusses posture and positioning anomalies that are associated with seated work and offers a short therapeutic exercise regimen.

Lighting

It is obvious that visual function, including reading, will be impaired by light that is too dim, by glare, or by too much or too little contrast. So the first step toward analyzing the visual ergonomics of any situation is to evaluate the lighting. Fortunately, it is relatively easy to measure light levels and compare them with standards that have been developed for reading or for virtually any other activity imaginable. Unfortunately, the quantitative science of measuring the amount of light (photometry) is cloaked in such a daunting welter of symbols, units, and mathematical relationships that most optometrists have consigned the subject to the purview of a few specialists.

CLINICAL PEARL

Visual function, including reading, will be impaired by light that is too dim, by glare, or by too much or too little contrast.

But this is not really necessary. In what follows we will define the relevant photometric concepts, discuss lighting standards, and show how to apply these standards to some common reading environments.

Photometric Concepts

There are five basic terms to understand in the photometric vocabulary—luminous flux, illuminance, luminous intensity, luminance, and reflectance—and six special units that are necessary to characterize these quantities:

General: lumen, candela
Metric: lux, apostilb
English: foot-candela, foot-Lambert

CLINICAL PEARL

There are five basic terms to understand in the photometric vocabulary—luminous flux, illuminance, luminous intensity, luminance, and reflectance.

Although optometrists use metric units in all other optics, a sufficient number of light meters are calibrated in English units to make it necessary to learn both systems. Fortunately, conversion from one to the other is exceptionally easy. There are other units, but a knowledge of the stilb, nit, etc. is not necessary to understand or apply photometry.

Luminous flux

The electromagnetic energy or radiant flux from a light source is given in watts of power. But the watt applies to all electromagnetic radiation, regardless of wavelength. It applies, for example, to x-rays, television transmission waves, microwaves, infrared and ultraviolet radiation, and all types of other electromagnetic radiation irrelevant to vision. In fact, the eye responds to only a small portion of the electromagnetic spectrum. It is most sensitive to light of 550 nm wavelength (yellow), less sensitive to short wavelength (blue and green) and long wavelength (orange and red) light, and it receives no visual sensation at all from radiation with wavelengths below 410 or above 730 nm. This is shown quantitatively by the familiar spectral sensitivity curve in Figure 5-1.

Clearly, radiant flux is inappropriate for dealing with vision. Instead, in photometry we use luminous flux, which carries the unit *lumen* (abbreviated lm). Luminous flux is radiant flux weighted by the spectral sensitivity curve. This means that only visible light is included, and light near the peak sensitivity of the eye is weighted more heavily. A lumen of luminous flux produces the same magnitude of

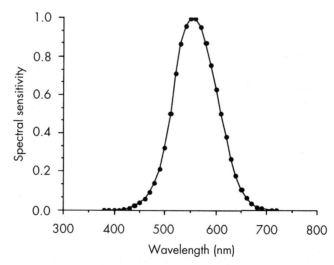

FIGURE 5-1 Spectral sensitivity curve. (Modified from Hecht S: Visual acuity and illumination, *Arch Ophthalmol* 57:565, 1928.)

"visual sensation" regardless of the wavelength of the light. From a purely photometric point of view, once we know how many lumens of flux come from a source we need concern ourselves with no other aspect of its spectrum. The customary symbol for luminous flux is F.

Illuminance (illumination)

Illuminance (sometimes called illumination) is a most important quantity in photometry because it is the only quantity that can be measured directly. It is defined as the amount of luminous flux incident on a surface per unit area (Figure 5-2) and is symbolized by E. Thus

$$E = F/A$$

where F is the amount of flux incident on an area A.

Suppose, for example, that 1000 lumens of flux falls on an area of 2 square meters. The illuminance of the area would be simply

$$(1000 \text{ lm})/(2 \text{ m}^2) = 500 \text{ lm/m}^2$$

The lumen/square meter is dimensionally the same as the *lux* (abbreviated lx), so the answer above could be, and usually is, given as 500 lx. The corresponding English unit is lumen/square foot, which is dimensionally the same as the *foot-candela* (abbreviated ft-cd). Because 1 square meter contains about 10 square feet, the conversion factor for the two units is approximately 10, and the answer to the above example in English units would be about 50 ft-cd. Some typical values for illuminance are given in Table 5-1.

Illuminance is measured with an illuminance meter (often simply called a light meter). Figure 5-3 is a schematic of an illuminance meter.

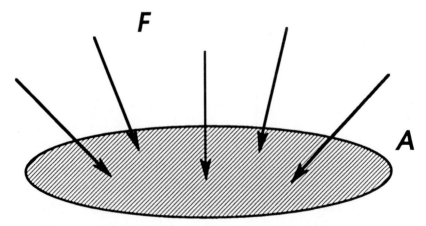

FIGURE 5-2 Illuminance is defined as incident flux per unit area, $E = F/A$.

TABLE 5-1
Typical Illuminance Values

Ground in bright sun	5000 ft-cd (50,000 lx)
Ground in overcast conditions	1000 ft-cd (10,000 lx)
Well-lit work surface 50 ft-cd	(500 lx)
Visual acuity chart 10 ft-cd	(100 lx)

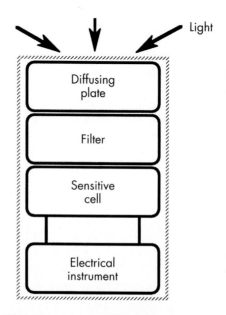

FIGURE 5-3 An illuminance meter.

Light incident on the meter head is diffused by a diffusing plate, typically a piece of translucent white plastic, which eliminates any directional sensitivity of the meter; thus a lumen of flux will register the same regardless of its angle of incidence. Meters with a proper diffusing plate are called *cosine corrected.*

Light passing through the diffusing plate passes through a filter on its way to a sensitive cell. The sensitive cell is a material that responds electrically to incident light. The classical selenium cell, for instance, generates a voltage when light strikes it—the more light, the more voltage. The cadmium sulfide cell found in many cameras, on the other hand, has a resistance that varies with the amount of incident light. The filter serves to remove or attenuate portions of the light spectrum so the combination of sensitive cell and filter will have a spectral response similar to that of the eye (see Figure 5-1). The electrical instrument turns the electrical response of the sensitive cell into a scale reading, either an analog reading with a moving needle or a digital reading with a light-emitting diode.

Figure 5-4 shows a typical light meter. Note the diffusing plate, clearly visible on top. To measure the illuminance of a surface, simply place the meter on the surface with its head parallel to the surface, adjust the scale switch until the needle settles somewhere near the center of the scale, and read the position of the needle on the scale, which corresponds to the position of the switch.

Luminous intensity

Light sources are either primary (which generate light energy) or secondary (which reflect light energy generated by primary sources). Tungsten and fluorescent bulbs are the most common primary light sources; walls, ceilings, clothing, etc., are all secondary sources.

Luminous intensity (or just intensity) characterizes the amount of luminous flux emitted by a small light source. Its unit is the candela (cd), and it is symbolized by I. Sometimes it is called candlepower.

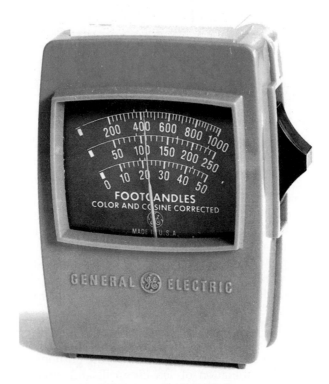

FIGURE 5-4 A typical light meter.

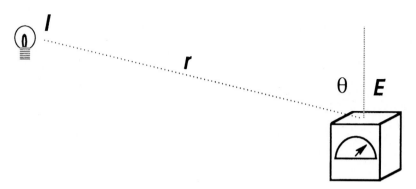

FIGURE 5-5 The inverse square law of photometry says that the meter illuminance E due to a light source of intensity I is $I\cos\theta/r^2$.

Intensity is analogous to charge in electrostatics or mass in gravitation. As in electricity and gravitation, there is an inverse square law of photometry that connects intensity and illuminance. With reference to the geometry of Figure 5-5, if a light meter is distance r from a light source of intensity I, and if the light meter is oriented so the normal to the diffusing plate (the normal being the line perpendicular to the plate) makes an angle (θ) with the line connecting the plate and the light source, then

$$E = I\cos\theta/r^2$$

The factor $\cos\theta$ means that the meter will measure the highest illuminance if it is aimed directly at the source and no illuminance at all if light from the source hits it at grazing incidence.

The intensity of a source can, and usually does, depend upon the source orientation. For example, more flux leaves the top of a light bulb than the bottom so the light bulb's intensity is greater from the top (Figure 5-6).

Luminance

Luminous intensity can adequately characterize the flux coming from a relatively small source, such as a light bulb viewed from a distance. Luminance characterizes the amount of light coming from an area of a large source, such as a fluorescent luminaire, a wall, or an item of clothing. Luminance is defined as light intensity of a unit-projected source area. In equation form

$$L = I/(\text{projected area})$$

where L is luminance and I is the intensity of the source along the line of sight. The usual metric unit for luminance is lux, and the English unit is foot-candela.

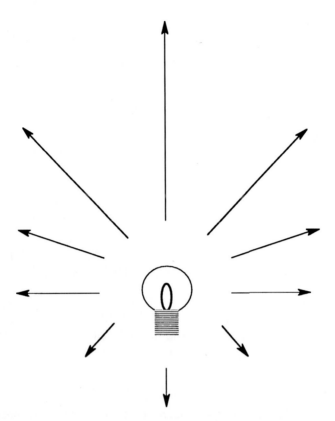

FIGURE 5-6 The luminous intensity of a light source varies with the angle of observation. Because more flux leaves the top of the light bulb than the bottom, the bulb has greatest luminous intensity when viewed from the top, less when viewed from the side, and least when viewed from the bottom.

As shown in Figure 5-7, the projected area is just the apparent area of a source subtended along the line of sight of an observer. "Projected area" is used in the definition of luminance because the area of the retinal image of an object is proportional to the object's projected area at the eye. Because the illuminance of the retinal image is the ratio of the flux reaching the image divided by the area of the image, and because the amount of flux reaching the retina depends on the intensity of the object, the illuminance of the retinal image is proportional to the luminance of the object (Figure 5-8).

The illuminance of the retina initiates the visual process. The perceived "brightness" of an object is in proportion to its retinal illuminance.

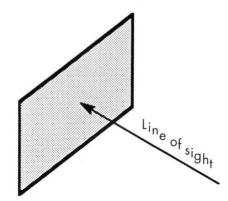

Line of sight perpendicular to area

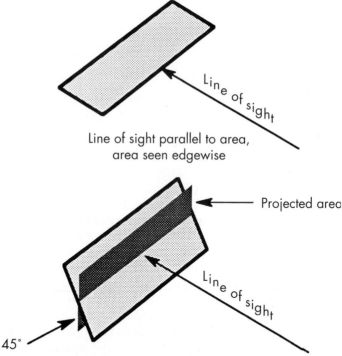

Line of sight parallel to area,
area seen edgewise

Area tilted 45° with respect to the line of sight,
projected area shown with dark shading

FIGURE 5-7 *Projected area* is the subtense of an area along the line of sight. If the line of sight is perpendicular to the area, the area and projected area are the same. If the line of sight is along the edge of the area, the projected area is zero. If an area is tilted 45° with the line of sight, the area will be cos 45° or 0.707 times the projected area.

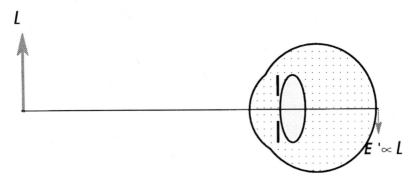

FIGURE 5-8 The illuminance (E') of the retinal image of an object is proportional to the luminance (L) of the object.

In fact, the illuminance of the image of *any* image-forming system is proportional to object luminance. For instance, the illuminance (E') of the image of a remote object of luminance L in a camera is given by

$$E' = (\pi/4)L/(f/\text{number})^2$$

where the f/number of an optical system is defined as

$$\frac{\text{focal length}}{\text{diameter of entrance pupil}}$$

The f/number (or f/stop) of a lens is written in the form f/4 to indicate that the f/number is 4. The f/number is useful because any two lenses with the same f/number setting will produce the same image illuminance (Figure 5-9).

Luminance can be measured with a special meter called a luminance meter, which is basically a camera system in which an illuminance meter replaces the film. The system is focused on the luminous object. Because E' is proportional to L, the illuminance meter, can be calibrated to read luminance directly (note that we are actually measuring an *illuminance* and inferring a *luminance* from that), the exposure meter built into a reflex camera is essentially a luminance meter.

Luminance also can be determined by devices that permit an observer to match the luminance of an object to that of another object of known luminance. In this case the subject is actually matching the retinal illuminances of the standard and unknown objects. The Goldman perimeter calibrates background luminance with an arrangement of this sort.

In general, the luminance of an object depends on the angle of observation. In fact, most sources, especially secondary ones, have the same luminance at all angles, which is why an object like a shirt, wall, or tablecloth does not appear brighter or dimmer when seen from different angles. Objects for which this is true are called Lambert radiators.

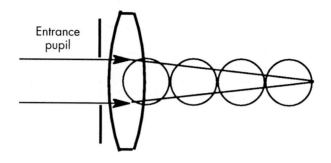

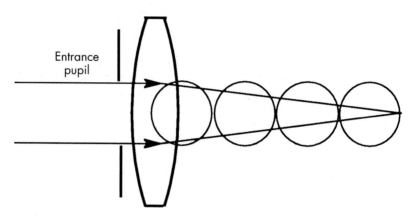

FIGURE 5-9 Both lenses above are f/4 and produce the same film illuminance.

This property makes it possible to determine the luminance of a Lambert radiator with an ordinary light meter—provided the source is large enough and has uniform luminance. Simply hold the light meter close to the surface with the diffusing head parallel to the surface, but not so close as to cast a shadow. The luminance is related to E_{meter}, the meter reading, by the equations

$$E_{meter} \text{ (lx)} = \pi L(\text{lx}) = L(\text{asb})$$

$$E_{meter} \text{ (ft−cd)} = \pi L(\text{ft−cd}) = L(\text{ft−L})$$

where the units for the quantities are in parentheses. These equations introduce the pesky Lambert units for luminance *apostilb* (asb) and *foot-Lambert* (ft-L). Lambert units were devised to eliminate multiplication and division by factors of $\pi = 3.14159$.

Suppose, for example, that a meter held above and parallel to the center of a carpet reads 100 lx. The luminance of the carpet would be

$100/\pi = 32$ lx or simply 100 asb. In English units the meter illuminance would be about 10 ft-cd, corresponding to a carpet luminance of 3.2 ft-cd or 10 ft-L.

Reflectance

Reflectance is an important property of secondary sources. It is defined as the ratio of light incident on an area to light reflected from that area. For a Lambert radiator, reflectance can be measured easily by taking the ratio of light meter readings with the meter aimed at the middle of the surface (but far enough from the surface to avoid shadows) to readings from the surface (Figure 5-10). The usual symbol for reflectance, ρ, can be given as a fraction (e.g., 0.7 or 70%).

There is a very simple relation between luminance, illuminance, and reflectance for a secondary Lambert radiator:

$$L(\text{asb}) = \rho E(\text{lx})$$

$$L(\text{ft-L}) = \rho E(\text{ft-cd})$$

For example, if the illuminance of an acuity chart is 500 lx and the reflectance of the chart is 80%, the luminance of the chart is (0.8)(500 lx) = 400 lx. In English units the illuminance would be about 50 ft-cd with luminance (0.8)(50 ft-cd) = 40 ft-L. And *this* is why they invented Lambert units!

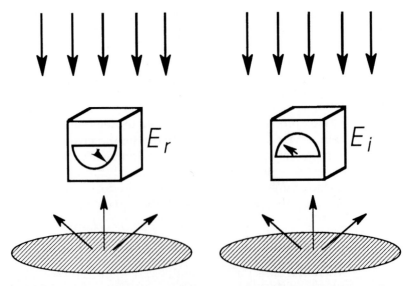

FIGURE 5-10 To measure reflectance, hold the meter above and parallel to the reflecting surface and take reading E_r. Reverse the direction of the meter and take reading E_i. The reflectance is the ratio of these two readings, $\rho = E_r / E_i$.

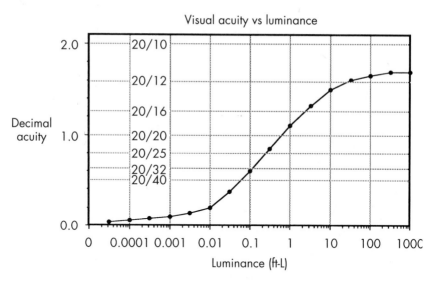

FIGURE 5-11 Visual acuity as a function of background luminance.

Lighting Standards

The luminance necessary for reading ordinary materials can be deduced from the curve in Figure 5-11, which gives a characteristic plot of visual acuity as a function of background luminance for a normal subject. The graph shows that acuity rises rapidly up to 100 asb (10 ft-L) and improves more slowly thereafter, very nearly reaching its maximum value at 1000 asb (100 ft-L) The curve suggests that the luminance in reading areas would be around 1000 asb (100 ft-L) and, because the reflectance of white paper is very high (nearly 100%, so $\rho \approx 1$), this would correspond to an illuminance of 1000 lx (100 ft-cd). And that is pretty much the case. The curve shows why acuity charts require a screen illuminance of 100 to 200 lx (10 to 20 ft-cd).[2] It also explains why beginning presbyopes have special problems in dim light. At low light levels they find it difficult to hold reading matter closer to compensate for their lower acuity.

Lighting standards for a great variety of activities are listed in the *Illumination Engineering Society (IES) Lighting Handbook*.[3] The IES recommendations are based primarily on the visibility of the task in question. Visibility can be thought of as a generalization of visual acuity. It depends upon the contrast, size, and details of the task. A task involving large high-contrast objects requires less light than one involving small or low-contrast objects. The IES establishes appropriate light levels, largely by determining experimentally the visibility of the task (using a visibility meter) and inferring an appropriate luminance from standard psychophysical data.[4] The end result is a table of illuminance values appropriate for various activities. A few typical recommendations are given in Table 5-2.

CLINICAL PEARL

Visibility can be thought of as a generalization of visual acuity. It depends upon the contrast, size, and details of the task. A task involving large high-contract objects requires less light than one involving small or low-contrast objectives.

IES lighting recommendations for several typical reading tasks are presented in Table 5-3. As would be expected from the acuity vs luminance curve, most recommendations are in the 200 to 500 lx (20 to 50 ft-cd) range. The exceptions are tasks with lower visibility due to lower contrast (e.g., text written with a no. 4 pencil) or greater detail (substandard-size music scores).

Glare and adaptation effects can degrade comfort and performance. Because individuals function best when visual tasks are performed against a uniformly lit background of the same average luminance as the task, the IES recommends the luminance ratios given in Table 5-4.

Walls and furnishings in reading areas should be matte reflectors with reflectances chosen to minimize large variations in luminance. The IES[3,4] and Harmon[5] both have compiled recommended reflectances for offices and classrooms. There are small variations, but generally these recommendations are quite consistent with one another. Table 5-5 gives a simplified compilation of reflectances.

TABLE 5-2
IES Illuminance Recommendations

Description	lx	ft-cd	Examples
It's pretty dark in here!	<100	<10	Discotheques, baseball seating, inactive library stacks, hospital corridors, restaurant dining areas
Good enough for walking around	100 to 500	10 to 50	Hotel lobbies, locker rooms, toilets, slaughterhouses
General tasks, including most reading	500 to 1000	50 to 100	Kitchens, hotel front desks, beveling glass
Critical reading, inspection, etc	1000 to 2000	100 to 200	Eye surgery, birthing rooms
Really critical or difficult applications	>2000	>200	Watchmaking, chicken sexing

Modified from Kaufman JE: *IES lighting handbook, application volume,* New York, 1981, Illumination Engineering Society of North America.

TABLE 5-3
IES Lighting Recommendations for Various Reading Activities

Reading matter	lx	ft-cd
Microfiche reader CRT screens	50 to 100	5 to 10
Mimeograph Photocopy (1st generation) Impact printer (good ribbon) Ink jet printer Ball-point pen Felt-tip pen 8- and 10-point type Glossy magazines Newsprint Typed originals Music (simple scores)	200 to 500	20 to 50
Ditto copy Photographs (moderate detail) Photocopy (3rd generation or later) Impact printer (poor ribbon or 2nd carbon) Thermal print No. 3 and softer leads Handwritten carbon copies Chalkboards 6-point type Maps Telephone books Music (advanced scores)	500 to 1000	50 to 100
Thermal copy (poor legibility) No. 4 and harder leads Music (substandard-size scores)	1000 to 2000	100 to 200

Modified from Kaufman JE: *IES lighting handbook, application volume,* New York, 1981, Illumination Engineering Society of North America.

TABLE 5-4
IES Recommended Luminance Ratios

Task to immediate surround (dark surfaces) 1 to 1/3
Task to immediate surround (light surfaces) 3 to 1
Task to remote dark surfaces 1 to 1/10
Task to remote light surfaces 1 to 10

Modified from Kaufman JE: *IES lighting handbook, application volume,* New York, 1981, Illumination Engineering Society of North America.

TABLE 5-5

Recommended Reflectances in Offices and Classrooms

Surface	Recommended reflectance (%)
Floor	30 ±10
Walls and partitions	60 ±10
Blackboard	<20
Blackboard surround	50 ±10
Desk tops and furniture	50 ±10
Ceiling	>80

The IES recommendations are developed for young persons with normal vision. Older persons generally need more light and also may require illuminances 50% to 100% greater than the baseline recommendations.[6] The visual needs of visually impaired individuals are difficult to predict, and it is helpful to provide variable-output light sources whenever possible.[7]

Measuring Light Levels

It is easy to measure the illuminance of a task. Simply place the light meter on and parallel to the work surface in question.

Measuring reflectance of a large surface is almost as easy (Figure 5-10). First, measure the illuminance of the surface with an illuminance meter. Then, turn the illuminance meter over until its head is parallel to the surface and the meter is near the center of the surface, close to the surface but not casting a strong shadow. The meter reading in this position divided by the surface illuminance is the reflectance. The light illuminating the surface during this measurement should not hit the surface at grazing incidence.

Luminance ratios can, of course, be measured with a luminance meter. But these are fairly expensive special-purpose instruments. If you do not wish to invest in one, you can use an SLR camera.[8]

1. Meter the work area.
2. Meter the immediate surround. If there is less than 3 stops of difference, all is well.
3. Meter the remote areas. If there is less than 4 stops of difference, all is well.

Room Surveys

There are two reasons for doing room surveys[9]—to calculate the average room illuminance (to verify engineering plans and specifications) and to survey the workstations (to verify compliance with these standards).

The first is done with an excruciatingly detailed form and is of interest to engineers. The second can be done much more simply and is of interest to health and safety officers, educators, and vision care professionals. Table 5-6 shows an example of an illuminance survey.

Typography

Typography is the style and appearance of printed matter. Although printers have learned, by centuries of experimentation, many of the lessons of print legibility, it is important for these questions to be answered in the less ambiguous arena of vision research. Much of the outcome of research has confirmed the validity of many printing conventions.[10] It is now well understood that reading comprehension and information processing derived from the printed word can be greatly influenced by typographical presentation.[11] Legibility research is concerned with the efficiency of information transmissibility of the printed word. For this reason, the study of typography is essential when considering the ergonomics of reading.

TABLE 5-6
Results of an Illumination Survey

Location	Light source	Illuminance (ft-cd)	IES Recommended average	Reflectance (%)	IES Recommended average (%)	Contrast (pass/fail)
Lecturer's desk	Overhead luminaires with sunlight through windows	130	>70	18	35-50	pass
Desk, front of class, window side		200		18		fail
Desk, rear of class, window side		150		18		pass
Desk, front middle of class		90		18		pass
Desk, center of class		110		18		pass
Desk, rear middle of class		100		18		pass
Desk, front of class, door side		100		18		pass
Desk, middle of class, door side		90		18		pass
Desk, rear of class, door side		90		18		pass
Blackboard				17	<20	
Blackboard surround				40	40-60	
Wall				44	40-60	
Floor				33	30-50	

Summary and recommendations: Illuminances fall within guidelines. Contrast is too great at one desk due to sunlight. Fix venetian blinds so that direct sun can be blocked off. Desk reflectances are slightly low, but surfaces are small and probably covered by higher reflectance student notebooks during use.

CLINICAL PEARL

Reading comprehension and information processing derived from the printed word can be greatly influenced by its typographical presentation.

Typography is equally important for the clinician. Within a relatively wide range, legibility may not be a significant issue for adult, experienced readers, but children learning to read or disabled readers who already confuse very visible, individual letters and words may be further impaired by poorly legible typography. Type that is too small or too large, that is set in lines too close together or too far apart, or with words that are too close together or too far apart, blunts the pleasure of reading and discourages all but the most persevering. Poor typography can produce stress and discomfort for the reader. There may be a category of patients who are best described as typography sensitive; that is, even when reading print in standard typographical formats, they experience visual difficulty by some as yet poorly understood mechanisms.

CLINICAL PEARL

Legibility may not be a significant issue for adult, experienced readers, but children learning to read or disabled readers who already confuse very visible, individual letters and words may be further impaired by poorly legible typography.

Black letter was the first typeface used in printing in Europe.[11] It is a heavy typeface with very broad stems and counters (the enclosed white space of a letter) and thick ornamental serifs (see Figure 5-12). Early printers attempted to use print type in the style of writing of the day. This was the typeface used by Gutenberg, which is still widely used in Germany.

It was disparagingly called "Gothic" by Italian scholars, although it had nothing to do with the Goths. Roman-style type with serifs, the predominant typeface used today, originated in Italy (Venice) in the fifteenth century. The reason for the change was that, as printing

Print with this typeface is more difficult to read than other typefaces.

FIGURE 5-12 Black letter or Gothic typeface.

spread from north of the Alps across Europe, printers had to copy the style of writing in the region.[11]

Research Methods

The classical period of research of legibility of print was during the 1920s, '30s and '40s. There were several experimental paradigms developed during this time. A brief description of each follows.

The visibility meter of Luckiesh and Moss[12] consisted of two filters, much like Polaroid filters, that when rotated varied the amount of light transmitted. To test for visibility of a letter or word, the filters were rotated, altering the luminance and contrast of the target until it could be correctly identified.

The distance method utilized a 3 m long wooden rail, much like Howe's ergograph, on which the test stimulus was placed in a small illuminated car that could be moved on the rail.[13] The target stimulus was placed at the far end of the rail and advanced in 10 cm increments. The farthest distance from the subject that the stimulus could be correctly identified was a measure of its visibility.

The short-exposure method utilized a conventional tachistoscope.[14] The target stimulus was presented for brief intervals ($\leq$ 100 msec). At these durations saccadic eye movements are not available to assist in identification. The percentage of correct responses at particular exposures established the target's visibility.

The focal variator developed by Weiss[15] displayed a visual stimulus that could be defocused to a known level without changing the size of the image. To determine visiblity of a stimulus, it was first displayed at maximum defocus (blur) and the blur was then decreased until the stimulus could be correctly identified.

Luckiesh and Moss[16,17] suggested that a reader's involuntary blink rate could be used as a measure of the readability (legibility) of text. The relationship was inverse (i.e., reduced readability increased the blink rate). However, Tinker[18,19] later investigated this relationship and found it to be invalid and unreliable.

The analysis of eye movement patterns during reading reveals the variations in a person's reading speed that can occur from one typographical arrangement to another.[20] Fixation duration and the number of individual fixations and regressions that occur when reading a selection provide objective evidence of the reader's proficiency when encountering text. An increase in any of these parameters strongly suggests that the reader is experiencing difficulty. In studying the legibility of print, eye movement measures are highly reliable and valid indicators of reading performance.

Perhaps the most intuitive method of investigating the visibility of print is the speed of reading. With this method, performance output is the dependent variable. The subject is engaged in the very activity that interests the investigator. Therefore, the rate of work has been considered the preferable measure of legibility. The supposition is that, all other things being equal, a typography that is read faster also should be easier to read.

During this classical experimental period there were two important tests used to measure reading. Their innovative design made them ideal as research tools for the investigation of text legibility.

The Chapman-Cook Speed of Reading Test consisted of 30 short paragraphs of 30 words each.[14] Each paragraph contained one word that was contextually inappropriate. The reader's task was to read the paragraphs and strike through the inappropriate words. Following is an example:

> When I am enjoying anything very much, time seems to go very quickly. I noticed this the other day, when I spent the whole afternoon reading a very uninteresting book.

The offending word is ~~uninteresting~~. For adults, comprehension measured in this fashion is nearly 100%. The number of paragraphs completed in a specified time was the measure of reading rate, and the determination of reading rate was uncontaminated by faulty comprehension influences. This method was considered at the time a purer measure than any other of the rate variable alone. The typical testing time was 1.5 minutes.

Tinker[14] also produced a similarly formatted reading test that extended allowable testing time to over 30 minutes. The Tinker Speed of Reading test consisted of 450 items of 30 words each. Following is an example:

> In Ohio there are many coal mines. They are so damp, dark, and dirty, and even dangerous at times, that we do not envy the musicians who work in them.

The correct response is ~~musicians~~.

There has been considerable research into the visibility of typography (i.e., the effects of typeface, line length, interlinear spacing, and margins) on reading performance. These efforts probably began with Javal[21] in 1878, who asked the hypothetical question concerning the relative visibility of letters. He postulated that the poor typography of the day contributed to the development of myopia, and he felt that Gothic type (black letters) with excessive spacing in printed materials was detrimental to good visual hygiene. He also advocated the use of yellow-tinted paper instead of white, which was thought to be less fatiguing to the eyes.

Legibility of Print

The following is a compendium of important concepts about the legibility of print.[22] Each statement reinforces the concept that even small changes in almost any printed detail have an effect on readers[10]:

1. The upper portion of letters carries more information for the identification of words than the lower portion. Also the more distinctive features present in the upper portion lead to less confusion between letters[14] (Figure 5-13).

CLINICAL PEARL

The upper portion of letters carries more information for the identification of words than the lower portion. Also the more distinctive features present in the upper portion lead to less confusion between letters.

---

2. Figure 5-14 describes some of the common components of printed words. Word shape or the block outline of words is important for their recognition. All-capital printing reduces reading speed more than any other single typographic factor[23,24] (Figure 5-15). This influence is indeed significant. For a 20-minute period, reading rate can be reduced by nearly 14%.

3. The perceived aesthetics or beauty of individual typefaces has a poor correlation with measured reading performance (rate). In a related issue, personal preferences or subjective opinions of readers concerning the ease of reading text are not always consistent with objective measures of reading performance.[25,26]

4. Research on the legibility of individual lower case letters has shown remarkable agreement over many studies.[27] The letters *d, m, p, q,* and *w* have a high degree of legibility; but *c, e, i, n,* and *l* have considerably less. Distinctive characteristics and a large area of enclosed white space within a letter contribute to legibility. All things being equal, the greater the enclosed white space of a letter (counter or inside bowl), the greater the legibility.[27]

   Heavy or long serifs diminish legibility. The horizontal dimension or overall size of a letter also contributes to its legibility. For example, *m* and *w* are more legible than either *i* or *l*. As an interesting fact, the dot of the letter *i* should be high over the stem

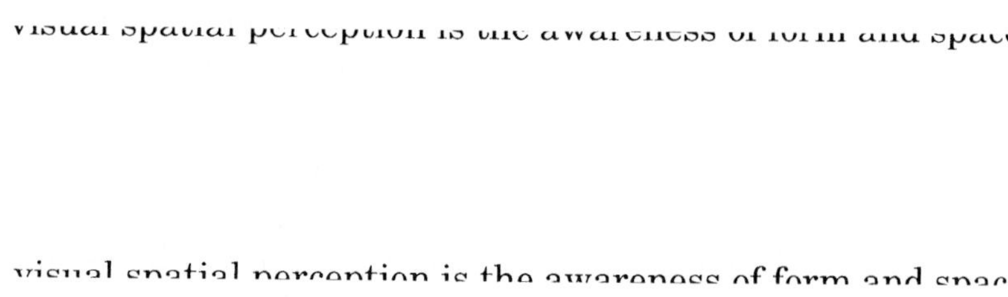

visual spatial perception is the awareness of form and space

visual spatial perception is the awareness of form and space

FIGURE 5-13 Note how the top half of a printed line carries more information for word identification than the bottom half.

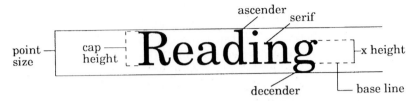

FIGURE 5-14 Standard features of Roman or serif type. The *x* height of a typeface refers to the size of the lowercase letters. Typefaces vary considerably in the ratio of *x* height to point size.

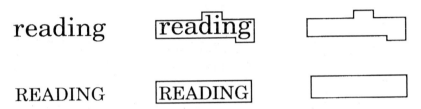

FIGURE 5-15 Block outlines of the word *reading* illustrate that lowercase print provides distinctive word shape information whereas all-capital printing provides none except for word length.

for maximum legibility, but the shape of the letter is of little consequence. A large, heavily dotted *i* adds to its legibility.[28]

5. Typefaces in common use are equally legible (as determined by reading rate), with the exception of black letter typefaces for relatively short-duration reading.[23]

6. Serifs are the small fine lines finishing off the main strokes of a letter at the end of roman letters. Sans serif typeface is read as quickly as serif (roman) typeface for short reading durations, but readers do not prefer it. With more extended reading, typefaces with serifs are preferable.[14] There are two classes of serifs, the top serif and the foot serif. They can take several design forms— bracketed, hairline, wedge, slab, or straight.

Three principal reasons have been advanced to explain the superiority of serif typefaces for word legibility.[10,11] First, the serifs link the letters together to form word units. The superiority of letter discrimination within words compared with discrimination of single letters is a well-known phenomenon. Second, serifs help to maintain adequate spacing between letters and emphasize the separation between words. Third, serifs help to avoid confusion by enhancing letter differentiation.

Roman letters (all capitals) with serifs first appeared in 1816. The serifs were called "English Egyptian" for the exotic appearance they gave letters.[11] The first lowercase serif letters were produced in London in 1835 and were referred to as "seven lines grotesque," primarily because of their "grotesque" appearance compared with their contemporaries. The grotesque reference was shortened to "grot," then to "sans serif," and finally to "sans."

7. Despite reader preferences to the contrary, bold typeface is as legible as normal type when measured objectively.[23]

8. Italic type slows reading by about 15 words per minute. This was found to be consistent with the subjective impressions of 96% of readers studied.[29,30]

9. Printing variables such as type size, line length (column width), and interlinear spacing (or *leading,* pronounced "ledding") are complex, interrelated, and interdependent for legibility.[23]

   The *point* is a unit measure of type size and interlinear spacing (leading) that equals 1/72 of an inch (1/12 of a pica). The *pica* is a unit measure of column width (line measure) that equals 1/6 of an inch. Leading is the amount of space between lines of type; it is measured in points.

   Common type sizes, 9- to 12-point, are equally legible.[14,23] But the relationship between type size and legibility is an inverse U-shaped curve. Smaller and larger type sizes cause reductions in reading rate. Reading print away from the perpendicular changes typeface size: 12-point type read at a 45° angle away from the perpendicular reduces the text to 8 point, a 33% reduction.

   The optimal line length for efficient reading should contain 10 to 12 words or 60 to 70 characters.[14,23] Again, shorter and longer lines of text reduce reading rate. Smaller line length actually increases the number of fixations required to read the line, and each fixation has a longer duration on each line. Larger line lengths increase the number of regressions.

   Interlinear spacing has an important effect on the legibility of text.[10] Legibility depends upon being able to recognize the ascenders and descenders of letters. If adjacent lines of text are squeezed together, the lines above and below "crowd" the visual system and the reader's attention. Too much space is also undesirable for legibility, for two reasons. First, the added white spaces around the text can be a glare source. Second, the oculomotor control system may have difficulty finding the beginning of the next line (causing frequent rereading or skipping of lines). Two-point spacing is apparently optimal. Paterson and Tinker[23] described a "safety zone," within which the limits of variation in line width and interlinear spacing may be used for a given type size without loss of legibility. Generally speaking, the greater the number of characters in a line of print, the larger the required interlinear space. For increased legibility the interlinear space (leading) should be greater than the spacing between the words.

10. Although unjustified lines were once considered an indication of ragged and sloppy printing, they apparently have little influence

on reading rate.[31] There has been at least one report[32] of poor readers who read unjustified text more quickly than justified text.

11. There have been a few curious attempts to make the presentation of text more efficient for reading. Kujus[33] suggested a modified boustrophedon text, which was thought to necessitate less eye movement and thus cause less visual fatigue by eliminating the need for large return sweeps. The following is an example:

> It has been suggested that reading
> fatiguing less be would way this in text

Presenting text in vertical columns, thereby eliminating the need for horizontal eye movements altogether, also has proven to be ineffectual at improving reading efficiency.[34] Even after 6 weeks of training, adults read vertically oriented text significantly more slowly than horizontal text. It remains to be seen if children exposed to reading in this format from the beginning of their education would demonstrate an affinity for vertical orientation.

Obliquely arranged or slanted lines of text are read more slowly than horizontal or vertical presentations.[14,35,36]

12. Indenting alternate lines of text slows reading a small amount (3% to 4%) compared with the regular arrangement, in which all lines except the first of a paragraph are block left.[23]

13. The importance of margins has been advocated in both preventing and creating visual fatigue. The most interesting explanations are oculomotor and ergonomic. The presence of a margin would prevent the eyes from swinging off the page when saccading along a text line. (This seems hardly convincing.) Conversely, the presence of narrow margins would reduce peripheral glare and color distractions.[37-39] (This seems more plausible.) Clinicians are aware of some glare-sensitive patients who complain of visual discomfort apparently caused by the overpowering whiteness of a page of print. The use of masks or filters might be beneficial for these patients.

For short reading periods, Paterson and Tinker[23] found little difference in reading rates between margined and unmargined text. A margin ratio of 1 (for the inner margin), 1.5 (for a head), 2 (for the foredge), and 2.5 (for the foot) is a conventional starting point, but the typical conditions of book production are so varied that any one formula would be senseless.[10]

Paterson and Tinker[23,40] measured 400 available textbooks and found that, on average, 50% of a page of print was taken up by margins; that is, the text portion occupied only 50% of the total page area. This relationship is not readily perceived by readers. In fact, readers generally overestimate the extent of text area by an average of 18%. (The most frequent estimate is 75%.)

14. Large books and bound volumes of journals have inner margins that are sufficiently small to present the text on a curve. The book

binding prevents the pages from lying entirely flat. Reading of curved text significantly reduces both the legibility of individual words and the reading rate.[41]

15. Professional journals and commercial magazines are usually printed in multiple-column formats. The effect on reading of single-versus multiple-column printing is related to the legibility issues of type size, optimal line widths, and leading. Reader preferences are clearly for the double-column presentation. Intercolumnar spacing also is to be considered. Text with any particular intercolumnar arrangement is read just as fast as any other.[23] However, readers prefer a rule (small vertical line [|]) between columns with 1/2 pica of space on each side, though this is rarely done.

16. Single digits also have different legibilities; 3, 5, 8, and 2 are regarded as having the lowest level.[13] Mathematical signs also vary in legibility; the more legible signs are =, Σ, and ; and the less legible ones are: $\pm$, $\div$, and π. Exponents (superscripts) and subscripts have lower legibility, probably because of their decreased size relative to that of numerals and letters in mathematical formulas.

17. When reading mathematics problems, people seem to fixate and scrutinize numerals individually, digit by digit, and hence find them more difficult to read than words. This has been determined by analyses of reading eye movements.[42,43] There is a much greater tendency to fixate each digit in a numeral than each letter in a word.

18. Mathematics problems with Arabic numerals are read faster than problems with numerals spelled out in words.[27,44,45] Mathematical tables are more legible if they have columns with groups of 5 numerals, 1 pica space between columns, and fewer columns.[46-48]

19. Typewriting is more legible than manuscript and cursive script, and manuscript is more legible than cursive script.[49-51] With cursive script, the only upper case letter that causes consistent difficulty for readers is *I*. In one study, pertaining to lower case letters, *r* and *n* were particularly difficult; those two letters and *e*, *a*, *d*, and *o* accounted for 50% of all cursive script illegibilities.[52]

20. Black print on white paper results in approximately 10% greater reading efficiency than the reverse contrast.[53,54]

21. There is an inherent superiority of black ink on white paper relative to colored inks or papers. Contrast may be the determining variable. When contrast is lowered by the use of colored paper or colored inks, the text becomes less legible.[55] These investigations studied asymptomatic, normally achieving adult readers. The effects of colored paper or inks in other categories of subjects (i.e., the reading disabled) remain contentious.

22. The characteristics of paper and ink also are important to consider from the standpoint of their effects on reading. Readers dislike

reading text on glossy paper, which can produce a veiling glare with poorly designed illumination sources.[23] If glare is present, reading efficiency is reduced. However, if glare is eliminated, there is not an appreciable difference between glossy and flat-finished papers.

Opacity is the quality of paper that prevents one side from showing through to interfere with the legibility of print on the other. Obviously, paper with insufficient thickness or opacity will have a detrimental effect on reading performance.

Although rarely mentioned in discussions of glare, ink also can contribute to glare production. Ink is meant to look glossy when dry. Heavy layers of ink increase gloss. Paper has a greater effect on ink gloss than the ink itself does. Glossy paper has good ink holdout (decreased absorption), which maximizes ink reflectance.

Video Display Terminals

No review on the ergonomics of reading would be complete without a discussion of the video display terminal (VDT). In recent years VDTs have become an integral part of many people's lives. Jobs that previously required little or no near work may now have VDT work associated with them. Today between 40 million and 50 million workers use VDTs in the workplace on a daily basis. In addition, more than 20% of households in the United States have a personal computer.

CLINICAL PEARL

In recent years the video display terminal (VDT) has become an integral part of many people's lives. Jobs that previously required little or no near work may now have VDT work associated with them.

With the proliferation of VDTs in the workplace and home, there has been an increase in visual complaints associated with their use. VDT workers report more ocular, visual, and systemic symptoms than people who have similar occupations requiring little or no VDT work.[56-60] The visual symptoms are more intense compared with those of non-VDT workers.[61] Visual complaints reported include eye strain, irritation, blurred vision, headaches, transient color vision problems, and discomfort.[62,63] Depending on the study, visual symptoms have been reported in 45% to 94% of groups studied.[64-68] Task-related variables (e.g., break time, work pressure, work interest, workplace ergonomics) influence the frequency and severity of reported symptoms.[69] One study[61] projected that almost 10 million eye examinations per year were performed on patients who presented primarily with symptoms related to VDT use.

There have been reports of long-term health problems associated with VDT use. However, little evidence exists to show that VDT workers are more likely to have ocular health problems than non-VDT workers with similar job descriptions.[70,71]

Before beginning work at a VDT, all persons should undergo a comprehensive vision examination with emphasis on functional skills, including (although not limited to) a thorough case history, distance and near visual acuity, color vision, stereopsis, keratometry, retinoscopy, subjective refraction at far and near, phoria and vergence measurements, amplitudes of accommodation and convergence, and an ocular health assessment. The history should include a detailed description of the symptoms noted, queries about the nature and type of VDT work activity, other job-related tasks (particularly near point ones), the amount and frequency of distance-near fixation changes required, the VDT working distance, sources of environmental illumination, and a description of the workstation.

CLINICAL PEARL

Before beginning work at a VDT, all persons should undergo a comprehensive vision examination with emphasis on functional skills, including (although not limited to) a thorough case history, distance and near visual acuity, color vision, stereopsis, keratometry, retinoscopy, subjective refraction at far and near, phoria and vergence measurements, amplitudes of accommodation and convergence, and an ocular health assessment.

Refractive Status

Refractive corrections are of utmost importance for persons working with a VDT. The electron gun system used to create the image on the screen does not produce a facsimile with the same quality as hard copy. But it does produce an electronic image, and this can be a problem with the older screens that are still used in many work areas (although less so with the newer high-resolution screens). Many of the complaints associated with VDT use may be attributed to the fact that a large portion of the population does not have adequately corrected vision.[72]

In correcting a VDT worker, it is important to know the working distance at which the screen is located. Most displays are located in the range of 20 to 26 inches, which is beyond the usual near point working distance. When prescribing, you should know the working distances to the screen, keyboard, hard copy, and any other material the patient may be using in performing the task. It also is important to consider the heights at which these objects are placed.

In correcting hyperopia and myopia, the prescribing considerations are much the same as for everyone else. The uniform prescription of low plus lenses has not been shown to be of general benefit.[73] Astigmatism for the VDT worker should be corrected in a very aggressive fashion. Small amounts of uncorrected astigmatism that would cause no problem for a non-VDT worker may cause asthenopic complaints for the VDT worker.

Presbyopia presents the most prescribing permutations in determining the best correction. Many presbyopic VDT operators are overcorrected in the near point addition relative to their actual working distance. To prescribe spectacles accurately for VDT use, you need to know the working distance to the screen and to all other important reference points at the workstation. Before prescribing, have the patient provide this information for you. A co-worker can measure the distances while the patient is seated at the workstation.

CLINICAL PEARL

Presbyopia presents the most prescribing permutations in determining the best correction.

In addition to determining add power, you need to consider the design of the near lens. A single-vision lens appropriate for the screen viewing distance may be best for the overall width of the working area, but it obviously limits the patient to one working distance. However, if the person's duties require distance fixation or, for example, greeting people walking into the work area, the single-vision lens has serious limitations. A bifocal lens with the segment prescribed for the screen-viewing distance may not be the appropriate power for other reading tasks. The height of the bifocal has to be raised to allow the patient to use it when viewing the screen. A frame should be selected that provides a sufficient B dimension to contain the bifocal segment. If the bifocal is not set high enough, the person's head will constantly have to be tilted backward (neck extension) to use it; with the segment set high enough to view the screen, it may get in the way when walking. A progressive lens provides clarity at all distances, but the patient may have difficulty with the narrow corridor of view that is provided at the distance of the screen.

All of these lens designs are currently worn by computer users and can be worn comfortably; unfortunately, however, there are other VDT users who will be uncomfortable with an improper spectacle. It is important to discuss with all patients the pros and cons of each lens design and to ascertain the design of their workstation and the types of tasks performed. In this fashion, it is possible to arrive at the best lens design for a particular patient.

There are no specific contraindications to contact lens wear for VDT workers. However, many of the environments in which VDTs are located are very dry with poor ventilation. The VDTs themselves emit heat, which can contribute to a low-humidity environment and cause problems for some lens wearers. This should be considered in the type of lens fit, materials, wearing time, and cleaning schedules selected for a patient. Some difficulties may be encountered by the reduction in blink rate that can occur with sustained concentration.

Binocular Vision

Binocular vision disorders account for a high percentage of the diagnosed vision problems in symptomatic VDT users. Consistent work at a VDT may cause a breakdown in normal binocular visual functions or exacerbate preexisting clinical or subclinical binocular vision dysfunctions.[74] Therefore, a full assessment of binocular vision skills is required, especially at near point. The lag, stability, facility, and amplitude of accommodation and vergence should be assessed.

CLINICAL PEARL

Binocular vision disorders account for a high percentage of the diagnosed vision problems in symptomatic VDT users. Consistent work at a VDT may cause a breakdown in normal binocular visual functions or exacerbate preexisting clinical or subclinical binocular vision dysfunctions.

Accommodative and vergence dysfunctions can be either primary or secondary. Primary dysfunctions occur in the absence of influential uncorrected refractive error. Binocular dysfunctions also can be secondary to the disrupting effects of uncorrected refractive error, including presbyopia. For example, uncorrected hyperopia increases the amount of accommodation for near point tasks and creates an esophoric tendency. The increased demands on accommodation and negative disparity vergence can disrupt normal self-regulatory behavior, creating the clinical portrait of an accommodative or vergence disorder.

The taxonomy of accommodative and vergence anomalies are presented in the boxes on p. 100. Accommodative disorders are classified into patterns of inadequate response to stimulation or relaxation, or both. Vergence disorders are typically classified according to the magnitude and direction of the distance and near point heterophorias.

An operationally based classification system of binocular dysfunctions is preferable because it clearly identifies a deficient subcomponent skill—which can lead to a more precise understanding of the nature of the defect and its relationship to the clinical signs and symptoms and to improvements in the efficacy of its treatment.

Accommodation Disorders

Accommodative insufficiency
Accommodative excess
Accommodative infacility
Ill-sustained accommodation
Accommodative instability

Vergence Disorders

Convergence insufficiency
Convergence excess
Divergence insufficiency
Divergence excess
Basic esophoria
Basic exophoria
Vergence instability

CLINICAL PEARL

An operationally based classification system of binocular dysfunctions is preferable because it clearly identifies a deficient subcomponent skill—which can lead to a more precise understanding of the nature of the defect and its relationship to the clinical signs and symptoms and to improvements in the efficacy of its treatment.

The subcomponent skills of accommodation and vergence are nearly completely analogous:

1. *Accuracy*—essentially a stimulus-response function; for a given accommodative or vergence demand, how accurately each system responds
2. *Amplitude*—or maximum range of response
3. *Facility*—or ease of making rapid and repeated changes in response of a predictable magnitude
4. *Sustainability*—the capacity to maintain an appropriate response over an extended period
5. *Consistency*—the ability to respond in a similar and/or predictable fashion to an array of stimulus conditions and demand levels
6. *Adaptability*—the capacity of slower or tonic operational accommodative and vergence mechanisms to activate during near point tasks; as tonic mechanisms increase output, there is a

concomitant reduction in the output of faster more reflexive mechanisms; a sufficient magnitude of this adaptation maintained at a consistent level is necessary for symptomless and efficient binocular function during reading

7. *Mutual interaction*—the magnitude of accommodative convergence/accommodation (AC/A) and convergence-accommodation/convergence (CA/C) ratios; this indicates how strongly one system can influence the output of the other

Binocular vision dysfunction related to VDT work or reading may be considered the result of reduced efficiency of feedback control processes.[75] Under stressful conditions the normal self-regulatory processes of oculomotor systems become disordered. Negative feedback systems are ignored, disconnecting the control systems for accommodation and vergence. This leads to less stable systems that cannot respond adequately to stimulus demands. Any accommodative or vergence problems discovered should be treated with lenses, prisms, or vision therapy as required.

CLINICAL PEARL

Binocular vision dysfunction related to VDT work or reading may be considered the result of reduced efficiency of feedback control processes.

After exposure to a high-contrast grating pattern, a small temporary spatial frequency–specific decline in contrast sensitivity occurs.[76] This adaptation in the horizontal and vertical meridians also occurs when viewing VDTs at the fundamental spatial frequency of the displayed text. With print reading the adaptation effects are probably smaller because the effective contrast is less than the negative contrast of a VDT.

The decrease in contrast sensitivity caused by adaptation could affect a worker who has to temporarily view low-contrast stimuli immediately following VDT operation. However, this would be highly unusual and very job specific. Although Lunn and Banks[77] suggested that it could affect accommodative control, the adaptation effects are small and probably of minor consequence because of changes in the viewing distance that alter the spatial frequency of the text display.

Longitudinal chromatic aberration affects the accommodative demand of the observer. The wavelength in focus on the retina varies with the level of accommodation. With an unaccommodated eye fixating a distance target, a wavelength of about 650 nm is in focus. At near working distances, the wavelength in focus for an appropriately accommodated eye is approximately 510 nm. This is why monitors with green phosphors are optimal for accommodation.[78]

Glare/Reflections

Even for the best-performing visual systems, complaints can arise from extrapersonal sources. It is necessary that you understand the workstation and any untoward effects that bad design can have on worker comfort and productivity.

CLINICAL PEARL

Even for the best-performing visual systems, complaints can arise from extrapersonal sources. It is necessary that you understand the workstation and any untoward effects that bad design can have on worker comfort and productivity.

The lighting that exists in an office is a major consideration in worker efficiency. Because VDTs are self-illuminated, they do not require additional lighting for their use. With many VDTs displaying negative contrasts, the room is too bright to allow for a recommended task/surround illumination ratio of 5:1. Often, the easiest way to solve the problem is by shutting room lights or removing bulbs from fixtures.

A related lighting consideration is glare. Glare represents one of the most significant problems facing VDT users. It arises from many sources, with improper lighting placement a significant contributor. When adjusting lighting, keep in mind that indirect types work best. Luminaires that reflect light off the ceiling or newer fixtures that channel light work better than rows of overhead fluorescent light tubes. When adding task lighting, be sure to shield the light source to avoid glare production.

Overhead lights, windows, work lights, the lighting in co-workers' work areas, and even light-colored blouses and shirts are potential sources of glare. A good method of determining what might be producing glare for an individual VDT screen would be to take a small mirror and, with the unit off, place the back of the mirror against the front of the screen; then move the mirror over the surface of the screen in a systematic fashion, looking into the mirror for any illuminated objects that come into view. Offending items (lights, windows, other objects) can then be identified as sources of glare and modified to be less offensive. VDTs should never face windows but should be perpendicular to them. Lights should be placed on the sides of the VDT, avoiding positions that are directly overhead, in front, or behind. Walls should be painted in neutral tones with a flat finish to decrease reflections. Windows can be fitted with pattern-free curtains or covered with a heavier drapery. If a glare source cannot be eliminated, its effect can be reduced in one of several ways. If the source is inducing veiling glare in the eyes, the patient may wear a cap with a bill or a visor, a hood may be fitted onto the terminal to shield the screen, or an antiglare screen may be used (i.e., mesh screens or the preferred multilayered optically coated glass screens); however, this will compromise brightness and contrast. Shiny objects are best kept away from the workstation. In fact, all surfaces in adjacent areas should have a dull finish to keep reflections to a minimum.

There are many spectacle tints available, purportedly for VDT use. But little evidence has been demonstrated that they improve comfort for the user. Pink tints have been advocated because they reduce crystalline lens fluorescence, which could have a veiling glare effect.

One spectacle modification that has been useful is an antireflection coating. Reflections from many sources, including spectacles, can cause problems for persons using a VDT. Lenses with an antireflection coating can reduce this to some degree. However, reflections are generally not a major source of discomfort because most occur with the screen.

Workstation Environment

Character color is another consideration for VDT users. A positive contrast provides better readability and comfort than a negative contrast.[79] In 10% to 20% of the population, colored letters on a black background have caused transient complementary colored afterimages based on the McCulloch effect.[80-84] In the United States, many early video screens used green characters on a dark background and patients often reported a rose or red-tinged appearance to the environment for a few hours after using the VDT. Interestingly, these aftereffects are usually stronger in amblyopic or suppressed eyes.[85]

The screen height should be adjusted so the top of the screen can be viewed with a 10° downward gaze. To accomplish this, the worker should place the top of the VDT cabinet at nose level. In this position, the top of the screen will be about 10° below primary gaze.

The keyboard should be detachable and of a dull finish to reduce reflections. It should also be directly in front of the VDT so the operator can shift gaze easily from one to the other.

If one word were to apply to the arrangement of the workstation and the features of the chair the operator is to use, it would be *adjustable*.[86,87] While the guidelines mentioned above work for most people, with adjustable chairs and screen heights the operator can move them and the task to positions that are individually preferable.

CLINICAL PEARL

If one word were to apply to the arrangement of the workstation and the features of the chair the operator is to use, it would be adjustable.

Flicker

Many people are sensitive to VDT screen flicker as the phosphors are refreshed. Flicker is caused by the decay of the phospher image before it can be refreshed by the electron beam. The flicker is often more apparent when the screen is at the periphery of the visual field as opposed to directly in front. Thus many people are sensitive to their co-workers' screen flicker rather than their own. The flicker sensation is usually not a problem if the refresh rate of the screen is 90 to 95 H_z or higher.[88,89] With modern screens, flicker is much less of a problem.

Posture and Positioning Considerations

Proper posture and positioning are essential in ergonomics. Postural and positioning anomalies associated with VDT work are a form of cumulative trauma disorder. Changes in posture occur gradually, advance insidiously, and persist beyond the workstation environment. VDT work demands static muscular contraction, which causes decreased circulation to muscles, making them susceptible to fatigue and injury. Bad posture creates muscular imbalances, which become habitual and irreversible without therapeutic intervention. When posture is neutral and the spine is supported, the effects of gravity are properly channeled. If positioning is poor, gravity exerts stress on the portion of the spine that is malpositioned. Unsupported sitting exerts greater pressure on the intervertebral discs than standing does.[90]

CLINICAL PEARL

Postural and positioning anomalies associated with VDT work are a form of cumulative trauma disorder. Changes in posture occur gradually, advance insidiously, and persist beyond the workstation environment.

A concept little understood by most people is that the position of one body part affects all other parts. The position or posture of the lower back affects the neck, and vice versa. The seating posture of the VDT worker is all important for proper efficiency. The position of one's body on a chair affects the entire musculoskeletal system. When seated, the back should be supported in a neutral position. Pressure is significantly reduced when the back rest is inclined to 110°. A 2 cm lumbar support is also desirable to maintain neutral lordosis. The depth of the seat should be 1 to 3 inches from the knee. The height of the chair should allow the worker's feet to rest comfortably on the floor. This posture normalizes the muscle tone of the lower extremities, freeing the upper extremities for access to the keyboard. The elbows and forearms require support to maintain a neutral posture, with the elbow flexed preferably between 70° and 90°, but never more than 135°. Slanting the VDT screen will assist in maintaining an upright posture.

A poorly designed seating system allows many variations in posture to occur, leading first to discomfort and muscle fatigue, then to muscle strain or injury, and finally to structural changes in the musculoskeletal system that may create chronic pain and disability.[91] Headaches, neckaches, and shoulder and lower back pain are common results. In addition, the circulatory and respiratory systems are frequently compromised.

CLINICAL PEARL

With a poorly designed seating system, many variations in posture can occur—leading first to discomfort and muscle fatigue, then to muscle strain or injury, and finally to structural changes in the musculoskeletal system that may create chronic pain and disability.

When the back is poorly supported, stress is placed on the head and neck. The body will seek a stable posture, falling forward at the head, which creates kyphotic adjustments in the spine and puts excess stress on the lower back to compensate for the weight of the head. This persisting posture will lead to shoulder rounding and a slouched posture. The stress occurring in the lumbar region radiates through the length of the spine, back to the head and neck area. The worker must reinforce his or her shoulder position, further adding to fatigue in this region.

A chair that is too deep is likely to create impingement of circulation at the knee joint and cause the worker to move away from the back of the chair. Moving forward to the edge of the seat limits the area of support for the trunk and provides less stability. This can lead to fatigue and lower back pain as the worker contracts and co-contracts the upper and lower trunk muscles for stabilization. It also forces the worker to move closer to the VDT screen, decreasing arm extension and creating a restricted posture of the fingers, elbows, and shoulders.

The height of the chair is extremely important. When the chair is too short, there is excessive hip and knee flexion. Here too circulation is compromised, leading to joint discomfort. When the chair is too high, the feet cannot touch the floor or are plantarflexed to toe touch. This is an uncomfortable position, and the worker is likely to move forward, which leads to the difficulties described previously.

Under situations of job stress, even with proper seating systems, things can go wrong. Muscle tightness increases, limiting movement and creating the assumption of a slouching position. Slouching can decrease chest expansion when breathing by nearly 40%, decreasing oxygen intake and creating muscular weakness and fatigue; this leads to further muscle tightness and possible injury.

Slouched sitting brings the head forward, decreasing range of motion in the upper extremities. The biomechanics at the shoulder and upper extremities are altered, making them less mechanically efficient.

This leads to shoulder protraction (forward movement) and rounding, which may compress the scapular nerve (innervating the rhomboids).[90] The resultant reduced innervation of the rhomboids contributes to further forward shoulder protraction, because the rhomboids are responsible for retracting the shoulders (adducting the scapulas). As the shoulders remain protracted, the pectoralis muscles tighten and undergo adaptive shortening, which prevents the shoulders and scapulas from returning to a neutral position. There is also an altered kinesthetic awareness of normal alignment. The same scenario occurs in the contralateral synergist of a paretic extraocular muscle. Even after the paresis resolves, the shortening or contracture remains. With chronic forward head position and shoulder protraction, nerve entrapments can occur. Running in the deep groove on the surface of the posterior arch of the atlas, the suboccipital nerves are very susceptible to entrapment. They primarily innervate muscles that move the head. This entrapment syndrome produces occipital headaches, limited range of motion of the neck, and even scalp numbness.

It is possible that these muscular aches and pains contribute to the large number of patients who present with visual discomfort. If a worker associates musculoskeletal discomfort with the performance of a highly demanding visual task, some of these symptoms may be referred to the eyes. Postural symptoms can also place the worker at-risk for the development or exacerbation of visual symptoms in the presence of questionable or inefficient visual skills.

Unless therapeutic exercises are undertaken, poor posture that develops during VDT work can remain when the individual resumes regular activity. The best possible course of action is to prevent these postural abnormalities. The following short 5-to-10-minute daily exercise regimen is designed to do so. However, any prevention program must also include a healthy lifestyle, with proper nutrition and proper rest.

> ## CLINICAL PEARL
> *Unless therapeutic exercises are undertaken, poor posture that develops during VDT work can remain when the individual resumes regular activity. The best course of action is to prevent these postural abnormalities.*

1. Neck:	Tuck chin to chest. Point chin to ceiling. Turn head to look over right shoulder, then left shoulder. Tilt head to right shoulder, then left shoulder. Repeat 5 times; increase to 10 to 15 repetitions.
2. Trunk flexion-stretch:	Stand against the wall, with arms over head and reach for the ceiling. Repeat 5 times.
3. Trunk rotation:	Sitting, clasp hands on left thigh. Raise arms together over right shoulder. Maintain fixation on hands throughout by moving head. Hold for 5 seconds. Lower hands to right thigh. Raise arms over left shoulder. Hold for 5 seconds. Repeat on opposite side. Repeat 5 times.
4. Breathing:	Sitting, lift one arm over head, breathing in deeply through the nose. Breath out through mouth while moving arm to right and then down. Repeat 5 times. Repeat on opposite side.
5. Shoulder shrug:	Shrug shoulders upward. Hold for 5 seconds. Repeat 5 times.
6. Shoulder circles:	Roll shoulders backward, then forward. Repeat repeat 5 times.
7. Elbow extension:	Straighten arms and shake fingers and wrists.
8. Trunk extension:	Sitting, arch back. Hold for 5 seconds.
9. Knee extension:	Sitting, straighten one knee. Hold for 5 seconds. Repeat on opposite side.
10. Ankle circles:	Sitting, lift foot off floor a few inches and make circles. Repeat five times in clockwise, and in counterclockwise, direction.

References

1. Hecht S: Visual acuity and illumination, *Arch Ophthalmol* 57:564-573, 1928.
2. Woo GCS, Long WF: Recommended light levels for clinical procedures, *Optom Month* 70:722-725, 1979.
3. Kaufman JE: *IES lighting handbook, reference volume,* New York, 1981, Illumination Engineering Society of North America.
4. Kaufman JE: *IES lighting handbook, application volume,* New York, 1981, Illumination Engineering Society of North America.
5. Harmon DB: *The co-ordinated classroom,* Grand Rapids, Mich, 1949, American Seating.
6. Lyons SL: *Management guide to modern industrial lighting,* ed 2, London, 1983, Butterworths.

7. Greenhalgh R (ed): *Light for low vision,* East Sussex, England, The Partially Sighted Society.

8. Long WF, Woo GCS: Measuring clinical light levels with photographic light meters, *Am J Optom Physiol Opt* 57:51-55, 1980.

9. Helms RN: *Illumination engineering for energy efficient luminous environments,* Englewood Cliffs, NJ, 1980, Prentice Hall.

10. McLean R: *The Thames & Hudson manual of typography,* London, 1980, Thames & Hudson.

11. Williamson H: *The methods of book design,* ed 3, New Haven, Conn, 1983, Yale University Press.

12. Luckiesh M, Moss FK: Visibility: its measurement and significance in seeing, *J Franklin Inst* 220:431-466, 1935.

13. Tinker MA: The relative legibility of modern and old style numerals, *J Exp Psychol* 13:453-461, 1930.

14. Tinker MA: *Legibility of print,* Ames, Iowa, 1963, Iowa State University Press.

15. Weiss AP: The focal variator, *J Exp Psychol* 2:106-113, 1917.

16. Luckiesh M, Moss FK: Frequency of blinking as a clinical criterion of ease of seeing, *Am J Ophthalmol* 22:616-621, 1939.

17. Luckiesh M, Moss FK: Boldness as a factor in type design and typography, *J Appl Psychol* 24:170-183, 1940.

18. Tinker MA: Reliability of blinking frequency employed as a measure of readability, *J Exp Psychol* 35:418-424, 1945.

19. Tinker MA: Involuntary blink rate and illumination intensity in visual work, *J Exp Psychol* 39:558-560, 1949.

20. Tinker MA: Reliability and validity of eye-movement measures of reading, *J Exp Psychol* 19:732-746, 1936.

21. Javal E: Hygiène de la lecture, *Bull Soc Med Publ:* 569, 1878.

22. Spencer H: *The visible word,* New York, 1968, Hastings House.

23. Paterson DG, Tinker MA: *How to make type readable,* New York, 1940, Harper.

24. Tinker MA, Paterson DG: Influence of type form on speed of reading, *J Appl Psychol* 12:359-368, 1928.

25. Tinker MA: Criteria for determining the readability of type faces, *J Educ Psychol* 35:385-396, 1944.

26. Tinker MA, Paterson DG: Studies of typographical factors influencing speed of reading. VII, Variations in color of print and background, *J Appl Psychol* 15:471-479, 1931.

27. Tinker MA: The relative legibility of the letters, the digits, and of certain mathematical signs, *J Gen Psychol* 1:472-496, 1928.

28. Ovink GW: *Legibility, atmosphere value, and forms of printing types,* Leiden, Netherlands, 1938, AW Sijthoff.

29. Tinker MA: Prolonged reading tasks in visual research, *J Appl Psychol* 39:444-446, 1955.

30. Tinker MA, Paterson DG: Influence of type form on speed of reading, *J Appl Psychol* 12:359-368, 1928.

31. Fabrizio R, Kaplan I, Teal G: Readability as a function of the straightness of right-hand margins, *J Topograph Res* 1:90-95, 1967.

32. Zachrisson B: *Studies in the legibility of printed text,* Stockholm, 1965, Almqvist & Wiksell.

33. Kujus H: Schrift und Auge, *Klin Monatsbl Augenheilkd* 126:220-229, 1955.

34. Tinker MA: Perceptual and oculomotor efficiency in reading materials in vertical and horizontal arrangements, *Am J Psychol* 68:444-449, 1955.

35. Tinker MA: Effect of angular alignment upon readability of print, *J Educ Psychol* 47:358-363, 1956.

36. Tinker MA: Effect of sloped text upon the readability of print, *Am J Optom Arch Am Acad Optom* 33:189-195, 1956.

37. Cohn HL: *Hygiene of the eye in schools,* London, 1886, Simpkin & Marshall.

38. Burt C: *A psychological study of typography,* London, 1959, Cambridge University Press.
39. Dearborn WF, Johnston PW, Carmichael L: Improving the readability of typewritten manuscripts, *Proc Natl Acad Sci USA* 37:670-672, 1951.
40. Paterson DG, Tinker MA: The part-whole proportion illusion in printing, *J Appl Psychol* 22:421-425, 1938.
41. Tinker MA: Effect of curved text upon readability of print, *J Appl Psychol* 41:218-221, 1957.
42. Terry PW: The reading problem in arithmetic, *J Educ Psychol* 12:365-377, 1921.
43. Terry PW: How numerals are read, *Suppl Educ Monogr,* no. 18, 1922.
44. Tinker MA: Numerals versus words for efficiency in reading, *J Appl Psychol* 12:190-199, 1928.
45. Tinker MA: How formulae are read, *Am J Psychol* 1:472-496, 1928.
46. Tinker MA: Readability of mathematical tables, *J Appl Psychol* 38:436-442, 1954.
47. Tinker MA: Legibility of mathematical tables, *J Appl Psychol* 44:83-83, 1960.
48. Tinker MA: Reading reactions for mathematical formulae, *J Exp Psychol* 9:444-467, 1926.
49. Bell HM: The comparative legibility of typewriting, manuscript and cursive script. I, Easy prose, letters, and syllables, *J Psychol* 8:295-309, 1939.
50. Bell HM: The comparative legibility of typewriting, manuscript and cursive script. II, Difficult prose and eye-movement photography, *J Psychol* 8:311-320, 1939.
51. Turner OG: The comparative legibility and speed of manuscript and cursive handwriting, *Element Sch J* 30:780-786, 1930.
52. Pressey LC, Pressey SL: Analysis of three thousand illegibilities in the handwriting of children and of adults, *Educ Res Bull* 6:270-273, 1927.
53. Paterson DG, Tinker MA: Studies of typographical factors influencing speed of reading. VI, Black type versus white type, *J Appl Psychol* 15:241-247, 1931.
54. Taylor CD: The relative legibility of black and white print, *J Educ Psychol* 25:561-578, 1934.
55. Tinker MA, Paterson DG: Studies of typographical factors influencing speed of reading. VII, Variations in color of print and background, *J Appl Psychol* 15:471-479, 1931.
56. Knave BG, Wibom RI, Voss M, et al: Work with video display terminals among office employees, *Scand J Work Environ Health* 11:457-466, 1985.
57. Frank AL: Effects on health following occupational exposure to video display terminals (40536-0084), Lexington, 1983, Department of Preventive Medicine and Environmental Health, University of Kentucky.
58. Ong CN, Hoong BT, Phoon WO: Visual and muscular fatigue in operators using visual display terminals, *J Hum Ergol* 10:161-71, 1981.
59. Rey P, Meyer JJ: Visual impairments and their objective correlates. In Grandjean E, Vigliani E (eds): *Ergonomic aspects of visual display terminals,* London, 1982, Taylor & Francis.
60. Smith MJ, Cohen BGF, Stammerjohn LW: An investigation of health complaints and job stress in video display operations, *Hum Factors* 23:387-400, 1981.
61. Rose L: Workplace video display terminals and visual fatigue, *J Occup Med* 29:321-324, 1987.
62. Haile KG: Visual difficulties from video display terminals, *South Med J* 78:887-888, 1985.
63. Dainhoff M, Happ A, Crane P: Visual fatigue and occupational stress in VDT operators, *Hum Factors* 23:421-438, 1981.
64. Hultgren GV, Knave B: Discomfort glare and disturbance from light reflections in an office landscape with CRP display terminals, *Appl Ergonom* 5:2-8, 1974.
65. Laubli T, Hunting W, Grandjean E: Visual impairments related to environmental conditions in VDT operators. In Grandjean E, Vigliani E (eds): *Ergonomic aspects of visual display terminals,* London, 1983, Taylor & Francis, pp 77-83.
66. Mariott IA, Stuckly MA: Health aspects of work with visual display terminals, *J Occup Med* 28:833-848, 1986.

67. Smith MJ, Stammerjohn B, Cohen B, et al: Video display operator stress. In Grandjean E, Vigliani E (eds): *Ergonomic aspects of visual display terminals*, London, 1983, Taylor & Francis.

68. Sheedy JE: Vision problems at video display terminals: a survey of optometrists, *J Am Optom Assoc* 63:687-692, 1992.

69. Collins MJ, Brown B, Bowman KJ, Caird D: Task variables and visual discomfort associated with the use of VDTs, *Optom Vis Sci* 68:27-33, 1991.

70. Murray WE, Moss CE, Parr WH, et al: *Potential health hazards of video display terminals*, U.S. Department of Health and Human Services, Publication no. 81-129 (N10SH), 1981.

71. Rose L: Workplace video display terminals and visual fatigue, *J Occup Med* 29:321-324, 1987.

72. Cakir A, Hart DJ, Stewart TFM: *Visual display terminals*, New York, 1980, John Wiley & Sons.

73. Dain SJ, McCarthy AK, Chan-Ling T: Symptoms in VDT operators, *Am J Optom Physiol Opt* 65:162-167, 1988.

74. Brozek J, Simonson E, Keys A: Changes in performance and in ocular functions resulting from strenuous visual inspection, *Am J Psychol* 63:51-66, 1950.

75. Garzia RG: Optometric factors in reading disability. In Willows DM, Kruk RS, Corcos E (eds): *Visual processes in reading and reading disability*, Hillsdale, NJ, 1993, Lawrence Erlbaum.

76. Greenhouse DS, Bailey IL, Howarth PA, Berman SM: Spatial adaptation to text on a video display terminal, *Ophthalmic Physiol Opt* 12:302-306, 1992.

77. Lunn R, Banks WP: Visual fatigue and spatial frequency adaptation to video displays of text, *Hum Factors* 28:457-464, 1986.

78. Sivak JG, Woo GC: Color of VDTs and the eye: green VDTs provide the optimal stimulus to accommodation, *Can J Optom* 45:130-131, 1983.

79. Radl GW: Experimental investigations for optimal presentation-mode and colours of symbols on the CRT-screen. In Grandjean E, Vigliani E (eds): *Ergonomic aspects of visual display terminals*, London, 1980, Taylor & Francis.

80. Greenwald MJ, Breenwald SJ, Blake R: Long lasting visual aftereffect from viewing a computer visual display, *N Engl J Med* 309:315, 1983.

81. Khan JA, Fitz J, Psaltis P, et al: Prolonged complementary chromatopsia in users of video display terminals, *Am J Ophthalmol* 98:756-758, 1984.

82. Walraven J: Prolonged complementary chromatopsia in users of video display terminals, *Am J Ophthalmol* 100:350-351, 1985.

83. Khan JA, Fitz J, Ide CH: Prolonged complementary chromatopsia in users of video display terminals letter, *Am J Ophthalmol* 99:736-737, 1985.

84. Seaber JH, Fisher B, Lockhead GR: Incidence and characteristics of McCollough aftereffects following video display terminal use, *J Occup Med* 29:727-729, 1987.

85. Seaber JH: Enhanced McCullough effects, *Invest Ophthalmol Vis Sci* 26(suppl):182, 1985.

86. Harwood K, Foley P: An insight into the video display terminal (VDT) "problem," *Hum Factors* 29:447-452, 1987.

87. Sheedy JE, Parsons SD: The video display terminal eye clinic: clinical report, *Optom Vis Sci* 67:622-626, 1990.

88. Nishiyama K, Brauninger U, de Boer H, et al: Physiological effects of intermittently illuminated textual displays, *Ergonomics* 20:1143-1154, 1986.

89. Bauer D: What causes flicker in bright background VDT's and how to cure it? In Grandjean E, Vigliani E (eds): *Ergonomics and health aspects in modern offices*, London, 1984, Taylor & Francis.

90. Lear CA, Pomeroy SJ: Office ergonomics. 1, The anatomy of seated work, *Phys Ther Forum*, October 7, 1994.

91. Lear CA, Pomeroy SJ: Office ergonomics. 3, Chair fitting considerations, *Phys Ther Forum*, October 28, 1994.

6

Refractive Status, Binocular Vision, and Reading Achievement

Ralph P. Garzia
Aaron S. Franzel

Key Terms

| visual acuity | binocular vision | visual efficiency |
| refractive status | research | correlates |

Reading disability is an unexpected difficulty in learning to read despite normal intelligence and the opportunity to learn with competent instruction. It cannot be attributed to general health problems, emotional disturbances, or sensory deficits. Generally accepted estimates of its prevalence in school-age children[1,2] range from 3% to 9% but may run as high as 20% to 25%.[3] Reading disability accounts for nearly 75% of referrals for learning disability, which the United States Department of Education estimates as 5% of the total school enrollment.[4]

Optometrists and educators have been interested in the relationship between vision and the acquisition of reading skill for nearly a century. The relationship is axiomatic. Visual processing is a fundamental part of the reading process. There can be little doubt that the initial phases of reading, before phonological encoding, before language processing, and before access to short- and long-term memory, are visual. Vision is certainly not obligatory for all types of reading-like activity, as evidenced by Braille reading in the visually impaired. However, in the more typical situation, visual processes (both peripheral and central) must operate automatically and effortlessly for facile reading. In this chapter we discuss the relationship between peripheral visual skills (i.e., refractive status and binocular vision) and reading achievement. The nature of this discussion will center around the ophthalmic and educational literature in this area.

Of course, what is of the utmost interest to professionals managing children who have reading disabilities is an answer to the question, "Do vision problems cause reading disability?" As with most cause-and-effect relationships in medicine and optometry, vision problems are neither a necessary nor a sufficient cause of reading disability. Reading disability can occur in the absence of significant vision problems. Not all persons with vision problems develop reading disability; rather, vision problems as a cause of reading disability are primarily contributory. The presence of anomalies of refraction and binocular vision, perhaps at some critical stage of reading development, enhances the possibility for reading disability.

CLINICAL PEARL

Vision problems are neither a necessary nor a sufficient cause of reading disability. Reading disability can occur in the absence of significant vision problems. Not all persons with vision problems develop reading disability; rather, vision problems as a cause of reading disability are primarily contributory.

Knowledge about visual skills and reading is important for optometrists because they are often the first professionals external to the educational system to evaluate a child with reading difficulties. Informed teachers and parents will request an evaluation of a child who is not making appropriate progress in reading acquisition; or they may request an evaluation concurrent with an educational diagnostic assessment. With increasing frequency, a vision evaluation is included as a component of the comprehensive-cross disciplinary assessment of a child. The anticipated goal for the optometrist is to establish the degree of involvement of visual disorders in the failure to reach expected reading achievement.

Refraction and Binocular Vision

The assessments of refractive status (with visual acuity) and binocular vision are standard features of a functional vision examination. Abnormalities of refractive status or dysfunctions of binocular vision reduce visual efficiency and form the core of learning-related vision problems. This means that they are capable of disturbing the visual environment in which reading instruction, and hence reading development, occurs.

Signs and Symptoms

Uncorrected refractive error, particularly hyperopia and anisometropia, and anomalies of binocular vision can produce a coterie of clinical signs and symptoms.

The clinical signs reported by teachers and parents include squinting, frowning, excessive blinking, eye rubbing, covering an eye, or tilting the head when reading. A very common observation is an excessively close reading distance. The clinician should be attentive to these signs during an examination, for they can be indicators of poor qualitative or stressful responses despite sometimes normal quantitative test results.

It is imperative that clinicians remember the difficult chore children have in understanding or describing the nature of their symptoms. This is compounded in reading-disabled children because of their limited expressive vocabulary and episodic memory. The caveat becomes: Limit reliance on symptoms as the dominant indicator of visual function and in the determination of a problem-oriented testing regimen. When the presenting problem or chief complaint is reading difficulty, assessments of refractive status and binocular vision should be done thoroughly. The most common ocular symptoms associated with reading are blur and diplopia. Asthenopia or localized eye discomfort can accompany the blur or diplopia or may be an independent occurrence. Headaches are also frequently reported. They are typically frontal and are initiated or exacerbated by reading.

CLINICAL PEARL

Limit reliance on symptoms as the dominant indicator of visual function and in the determination of a problem-oriented testing regimen. When the presenting problem or chief complaint is reading difficulty, assessments of refractive status and binocular vision should be done thoroughly.

The prevalence rate of signs and symptoms of uncorrected refractive error or binocular vision anomalies among reading-disabled children is largely unknown at this time. In a report by Meier,[5] classroom teachers observed facial grimacing (including squinting) in 28% of disabled readers, head forward or tilted to one side when reading in 18%, close working distance in 17%, and eye rubbing when reading in 14%.

Other symptoms that can occur are more of a perceptual nature. These range from illusory text movement to distortions of letters, words, or entire lines. Text movement may be in the form of oscillations or even words "jumping around." Individual letters may be seen as misshapen, deformed, or ill proportioned to the point of hindering their identification. Words appear to be overlapping or irregularly spaced.

Behavioral manifestations of uncorrected refractive error or binocular vision anomalies are frequently overlooked. For example, if sustained near work causes asthenopia, some children will learn to limit such activity. This will gradually become a habitual pattern of avoidance and may be construed in the classroom as inattention. Children with vision problems have more difficulty in coming to attention and sustaining attention than children with normal visual efficiency.[6] Distractible children or those labeled with attention-deficit disorder may literally be unable to stay focused on the task because of visual constraints. Children with preexisting attentional deficits may be particularly at risk for the "distracting" effects of visual inefficiency.

In summary, children diagnosed with refractive or binocular vision anomalies should be carefully managed and promptly treated. The effectiveness of any treatment should be assiduously monitored.

Interactions

Uncorrected refractive error, particularly hyperopia and anisometropia, and binocular vision anomalies can have an impact on the reading process either in isolation or, more commonly, in combination. Their specific effect on reading depends on the nature and severity of the visual problems and the particular stage of reading development at which they occur. Vision can be a dominant factor in the genesis of a reading disability, an insignificant factor, or more commonly a contributory factor of variable degree. This is for you to estimate and to provide counsel regarding for parents and teachers.

With the exception of significantly reduced visual acuity and perhaps diplopia, there is no conceptual framework to suggest that vision problems have a direct impact on the reading process. Rather, it is understood that the effects are indirect. There are two major hypothetical modes of influence.

First is the so-called Matthew effect.[7] Ocular discomfort during reading reduces the amount of time in reading activity by avoidance. The visually symptomatic child who reads less will have diminished opportunity to develop vocabulary and reading skill. From a behavioral perspective, the child associates reading with discomfort, further contributing to a dislike of or frustration with reading. Children who are not limited in their reading activity because of a vision problem will read more, expand their vocabulary and reading skill, and read even better and enjoy it more (leading to more and better reading).

Second is the area of attention allocation. Blurred or diplopic text, or discomfort associated with visual inefficiency, may interfere with automatic information processing required for successful reading.[8] This concept presumes that attentional resources have a limited capacity. With efficient visual function, the allocation of attention can remain at the semantic level to maximize reading comprehension. It will not be depleted by the need for volitional control of visual functions. Optically degraded text has an adverse effect on the speed of word recognition.[9] This has been corroborated electrophysiologically with event-related potentials.[10] Reduced speed of word recognition slows the entire reading process. If attention has to be directed to the word-recognition process, then ongoing reading comprehension will be hampered. Correcting significant hyperopia (>2.00), a condition with the real potential for evoking near point blur, has been found to enhance speed of word recognition measured tachistoscopically.[11]

CLINICAL PEARL

Blurred or diplopic text, or discomfort associated with visual inefficiency, may interfere with automatic information processing required for successful reading.

Research on Vision and Reading

For more than six decades, there has been a considerable literature devoted to answering the epistemological question regarding the role of vision anomalies in the genesis of reading disability. The essential questions were two. First, is there a higher prevalence of vision anomalies among reading-disabled children compared with normal achievers? Second, is there a relationship between the magnitude or severity of the vision anomaly and the extent of reading disability? At their essence these are cause-and-effect questions.

However, these research endeavors are honeycombed with confusion and misunderstanding. The very complex and poorly understood nature of the reading process itself, a considerable naiveté about vision, experimental design flaws, the misapplication of statistics, and experimenter biases have all contributed. Unfortunately, this confusion has led to the belief that refractive status and binocular vision have a minor and irrelevant influence on reading achievement. This has been extended to the patient-care domain by the inattention directed to visual efficiency in children experiencing difficulty learning to read.

CLINICAL PEARL

Research endeavors are honeycombed with confusion and misunderstanding. The very complex and poorly understood nature of the reading process itself, a considerable naiveté about vision, experimental design flaws, the misapplication of statistics, and experimenter biases have all contributed.

There have been primarily two experimental approaches to address the two fundamental questions stated previously—the case-control study and the correlational study. Prevalence rates of refraction or binocular vision functions or abnormalities (or arbitrarily defined levels of performance) were compared between a poor-reading group and a control group of normal readers. Presumably, a different distribution of refractive status or a greater prevalence of binocular vision anomalies between the two groups would reinforce the causal argument for vision. There are inherent difficulties in the use of case-control study designs because of the question of risk.[12] These studies in actuality look backward, from effect to cause. Children eligible for the study are known to have the effect (i.e., reading disability) or not. The question is to determine if the suspected cause of the reading disability (i.e., vision problems) is present. In a case-control study, the children have already sorted themselves out and the experimenter tries to figure out how and why. After the reading disability has already developed, investigators look back to see how many of the children also have vision problems. This is an answer to a question that no one has asked, and it is irrelevant. Parents and teachers can only be told that a reading-disabled child is at increased risk for a certain vision disorder. A case-control study identifies the risk of vision anomalies having been present among the children with a reading disability and among the controls.

In a case-control study the number of experimental subjects is contrived depending on the resources of the experimenter, the availability of subjects, etc. The number of controls is also quite arbitrary. This makes case-control studies vulnerable to a number of biases.[12] Therefore risks can never be determined in absolute terms. Assume a population where 40% of good readers and 80% of poor readers have vision problems. A case-control study with 100 subjects in each group would have 80 poor readers among 120 vision-problem patients. This is an estimated risk for reading disability among vision-problem patients of 66.7% (80/[80+40]). In a study with 1000 controls, the risk of reading disability among vision problems would appear to be reduced, to 16.7% (80/[80+400]).

Instead of case-control studies, cohort studies are needed in which an experimental group with vision problems and a control group without vision problems are followed for the development of reading disability. With a cohort study, the risk for reading disability can be determined in those exposed to the cause—those with and those without vision anomalies—and thus allows the development of a risk ratio in which the prevalence/incidence of reading disability can be calculated.

The second prominent research design has been the correlational study. This design, by its very nature, cannot attribute causation. In correlational studies quantitative measures of a visual function are related to reading level in a designated sample. A correlation coefficient, usually the Pearson r, is calculated. A significant positive correlation demands that the more profound the reading disability is the greater will be the associated visual abnormality. However, this is often an untenable situation from a clinical viewpoint. For instance, most would agree that the difference between 2 and 4 prism diopters (Δ) of near point exophoria is not clinically significant in defining a visual dysfunction. In actuality, for this particular example, 2 Δ of exophoria is more deviant from the normal level of 6 Δ. Yet, a correlational statistic would demand that the higher exophoria be associated with poorer reading. Likewise, there is no logic in the proposition that higher levels of any visual finding should necessarily be more strongly correlated to lower levels of reading achievement. The correlational approach to understanding the relationship between vision and reading is undeniably the wrong approach.[13] Clinical experience has taught that the magnitude of an individual test result is not necessarily the singular determinant of visual efficiency. Visual inefficiency is based not on minor differences from the norm but on when some threshold level of dysfunction is reached.

By way of a specific example of the limited effectivity of correlational research, Robinson[14] correlated reading scores and visual skills for 100 pupils each from elementary grades 1 through 8. Visual acuity, refractive error, stereopsis, vertical and lateral heterophoria, and vergence ranges were determined. Correlation coefficients were small and in the range from +0.25 to −0.25 (consistent with the majority of published correlational studies). However, when a subsample of the best readers (2 grades above expected) and the poorest readers (greater than 1.6 grades below) were compared, significant differences materialized. Compared with the better readers, the poorer readers were more hyperopic, had lower vergence ranges, and had phorias that deviated significantly from the normal range.

The variability of the visual functions under investigation is another influence. For instance, refractive error distribution for children entering school is decidedly leptokurtic (the same is true of distance horizontal heterophoria). The range and variability of refractive status are necessarily limited in this age group. The low variability in refractive error relative to the variability among other factors that determine reading skill (e.g., language ability) means that refractive error will not be as strongly related to individual differences in reading skills despite its potential importance as an underlying factor in every child's reading performance. If the variability in one factor is restricted, then other factors will necessarily be more strongly related to differences in reading achievement.

Another difficulty encountered in studies relating vision and reading is the use of arbitrary and/or nonuniform criteria for designating normal and abnormal visual function. A recent example is the publication of Helveston, Weber, Miller, et al.[15] In an evaluation of 1910 first, second, and third grade children, they found the prevalence of binocular functions to be no greater among below-average readers than among average and above-average readers. Concerns about their conclusions are raised both by the selection of tests used to evaluate visual functions and by their apparently arbitrary criteria for normal function. For example, a Titmus stereoacuity of 140 seconds, a near point convergence of 10 cm, and an accommodation amplitude of 11 D (independent of age) were all considered normal findings. Most optometrists would unequivocally reject these criteria in this age group.

CLINICAL PEARL

Another difficulty encountered in studies relating vision and reading is the use of arbitrary and/or nonuniform criteria for designating normal and abnormal visual function. Few studies have used comprehensive clinical testing or complete diagnostic classification.

Few studies have used comprehensive clinical testing or complete diagnostic classification of visual function. There has been an over reliance on the analysis of individual tests. This approach facilitates data collection, but it has seductively led to viewing each visual function separately, presumably neither interrelated with nor interdependent on other visual functions. This is decidedly different from the usual clinical approach of grouping data and collectively evaluating them in a syndromic framework.

Previous research efforts have been hampered by definitional complications surrounding reading disability. There are a myriad of contributors to reading disability,[16] including physical, cognitive, language, emotional, environmental, and educational factors. There are almost certainly complex interactional effects among these factors that determine an individual child's specific reading ability. This important issue was ignored in many older studies. Selection criteria or quantitative measures of reading ability were inconsistently reported. Children were nominally identified as reading disabled. On an encouraging note, this has been addressed more faithfully in recent research.

One frequently neglected point is the timing of the vision disorder. Refractive changes and binocular vision anomalies are not static phenomena. The shift in refractive error from hyperopia toward myopia during the school years is well established. Binocular vision disorders have periods of remission and exacerbation. Nonstrabismic binocular vision anomalies are not congenital. They usually first appear during the early elementary grades, when near point demands increase. A preclinical reduction of binocular function might be present earlier, but it does not become manifest until suitable environmental conditions are present. A considerable amount of sensitivity in testing and diagnosis is required to detect binocular anomalies in this preclinical phase. Usually a single test, performed in isolation, is insufficient. A child selected for participation in a study of reading disability in the third grade may have had a significant uncorrected hyperopia in kindergarten or first grade that interfered with the acquisition of reading skills. However, through the course of ocular development the amount of hyperopia decreased while the reading difficulties persisted. Conversely, a normally achieving child may have been in the initial stages of a binocular vision dysfunction that had insufficient time to become an impediment to reading. The same increases and decreases in reading ability occurred and the same arguments can be made. These are intrasubject variations but they are intensified by the reliabilities, or lack thereof, among testing instruments.

Most of the published studies reporting negative results have lacked sufficient power to detect an actual difference (if one truly existed).[17] The power of a study is the likelihood that it will detect a statistically significant difference if one exists. The failure to detect a difference when one exists is called a Type II or β error. Power is $1 - \beta$ (or 80%), with $\beta = 0.2$, which is an acceptable value. (False rejection of the null hypothesis is termed a Type I or α error. By tradition α is set at 0.05. This means that there are 5 chances in 100 of rejecting the null hypothesis when chance alone is operating.) If a study has a power of 80% in detecting a specified difference between reading disabled and controls, there is an 80% likelihood that a statistical significance will be proved.

The power of a study is determined by the interaction of several factors—the magnitude of the outcome variable, the magnitude of the expected differences between experimental and control groups, and the size of the samples. When the magnitude of the clinical effect decreases, the chances of a Type I or Type II error increases. When the expected differences between groups decrease, the chances of a Type II error increase. Larger sample sizes are required to meaningfully detect a significant difference between groups. For example, Ygge et al.,[18] comparing disabled readers and a control group across a large number of tests of binocular vision, concluded that reading-disabled students did not differ statistically from a control group in binocular function. They reported a 23.2% prevalence rate of horizontal heterophoria in the control group. For $\alpha = 0.5$ and $\beta = 0.20$, to detect a 20% increase in the reading-disabled group, a sample size greater than 1500 would be required in each group. Their subjects numbered 86 for each group.

A review of the literature in this field will find appalling examples of egregious experimenter bias,[19] even to the point of ignoring positive results.[20]

Correlates Between Vision and Reading

In an extensive study-by-study narrative review of the literature, Simons and Grisham[21,22] concluded that there is a relationship between a child's refractive status and binocular vision and reading. This was further supported by a metanalysis of the same literature.[23] In the remaining part of this chapter we will review the literature. We must admit a certain amount of confirmatory bias in this discussion.

Visual Acuity and Refractive Status

There is little reason to suspect that distance visual acuity influences reading performance, except as it mirrors dysfunction in accommodation and vergence control. Most of the published research corroborates this.[24] Paradoxically, there has been little attention directed to near point visual acuity and reading. In a substantive well-controlled report, published in 1935, Fendrick[25] used a modified Jaeger chart to measure near point visual acuity and found a higher prevalence of reduced near acuity among reading-disabled subjects ($p < 0.05$ for binocular acuity).

CLINICAL PEARL

There is little reason to suspect that distance visual acuity influences reading performance, except as it mirrors dysfunction in accommodation and vergence control.

In a more recent study from Sweden[26] disabled readers were found to have a lower prevalence of best corrected visual acuity at the 20/20 level than occurred in controls. The effects were noted for distance and near fixation, and monocularly as well as binocularly. At near point nearly all of the control subjects could obtain at least 20/20 acuity. However, a significant number of reading-disabled subjects (approximately 10%) could not.[26]

It has been known for some time that reading-disabled children have reduced contrast sensitivity for low spatial frequency gratings.[27] These studies have been conducted under laboratory conditions with briefly displayed stimuli. Of note from the Swedish study, Ygge et al.[26] demonstrated these contrast deficiencies with clinical measures. Using the near point Vistech test with best corrected visual acuity, reading-disabled subjects were found to have reduced contrast sensitivity for the 1.5 and 3.0 c/deg gratings. Contrast sensitivity reductions were also found for the highest spatial frequency grating tested (18 c/deg). Although this latter result is somewhat surprising and atypical, it probably reflects the reduced near point visual acuity in reading-disabled children.

There is substantial consistency among studies of refractive status and reading ability. None have reported an association of hyperopia with good reading and myopia with poor reading. Myopia appears to be associated almost completely with normal or above-normal reading achievement.

CLINICAL PEARL

There is substantial consistency among studies of refractive status and reading ability. None have reported an association of hyperopia with good reading and myopia with poor reading. Myopia appears to be associated almost completely with normal or above-normal reading achievement.

Thomas H. Eames, optometrist, physician, and educator, has contributed considerably to the understanding of the relationship between refractive status and reading. In a series of reports,[28-30] including more than 1000 reading-disabled children in one study alone, he found significant differences in the prevalence of hyperopia between reading disabled and control groups. These results were present even with IQ controlled.

In a related study, Eames[31] divided third and fourth grade children into three groups according to refractive error—emmetropes, myopes, and hyperopes. Among the good readers there were no differences in reading achievement across the three refractive groups. Among the poor readers, however, the hyperopes had the lowest reading levels.

Young[32] compared refractive error and reading achievement with refractive error as the independent variable in 316 eyes. Hyperopia was defined as more than +0.75 D, myopia as any amount. There was a significant difference between hyperopes and myopes. The myopes were better readers than the hyperopes and generally better readers than the emmetropes. Overall, these results provide an effective argument for hyperopia as a risk factor in reading disability.

In two recent reports[33,34] the interactions between refractive status and visual perceptual-motor development were reported. Although not investigations of reading per se, they did show that children with visual perceptual-motor delays were at risk for reading underachievement. In the first study of a sample of 712 children aged 6 to 12 years, only 18% with less than 1.25 D of hyperopia displayed age-appropriate visual-motor skills, in contrast to 74% of the emmetropic and myopic children.[33] In a second and related study of 48 6-to-12-year-old hyperopes with more than 2.25 D, the children who were corrected before their fourth birthday manifested fewer visual-motor delays than did those corrected later.[34]

The prevalence of at least 1.00 D anisometropia has been found[35] to be higher among reading disabled. Among anisometropes, Eames found a significantly higher percentage of children who were 3 or more months below expected reading level compared with an isometropic group. Of commensurate importance, after refractive correction, the anisometropic group demonstrated greater relative gains in reading achievement over a 6-month period. The efficacy of refractive correction, particularly hyperopia, on reading progress was also noted by Farris.[36] Seventh grade students wearing a spectacle correction for hyperopia made more substantial gains in reading over a 1-year period than an uncorrected hyperopic control group did.

In the previously described Swedish study, Ygge et al.[26] found no significant refractive differences between reading-disabled and control groups.

Binocular Vision

Monocular reading

The capacity to read better under monocular conditions would argue that binocular vision has some negative effect on reading efficiency. Birnbaum and Birnbaum[37] found that second and fourth grade children were able to read monocularly somewhat faster and with reduced error rates compared with binocular reading. Stein and Fowler[38] found improved reading ability in excess of expected maturational improvement after a 6-month period of monocular occlusion for all reading and close work in a group of children with poor divergence ranges. Children with unstable binocular vision have been found[39] to read word lists more accurately with one eye occluded.

Heterophoria

Eames's 1935 study[29] found a nearly four times greater prevalence of exophoria in a reading-disabled group compared with controls. In a later study[30] he found a greater median magnitude of exophoria among disabled readers. Unfortunately, no heterophoria testing method was described in either study.

Good[40] matched an experimental group with a control group in age, sex, school experience, and IQ. The experimental group consisted of 25 elementary-school children who had been selected by teacher observation and whose reading level was confirmed by a reading test. No members of the control group, but 40% of the reading-disabled, had a lateral imbalance of 3 Δ or more.

Others authors,[25,26,41,42] however, have found no significant differences in heterophoria between reading-disabled and controls.

Vergence

Results of clinical measurements of fusional vergence ranges have been mixed, some[42,43] showing decreased ranges in the reading-disabled and some[26] no significant differences. Vergence facility over a 20 Δ range has been found[44] to be significantly slower in a group of disabled readers compared with controls.

Stein, Riddell, and Fowler[45] measured vergence responses with a synoptophore. Vergence eye movements were recorded by the infra-red photoelectric method. Vergence changes were introduced at the rate of 0.5°/second. All of the control group, but only 36% of the disabled readers, achieved at least 20° and 5° of positive and negative fusional vergence respectively. One important aspect of this study was that vergence eye movements were objectively monitored. Disordered vergence control was exhibited in the disabled readers not only in their limited range of vergence but also by the nature of their vergence responses. Instead of a consistent response of disjunctive eye movements when the stimulus changed, the reading-disabled subjects intermittently exhibited conjugate eye movements.

No differences in fixational vergence errors (fixation disparity) occurred between the reading-disabled and controls when binocularly fixating individual words[46] or a Mallett unit.[42] However, with the eyes dissociated while viewing a Maddox wing, fixational instability was more frequently noted among reading-disabled.[42] In a related effect, increasing convergence demand creates a greater degree of destabilization of fixational eye movement control among reading-disabled than among normal readers.[43]

Investigating the temporal properties of vergence responses has supported the disordered vergence argument. Hung[47] compared the vergence responses of two young adult subjects who had a documented history of reading disability with two control subjects. Eye movements were recorded by the infrared photoelectric method. Disparity was induced with ramp velocities of 1.33° to 32.0°/second. Step displacements of a maximum of 4° were also presented. The two reading-disabled subjects showed generally slower peak-velocity vergence movements than the controls did. They also had slower responses (peak velocity) to both convergent and divergent step stimuli.

Accommodation

A number of studies[48-53] have concluded that accommodative disorders occur frequently in reading-disabled children. However, these studies were conducted without accompanying control groups or well-defined performance criteria. Other, larger, studies of a variety of visual functions using control groups[18,54] have not found significant reductions in the amplitude of accommodation among reading-disabled subjects. Evans, Drasdo, and Richards[42] found reductions in the amplitude of accommodation but not accommodative lag or near-far facility.

Efficacy of orthoptics

If a binocular vision dysfunction can have a deleterious effect on reading, then its improvement or elimination should lead to improved reading. Carrying this argument one step further, if binocular function is important to reading efficiency then enhancement of function with orthoptics should also be beneficial, even in the absence of a clearly demonstrable clinical problem. At least that was the logic behind two important intervention projects[55,56] conducted many years ago. Both studies were noteworthy because of good experimental design and their multidisciplinary nature.

In one study,[55] conducted at the University of Nebraska, 98 entering freshman were evenly divided into three groups, matched in reading and other psychoeducational areas. Group A received 6 weeks of orthoptics (3 half-hour sessions/week) followed by 3 weeks of reading instruction (2 hours/week). Group B received 6 weeks of similar reading instruction followed by 3 weeks of orthoptics. Group C received only reading instruction. The therapy emphasized instrument-based antisuppression, vergence, and ocular motility activities.

At the conclusion of the experiment, all three groups improved in reading rate and comprehension. However, those receiving orthoptics made greater gains than those receiving reading instruction alone. Of particular interest, the therapy made the most significant changes in students who had the highest scholastic aptitude potential as determined by preadmissions tests relative to their initial reading levels. These subjects had a discrepancy between reading achievement and academic potential. In was concluded that in this group orthoptics eliminated a visual deficiency that had acted as a limiting factor in the development of reading ability. These results were reported in detail in the educational literature by Worcester.[57]

In the second study,[56] conducted by the Department of Psychology of North Carolina State University, poorly achieving sophomore college students were placed in four groups matched for IQ and reading test scores. Group A received only orthoptics (three 45-minute sessions a week for 8 weeks), Group B orthoptics and vocational counseling, and Group C counseling only. Group D served as the control group. Orthoptics emphasized instrumentally based antisuppression, vergence, and ocular motility activities. Reading rate, but not comprehension, improved significantly (approximately 30% mean gain) for the orthoptics groups.

These studies were conducted with adult subjects. Four intervention studies with children have appeared in the literature since then.[58-61] Unfortunately, three of these[58-60] are of limited value primarily because they lacked a control group. The fourth[61] offers greater potential for evaluating the effects of orthoptics on reading achievement. Atzmon et al.[61] randomized a group of 124 reading-disabled children into two groups. The experimental group received orthoptics but no remedial reading; the control group spent an identical amount of time in remedial reading instruction but received no orthoptics. (A no-treatment control group was lost because of the ethical and political issues necessary for denying treatment.) Randomization occurred after the children were matched in IQ, reading rate and comprehension, and vergence ranges. Teachers and therapists were largely unaware of a child's group placement. Each child in the experimental group received between 35 and 40 individual therapy sessions for a period of 2 to 3 months. The control group received a similar amount of remedial reading instruction. After this interval, both the experimental and the control group showed significant and equal increases in reading performance measured with the same standardized tests. In other words, orthoptics and reading instruction produced the same results. Unfortunately there was not a no-treatment group to use in judging the true effectiveness of these interventions.

Overall indices of visual function

Trying to avoid the multiple-comparison problem caused by analyzing a series of individual and presumably independent binocular functions and engaging in "data dredging," some authors have attempted to combine a large data set into an overall index of visual and binocular function.

CLINICAL PEARL

Trying to avoid the multiple-comparison problem caused by analyzing a series of individual and presumably independent binocular functions and engaging in "data dredging," some authors have attempted to combine a large data set into an overall index of visual and binocular function.

Park and Burri[62] evaluated visual acuity, cycloplegic refraction, heterophoria (cover test, Maddox rod), and vergence ranges. Overall, 14 skills were evaluated. Each deviation from normal was considered a "defect." Children with greater reading abilities had a lower number of defects; and the lower the reading scores, the more likely it was that the child had an ocular defect. After developing a composite visual profile, Park and Burri[63] found a significant correlation coefficient between reading expectancy level and total eye score.

In arguably the most compelling research effort to explore the relationship between vision and educational performance, O'Grady[64] reported the results of a joint study conducted by the Education Department of Tasmania with local optometrists. A random sample of 227 second grade children was selected from 74 schools. The students were given a series of educational tests and a comprehensive office-based visual examination, including accommodative facility and fixation disparity but not vergence ranges. Each visual examination was provided by one of 26 optometrists. The vision tests were selected and standardized by the participating optometrists. The visual status of each child was categorized as normal, borderline, or suspect with a full examination recommended. Following the examination, 16.2% of the sample were judged as requiring additional vision care. Although four individual vision variables discriminated educational performance, the most interesting conclusion was that optometric recommendations based on the overall assessment of vision status were significantly related to reading and mathematics performance. Children in the suspect category were found to perform significantly more poorly on educational tests than the other children.

Instrument-based testing

The ubiquity of vision-screening instruments and their relative ease of operation have led to their use in the study of vision and reading. Instruments like the Bausch & Lomb Ortho-Rater, the Keystone Visual Skills Survey, and the American Optical Sight-Screener allow a rapid assessment of visual skills. Perhaps their greatest advantage, however, has been the compression of optical infinity, so that a 20-foot fixation distance is not required. With these instruments visual acuity, lateral and vertical heterophorias, suppression, fusion, and stereopsis can be studied. Some authors[21,65] have questioned the reliability of instrumentally based vision testing, and this certainly contributes to the lack of consistency in research conclusions. However, others[14,66] have found good short-term and long-term test-retest reliability for the Visual Skills Survey.

There are important differences between instrumental and standard methods of testing visual functions. The phenomena of induced convergence and myopia are well recognized with instrumental testing. Both of these effects shift the horizontal heterophoria toward esophoria. Unfortunately, there is significant intersubject variation, and because of this a few small but significant differences in horizontal heterophoria may be overlooked. Measurements of monocular visual acuity at distance and near point are typically performed binocularly and as such are influenced by suppression. This is not necessarily bad from a clinical standpoint, but it may confuse comparisons intended for visual acuity alone.

CLINICAL PEARL

There are important differences between instrumental and standard methods of testing visual functions. The phenomena of induced convergence and myopia are well recognized with instrumental testing.

The results of Robinson's study[14] were described earlier. Kephart[67] established a criterion level of performance on the Ortho-Rater Test battery, such that the results in a group of children who fell below that level tended to be lower test scores on the Stanford Achievement Test. Subsequently, he tested 250 students who were not involved in the initial phase of the study. They were divided into two groups based on reading achievement scores and then administered the Ortho-Rater Test. Of the students who scored above the previously determined visual criteria, 46% were in the higher reading group and 28% in the lower reading classification. This difference was statistically significant.

Wirt, Morgan, and Floyd[68] used a similar criterion-based minimal visual performance profile, but it is quite likely that the students who established these criteria also were in the experimental group.

Steinbaum and Kurk[69] developed a composite score of vision status on the Keystone Visual Skills Test battery for fifth and sixth grade students. Three descriptive levels of visual skills were defined— passing, failing, and marginal. Reading performance was classified in a similar manner. Consistent with the results of Robinson[14] and Kephart,[67] better readers were found with significantly greater frequency in the highest vision score category and poorer readers were clustered in the lowest vision category.

In another study using composite visual efficiency scores derived from components of the Keystone Visual Skills Test, Glatt and Glatt[70] compared the scores to standardized reading test results. Visual efficiency scores were determined by assigning 10 points for each "expected" response, 5 points for each "doubtful" response and 0 points for an "unsatisfactory" response. The correlation coefficient between vision scores and reading achievement was only +0.15. But of the 255 subjects who scored in the lowest 60% of reading, 87% were below average on visual efficiency.

Kephart, Manas, and Simpson[71] found a significant relationship between scores on the Keystone Visual Skills Test and school achievement in kindergarten students. A detailed 5-point grading scale was applied to each subtest of the Visual Skills Test. A factor analysis followed that determined nine tests to have the highest discriminatory potential. Subsequently, these tests were administered to a group of 45 children, with significant correlation coefficients found between school performance and vision performance.

Negative associational results were reported by Edson, Bond, and Cook.[24] Unfortunately, data and statistical analyses were not published with the paper, making discourse on the conclusions impossible. Swanson and Tiffin[72] and Stromberg[73] divided college students into poor and good reading groups. Visual efficiency was determined with a Keystone Telebinocular using a Betts slide series. In both studies no significant differences were found in fusional and heterophoria measurements between the two reading groups.

Summary

Visual skills are related to reading achievement. An analysis of the literature on the subject indicates that refractive error (in particular, hyperopia and significant anisometropia), exophoria, and disordered vergence are associated with reading underachievement. Supporting evidence can be found from studies considering overall indices of visual function, monocular versus binocular reading, correction of refractive error, and efficacy of orthoptics. The question of causation remains. We recommend that future studies of vision and reading be of the cohort or intervention variety. Any further case-control studies are likely to add to the confusion and should be disregarded.

CLINICAL PEARL

Visual skills are related to reading achievement. An analysis of the literature on the subject indicates that refractive error (in particular, hyperopia and significant anisometropia), exophoria, and disordered vergence are associated with reading underachievement.

Other visual functions have not been thoroughly investigated but have the potential for adversely influencing reading proficiency. Any visual assessment of the child having difficulty reading must include not only tests of visual acuity and refractive status but also tests of binocular vision. Visual abnormalities or dysfunctions encountered should be managed aggressively, with the goal of maximizing visual efficiency.

> **CLINICAL PEARL**
>
> *Any visual assessment of the child having difficulty reading must include not only tests of visual acuity and refractive status but also tests of binocular vision. Visual abnormalities or dysfunctions encountered should be managed aggressively, with the goal of maximizing visual efficiency.*

References

1. Yule W, Rutter M, Berger M, Thompson J: Over- and under-achievement in reading: distribution in the general population, *Br J Educ Psychol* 44:1-12, 1974.
2. Shaywitz SE, Shaywitz BA, Fletcher JM, Escobar MD: Prevalence of reading disability in boys and girls: results of the Connecticut Longitudinal Study, *JAMA* 264:998-1002, 1990.
3. Stedman LC, Kaestle CF: Literacy and reading performance in the United States, from 1880 to the present, *Read Res Q* 22:8-46, 1987.
4. McCormick S: *Remedial and clinical reading instruction,* Columbus, Ohio, 1987, Merrill Publishing.
5. Meier JH: Prevalence and characteristics of learning disabilities found in second grade children, *J Learn Disabil* 4:1-16, 1971.
6. Borsting E: Measures of visual attention in children with and without visual efficiency problems, *J Behav Optom* 2:151-156, 1991.
7. Walberg HJ, Tsai S: Matthew effects in education, *Am Educ Res J* 20:359-373, 1983.
8. LaBerge D, Samuels SJ: Toward a theory of automatic information processing in reading, *Cogn Psychol* 6:293-323, 1974.
9. Perfetti CA, Roth SF: Some of the interactive processes in reading and their roles in reading skill. In Lesgold AM, Perfetti CA (eds): *Interactive processes in reading,* Hillsdale, NJ, 1981, Lawrence Erlbaum.
10. Fagan JE Jr, Westgate TM, Yolton RL: Effects of video display character size, clarity, and color on P-300 latency, *Am J Optom Physiol Opt* 63:41-51, 1986.
11. Eames TH: The effect of glasses for the correction of hypermetropia and myopia on the speed of visual perception of objects and words, *J Educ Res* 42:534-540, 1949.
12. Andersen B: *Methodological errors in medical research,* Oxford, 1990, Blackwell Scientific Publications.
13. Solan HA: Vision and reading: an oversimplification, *J Behav Optom* 2:58, 1991.
14. Robinson HM: Visual efficiency and reading status in the elementary school. In Robinson HM, Smith H (eds): *Clinical studies in reading,* Chicago, 1968, University of Chicago Press.
15. Helveston EM, Weber JC, Miller K, et al: Visual function and academic performance, *Am J Ophthalmol* 99:346-355, 1985.
16. Bond G, Tinker M, Wasson B, Wasson J: *Reading difficulties: their diagnosis and correction,* Englewood Cliffs, NJ, 1984, Prentice-Hall.
17. Javitt JC: When does the failure to find a difference mean that there is none? *Arch Ophthalmol* 107:1034-1040, 1989.
18. Ygge J, Lennerstrand G, Rydberg A, et al: Oculomotor functions in a Swedish population of dyslexic and normally reading children, *Acta Ophthalmol* 71:10-21, 1993.
19. Blika S: Ophthalmological findings in pupils of a primary school with particular reference to reading difficulties, *Acta Ophthalmol* 60:927-934, 1982.
20. Norn MS, Rindziunski E, Skydsgaard H: Ophthalmologic and orthoptic examinations of dyslexics, *Acta Ophthalmol* 147:147-160, 1969.

21. Grisham JD, Simons HD: Refractive error and the reading process: a literature analysis, *J Am Optom Assoc* 57:44-55, 1986.
22. Simons HD, Grisham JD: Binocular anomalies and reading problems, *J Am Optom Assoc* 58:578-587, 1987.
23. Simons HD, Gassler PA: Vision anomalies and reading skill: a metanalysis of the literature, *Am J Optom Physiol Opt* 65:893-904, 1988.
24. Edson WH, Bond GL, Cook WW: Relationships between visual characteristics and specific silent reading abilities, *J Educ Res* 46:451-457, 1953.
25. Fendrick P: *Visual characteristics of poor readers*, New York, 1935, Teachers College, Columbia University.
26. Ygge J, Lennerstrand G, Axelsson I, Rydberg A: Visual functions in a Swedish population of dyslexic and normally reading children, *Acta Ophthalmol* 71:1-9, 1993.
27. Lovegrove WJ, Garzia RP, Nicholson SB: Experimental evidence for a transient system deficit in specific reading disability, *J Am Optom Assoc* 61:137-146, 1990.
28. Eames TH: A comparison of the ocular characteristics of unselected and reading disability groups, *J Educ Res* 25:211-215, 1932.
29. Eames TH: A frequency of physical handicaps in reading disability and unselected groups, *J Educ Res* 29:1-5, 1935.
30. Eames TH: Comparison of eye conditions among 1,000 reading failures, 500 ophthalmic patients, and 150 unselected children, *Am J Ophthalmol* 31:713-717, 1948.
31. Eames TH: The influence of hypermetropia and myopia on reading achievement, *Am J Ophthalmol* 39:375-377, 1955.
32. Young FA: Reading, measures of intelligence, and refractive errors, *Am J Optom Arch Am Acad Optom* 49:257-264, 1963.
33. Rosner J, Rosner J: Comparison of visual characteristics in children with and without learning difficulties, *Am J Optom Physiol Opt* 64:531-533, 1987.
34. Rosner J, Rosner J: Some observations of the relationship between the visual perceptual skills development of young hyperopes and age of first lens correction, *Clin Exp Optom* 69:166-168, 1986.
35. Eames TH: The effect of anisometropia on reading achievement, *Am J Optom Arch Am Acad Optom* 41:700-702, 1964.
36. Farris LP: *Visual defects as factors influencing achievement in reading*, Berkeley, 1934, University of California.
37. Birnbaum P, Birnbaum MH: Binocular coordination as a factor in reading achievement, *J Am Optom Assoc* 39:48-56, 1968.
38. Stein J, Fowler S: Effect of monocular occlusion on visuomotor perception and reading in dyslexic children, *Lancet* 2:69-73, 1985.
39. Cornelissen, P, Bradley L, Fowler S, Stein J: Covering one eye affects how some children read, *Dev Med Child Neurol* 34:296-304, 1992.
40. Good GH: Relationship of fusion weakness to reading disability, *J Exp Educ* 8:115-121, 1939.
41. Park GE: Functional dyslexia (reading failures) vs normal reading, *Eye Ear Nose Throat Month* 45:74-80, 1966.
42. Evans BJW, Drasdo N, Richards IL: Investigation of accommodative and binocular function in dyslexia, *Ophthalmic Physiol Opt* 14:5-19.
43. Eden GF, Stein JF, Wood HM, Wood FB: Differences in eye movements and reading problems in dyslexic and normal children, *Vision Res* 34:1345-1358, 1994.
44. Buzzelli AR: Stereopsis, accommodative and vergence facility: do they relate to dyslexia, *Optom Vis Sci* 68:842-846, 1991.
45. Stein JF, Riddell PM, Fowler S: Disordered vergence control in dyslexic children, *Br J Ophthalmol* 72:162-166, 1988.
46. Cornelissen P, Munro N, Fowler S, Stein J: The stability of binocular fixation during reading in adults and children, *Dev Med Child Neurol* 35:777-787, 1993.
47. Hung GK: Reduced vergence response velocities in dyslexics: a preliminary report, *Ophthalmic Physiol Opt* 9:420-424, 1989.

48. Hammerberg E, Norn MS: Defective dissociation of accommodation and convergence in dyslectic children, *Acta Ophthalmol* 50:651-654, 1972.
49. Hoffman LG: Incidence of vision dificulties in children with learning disabilities, *J Am Optom Assoc* 1:447-451, 1980.
50. Marcus SE: A syndrome of visual constrictions in the learning disabled child, *J Am Optom Assoc* 45:746-749, 1974.
51. Park GE: Reading difficulty (dyslexia) from the ophthalmic point of view, *Am J Ophthalmol* 31:28-34, 1948.
52. Sherman A: Relating vision disorders to learning disability, *J Am Optom Assoc* 44:140-141, 1973.
53. Wold RM, Pierce JR, Kennington J: Effectiveness of optometric vision therapy, *J Am Optom Assoc* 49:1047-1054, 1978.
54. Bettman JW, Stern EL, Whitsell LJ, Gofman HF: Cerebral dominance in developmental dyslexia, *Arch Ophthalmol* 78:722-729, 1967.
55. Peters HB: The influence of orthoptic training on reading ability. II, The problem, study, and conclusions, *Am J Optom Arch Am Acad Optom* 19:152-176, 1942.
56. Olson HC, Mitchell CC, Westberg WC: The relationship between visual training and reading and academic achievement, *Am J Optom Arch Am Acad Optom* 30:3-13, 1953.
57. Worcester DA: The influence of orthoptic training on the reading ability of college freshmen, *J Exp Educ* 9:167-174, 1940.
58. Atzmon D: Positive effect of improving relative fusional vergence on reading and learning disabilities, *Binoc Vision* 1:39-43, 1985.
59. Haddad HM, Isaacs NS, Onghena K, Mazor A: The use of orthoptics in dyslexia, *J Learn Disabil* 17:142-144, 1984.
60. Masters MC: Orthoptic management of visual dyslexia, *Br Orthopt J* 45:40-48, 1988.
61. Atzmon D, Nemet P, Ishay A, Karni E: A randomized prospective masked and matched comparative study of orthoptic treatment versus conventional reading tutoring treatment for reading disabilities in 62 children, *Binoc Vis Eye Muscle Surg Q* 8:91-106, 1993.
62. Park GE, Burri C: The relationship of various eye conditions and reading achievement, *J Educ Psychol* 34:290-299, 1943.
63. Park GE, Burri C: The effect of eye abnormalities on reading difficulties, *J Educ Psychol* 34:420-430, 1943.
64. O'Grady J: The relationship between vision and educational performance; a study of year 2 children in Tasmania, *Aust J Optom* 67:126-140, 1984.
65. Simons HD, Grisham JD: Vision and reading disability: research problems, *J Am Optom Assoc* 57:36-42, 1986.
66. Robinson H: An analysis of four visual screening tests at grades four and seven, *Am J Optom Arch Am Acad Optom* 30:177-187.
67. Kephart NC: Visual skills and their relations to school achievement, *Am J Ophthalmol* 36:794-799, 1953.
68. Wirt SE, Morgan CL, Floyd W: Achievement of grade school pupils in relation to visual performance, *Yearbook-Clarement College Reading Conference*, pp 59-66, 1947.
69. Steinbaum M, Kurk M: Relationship between the Keystone Visual Skills Test with reading achievement and intelligence, *Am J Optom Arch Am Acad Optom* 35:173-181, 1958.
70. Glatt LD, Glatt MM: Visual efficiency in the classroom, *Opt J Rev Optom* 93:37-39, 52, 1956.
71. Kephart NC, Manas L, Simpson, D: Vision and achievement in kindergarten, *Am J Optom Arch Am Acad Optom* 37:36-39, 1960.
72. Swanson DE, Tiffin J: Betts' physiological approach to the analysis of reading disabilities as applied to the college level, *J Educ Res* 29:433-438, 1936.
73. Stromberg EL: The relationship between lateral muscle balance and the ductions of reading speed, *Am J Optom* 14:415-420, 1937.

7

Eye Movements and Reading

Jack E. Richman
Ralph P. Garzia

Key Terms

eye movements	smooth pursuits	attention-deficit
ocular motility	magnocellular	disorder
attention	pathway	phonological coding
saccades	hyperactivity	naming

Reading is one of the most intricate processes that children and adults alike must master as the basis for understanding all written language. It entails recognition, decoding, and phonological and syntactic awareness of hundreds of squiggly and straight lines we call printed words. An integral component of reading is movements of the eyes across the page of print.

Components of Reading Eye Movements

There are two major components of reading eye movements, fixations and saccades. What determines the length of time an eye fixates before the next saccade is initiated? What determines where and how far the saccade will travel? During the fixation interval, visual information is transmitted for higher-level processing of word identification and recognition. The duration of fixation (and the decision of when to move the eyes) is determined on the basis of language and cognitive factors.[1,2] Where to move the eyes is based on low level parafoveal visual perceptual information that uses the spaces between words to calculate word length and hence saccade length.[3] There is a preferred "landing site" for the first saccade on a word.[4] This preferred viewing position falls just left of the word's center. The goal of the saccade is to land in the optimal position for the fastest word recognition.[5]

As reading skill improves, eye-movement patterns show marked changes.[6] The number and duration of fixations decrease, saccades become longer, and the number of regressions decreases. A first grade child reading a 10-word line will average 22 fixations, lasting for about 330 msec, and make over 5 regressions.[6] In contrast, an adult will average 9 fixations, each lasting about 240 msec, and make 1.5 regressions.[6] The average saccade length is 1° to 2° (about 8 character spaces), but it may range from 0.5° to 4°. The duration of the saccadic eye movement is 10 to 30 msec. As the number and duration of fixations decrease, reading rate increases and reading becomes more efficient with expanded comprehension.

CLINICAL PEARL

As reading skill improves, eye-movement patterns show marked changes. The number and duration of fixations decrease, saccades become longer, and the number of regressions decreases.

The ability to move the eyes to an appropriate location in a word seems to be fully developed by the first year of formal reading instruction.[7] As reading skill develops, there is a reduction in the frequency of refixating a word (i.e., making a short saccade to a further rightward portion of the fixated word). Refixating a word probably is related to the ability to identify and recognize the word on the first fixation.

Regressions are believed to provide an opportunity to review a word, glance back at an interesting detail, or verify a specific fact. In adult readers about 15% of the saccades are regressions, while in beginning readers as many as 40% are.[6] Reading eye movements also include larger return sweep saccades to place the eyes at the beginning of the next line of print.

When eye movements are recorded, one discovers a substantial difference in the pattern of fixations and saccades, even in normal readers. These differences are often related to many factors, including text difficulty, print size and spacing, and the experience of the reader.

Reading eye movement behaviors tend to closely parallel the condition of concurrent perceptual and cognitive processes.[8] The perceptual processes of reading include perceptual span and word identification. Cognitive processes include semantic and syntactic processing and comprehension.

Eye Movement Differences Between Normal and Disabled Readers

Many studies have reported differences in reading eye movements as a function of reading ability.[9,10] Disabled readers tend to exhibit a greater number of fixations of increased duration, shorter average saccade lengths, and a higher proportion of regressions for their age and reading level than normal readers do.[11] However, there is a wide variation in the eye movement patterns of poor readers. In fact, the overall impression one gets from reviewing these patterns is that they are erratic, irregular, inconsistent from line to line, and idiosyncratic.[12-16] Although disabled readers do show abnormalities of eye movement patterns, most authorities agree that they reflect the underlying language-based word-decoding disabilities seen in poor readers and the condition of concurrent perceptual and cognitive processing.

CLINICAL PEARL

Disabled readers tend to exhibit a greater number of fixations of increased duration, shorter average saccade lengths, and a higher proportion of regressions for their age and reading level than normal readers do.

Some writers[17] have suggested that a basic saccadic dysfunction causes reading disability; others[18-20] disagree. The positive results reported by Pavlidis[17] for sequential saccades to nonlanguage stimuli have not been replicated.[18-20] In addition, there appears to be considerable overlap in the accuracy of saccades of normal and disabled readers. After reviewing the literature, Garzia and Peck[21] concluded that there probably are no significant differences in saccadic main sequence (the relationship between saccadic amplitude to peak velocity and duration) between disabled and normal readers. Disabled readers can be found who have normal saccadic function and, conversely, normal readers can be found with saccadic dysfunction. However, a number of case studies[14-16] have demonstrated that some disabled readers have particular difficulty with the programming and execution of return sweep saccades. There is some evidence[21,22] to suggest that the principal and more universal oculomotor dysfunction in disabled readers may be decreased fixation maintenance.

Eye Movements, Attention, and Reading

Perhaps there is a fundamental skill that is basic to all reading and learning tasks—attention. Attention plays an important role in all stages of problem solving and learning.[23] If children are to learn, they must attend to and focus on the relevant elements of the learning task. There are three obvious and interrelated behavioral manifestations of attentional deficits.[24,25] The first is hyperactivity, in which the child has an excessive level of motor activity, particularly in the preschool and early school-age years. Hyperactivity can prevent a child from staying at one task or maintaining orientation to the task long enough to complete it. Second is distractibility, which describes the child who cannot maintain attention on a task. He or she responds to extraneous internal or external stimuli or is unable to select the relevant stimulus among alternatives. There is a failure to maintain and sustain on-task attention. The third attentional deficiency is impulsivity. Impulsive children do not pause for appropriate analysis before responding. This often produces inaccurate responses in basic learning and reading tasks. All of these ostensible manifestations of attentional deficits can adversely influence reading ability.

CLINICAL PEARL

There is a fundamental skill that is basic to all reading and learning tasks—attention. Attention plays an important role in all stages of problem solving and learning.

However, just as significant are disturbances of low-level *visual* attentional processes that can disrupt proper eye movement control during reading. Morrison's model of eye movement control in reading[26] plays a prominent role for visual attention in directing saccades. The model proposes that words are processed one at a time by an attention mechanism. At the successful identification of the fixated word, attention is shifted to the next word, which automatically signals the oculomotor system to execute a saccade to that word. Not only visual attention must be appropriately directed and sustained, it also must be efficiently shifted from one spatial locus to another in the proper temporal sequence. Steinman, Steinman, and Garzia (Chapter 11) have demonstrated that disabled readers exhibit anomalous spatial-temporal distributions of visual attention.

Important new information about the nature of oculomotor control and attention in reading has emerged from investigations of express saccades. Express saccades are very short latency saccades—approximately 100 msec—that typically occur when there is a gap between the offset of the fixation target and the appearance of the saccadic stimulus. Fischer et al.,[28-32] in their "gap" paradigm experiments, have reported that reading-disabled children produce more express saccades than normal readers do.

Because of their shorter latency, express saccades are made with little time for central processing and decision-making mechanisms. Several explanations have been advanced for the occurrence of express saccades, of which the best known is Fischer's attentional disengagement model.[28-32] The attentional disengagement model suggests that express saccades are most likely to occur when attention has been disengaged from the locus of fixation before the presentation of a potential saccade target.

According to Fischer's model, attention is in either the engaged or the disengaged state. In the gap condition the fixation point disappears for a period before the target stimulus appears. The absence of the fixation point promotes the shift of attention from an engaged to a disengaged state, resulting in a more rapid preparation to execute a saccade. The high frequency of express saccades in reading-disabled subjects suggests that they may not be in a state of engaged attention during the fixational period of reading, which may decrease their accuracy in processing text. The premature initiation of saccadic eye movements may lead to the need for regressions in order to reacquire information. The resulting increased number of eye movements may produce confusion or disrupt the normal integration of information.

CLINICAL PEARL

The high frequency of express saccades in reading-disabled subjects suggests that they may not be in a state of engaged attention during the fixational period of reading.

Related to the role of visual attention in reading eye movement control is the concept of perceptual span. Perceptual span is defined as the number of words "visible" during each fixation and is calculated by dividing the number of words read by the number of fixations.[9,33,34] With this method the perceptual span is much larger for adult than for beginning readers. The span is 1.11 words for adults and less than half a word for first grade children. The perceptual span represents the spatial extent of the use of parafoveal information (word shape and length and the initial letters) as a preview effect for both facilitated word recognition and the guidance of eye movements. The more mature and faster reader has become very proficient in using this information. Using a moving window technique that restricted the field of view to only five characters, Rayner[35] found that reading rate was reduced by 38% in beginning readers, but by over 65% in adults. An accepted explanation for this phenomenon is that young readers focus all their attention on foveal word processing and do not fully utilize parafoveal information. Thus limiting their field of view has a relatively small effect. However, if the perceptual span is artificially restricted in adult readers, their reading performance is dramatically affected because they cannot take the accustomed full advantage of parafoveal information under these conditions.

CLINICAL PEARL

The perceptual span represents the spatial extent of the use of parafoveal information (word shape and length and the initial letters) as a preview effect for both facilitated word recognition and the guidance of eye movements.

The reader who practices reading without deficiencies in eye movement control, attentional processes, or cognitive language functioning will develop efficient reading with little conscious attention or awareness of the process. With this experience words are recognized more automatically, allowing greater attention to be directed to comprehension. This ease in controlling the eyes and perceiving the words in an unconscious, effortless manner is called automatic cognitive processing or automaticity.[36,37] When there are impediments or delays in automatic processing, the child must devote an increased amount of time, attention, and effort to reading tasks and task components that others have mastered long ago.

Signs and Symptoms of Eye Movement Dysfunction

Patients with and without reading disorders often present with a relatively wide range of signs and symptoms associated with an eye movement disorder (see the box on p. 139). The eye movement disorder may be so severe or frequent that it creates a feeling of general ocular discomfort and limits the patient's ability to read effortlessly for more than a few minutes.

These symptoms may be considered the outcome of a lack of properly developed automatic processing—caused by breakdowns or delays in attention, oculomotor control, or language function. Symptoms are the end product of this chain of events that leads to increased time to complete reading tasks. It is then that the reader's awareness of these inefficiencies is reported as symptoms. Interestingly, breakdowns in accommodative or binocular functioning often have similar effects and produce concomitant symptoms during reading.

Signs and Symptoms of Reading Eye Movement Dysfunction

Loss of place
Need for finger or marker to keep place
Return sweep confusion
Rereading words or lines
Word omissions, additions, or transpositions
Illusory text movement
Reduced reading rate
Generalized visual discomfort or fatigue

Therefore the clinical assessment of symptoms related to reading needs to be multifactoral. Attention, automaticity, eye movement control systems, and binocularity require explanation and factoring. A simple assessment of ocular motility isolated from these other factors will lead to erroneous clinical decision making.[38] It is from this frame of reference that we will explore different methods used for assessing eye movements as they relate to reading performance.

Eye Movement Assessment

As indicated previously, attention and attention-related processes are involved in eye-movement control, particularly the maintenance of fixation and smooth pursuit. Clinicians frequently question the importance of testing smooth pursuit eye movements in disabled readers, primarily because only saccades are required for reading. However, recall that the magnocellular (M) pathway originating in the retina projects to the middle temporal area of the extrastriate cortex (MT). Area MT is involved in the control of smooth pursuit eye movements. Cells here are responsive to the speed and direction of moving stimuli. Experimental lesions of area MT in monkeys produce a scotoma for motion.[39] Within the affected visual field the speed of a moving target cannot be calculated, resulting in an inability to initiate a smooth pursuit to target motion.

CLINICAL PEARL

Attention and attention-related processes are involved in eye-movement control, particularly the maintenance of fixation and smooth pursuit.

The posterior parietal cortex receives projections from area MT. Unlike the neurons in MT, posterior parietal neurons are more concerned with the nature of a moving target and less with its inherent speed or direction.[40] Therefore this cortical area is probably related more to selective visual attentional processes required to pursue a moving target than to the neurophysiological control of smooth pursuit eye movements themselves.[41] Parietal lobe injuries have been shown[42] to cause abnormal visual attention. The posterior parietal lobe is also involved in shifts of visual attention.[43] And the parietal lobe is important in generating a continuously accurate representation of visual space before, during, and after eye movements. Neurons in the parietal lobe anticipate the retinal consequences of intended eye movement.[44]

The M pathway has been found[45-47] to be defective in reading-disabled subjects. Therefore testing smooth-pursuit eye movements is an important index of M-pathway integrity, including the processes of maintaining and shifting visual attention, which are essential for efficient reading.[48]

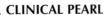

CLINICAL PEARL

Testing smooth-pursuit eye movements is an important index of M-pathway integrity, including the processes of maintaining and shifting visual attention, which are essential for efficient reading.

Children described as distractible or impulsive exhibit difficulties sustaining attention. This sustained attention, also called vigilance, is the readiness to respond to novel stimuli.[49-51] A child who is inattentive to classroom tasks is described as distractible and engaging in excessive "off-task looking." This off-task looking behavior is considered an essential sign in the diagnosis of attention deficit disorder.[52] Richman[53] found "off-task looking time" (the amount of time fixation was not directed to the task) and "off-task fixations" (the number of times fixation shifted off task) to be significantly related to classroom observations of short attention span, distractibility, and impulsive decision-making style.[53]

Off-task fixations can be observed during a comprehensive vision examination in many children with reading or learning disorders. For example, when steadiness of fixation is requested for cover tests, retinoscopy, or opthalmoscopy, the child may sustain fixation for only a few seconds. When smooth pursuits are measured, the clinical judgment of adequate or inadequate performance is based on the number of off-task fixations.[54]

The biomicroscope is frequently overlooked in the evaluation of off-task fixational patterns, even though it provides a means of evaluating fixation with control of illumination and magnification. This can be especially useful for the detection of minute levels of nystagmus or fixational drift patterns. Other common clinical instruments are also useful—the direct ophthalmoscope and the keratometer, which are sensitive to very small fixational drifts. Indeed, "off-task looking time" and "off-task fixations" during an assessment of eye movements more likely indicate attentional dysfunction than difficulty with oculomotor control per se. If these clinically observed behaviors are related to inappropriately sustained attention during eye movement tests, then it is necessary to ascertain if the child has a primary oculomotor dysfunction, an attentional dysfunction, or both.

CLINICAL PEARL

"Off-task looking time" and "off-task fixations" during an assessment of eye movements more likely indicate attentional dysfunction than difficulty with oculomotor control per se.

Several simple modifications of presently used clinical tests may give more insight into attentional functioning. First, have the child look at a fixation target (letter or number) across a fully lit room. Ask him or her to "Please look at this letter and don't take your eyes off of it. I am going to time you to see how long you can do this." (Test time is usually a minimum of 30 seconds.) Observe the child's eyes and note the number of times they are "off task." (This is applicable in children age 6 and older.) Children with attention deficits often have difficulty holding fixation steady for the full 30 seconds. Another modification is to increase the time of smooth pursuit testing. Usually the testing of ocular motility with the physiological H pattern takes less than 10 seconds. By increasing this to 60 seconds, you will be assessing the child's ability to sustain attention on a low-interest target for a significantly longer time. Observe the number of off-task fixations. Formal measures of sustained visual attention using continuous performance tests are available commercially,[55,56] with computerized versions also available.[57]

If smooth pursuits are saccadic with many off-task fixations, the child should be retested using attention-engagement procedures. These increase the attentional focus on a task by the use of increased sensory interaction. For example, demanding verbal picture, word, letter, or number identification enhances the engagement of attention. Tactual support can be provided with finger pointing or corollary arm movements with the target. If performance improves (i.e., less off-task fixations), this is positive indication that there is an important attentional element in the eye movement behavior. The change may then be considered relative to other clinical test results, symptoms, and the presenting history of classroom performance.

There are three classes of eye movement testing methods. Each will be discussed.

Electronic methods

Electronic instrumentation for assessing eye movements has been available for years. Its primary advantage is the objective documentation of basic eye movement components during reading (i.e., saccade length and velocity, fixation duration, and number of fixations and regressions). Several techniques are employed today that capture the dynamic characteristics of eye movements—including high-magnification biomicroscopic videography, fundus videography, direct-current electrooculography, and infrared limbal reflection oculography. Though quite accurate, these procedures are generally expensive, time consuming, and not clinically efficient. Ciuffreda and Tannen[58] offer a detailed discussion of the procedures and their strengths and weaknesses.

Chairside observational techniques

As an alternative to electronic measurements, many optometrists utilize highly subjective rating scales or insufficiently standardized procedures based on gross observations of eye movements. For example, the simple use of looking back and forth between two targets such as pencils has been helpful in objectively evaluating saccadic function. Ordinal scales may be used in an attempt to quantify and evaluate the quality of saccadic movements.[57] In one test gaining popularity, the NSUCO oculomotor test,[54] the patient's saccades are graded during five cycles of movement and smooth pursuits for two rotations in each direction. This test has good inter-rater and test-retest reliability, with a clear developmental trend for improvement of saccadic skill.

Visual-verbal naming tests

The need for a practical, inexpensive, and quantitative alternative to chairside testing procedures led to the development of visual-verbal naming tests. These, of course, do not directly measure eye movement patterns during reading but, rather, seek to assess oculomotor function indirectly in a simulated reading situation. Eye movement performance is based on the accuracy and time required to recognize and correctly name a series of single numbers arranged horizontally. The Pierce Saccade Test,[60] King-Devick,[61] and NYSOA-KD[62] are examples that have been widely applied. Developmental trends are evident in response accuracy and time. If there are significant delays in the time required to complete the task, or if excessive errors occur, then the presumption is made that an eye movement dysfunction is responsible. On the surface, these tests appear to have merit in terms of their psychometric design, repeatability, and practicality. Unfortunately, questions of validity have been raised because eye movements are not measured directly but are inferred from the total time to complete the test. The question arises, "What contributions do eye movements actually make to performance on naming tasks?"

A number of other confounding variables introduced into naming tests can significantly affect their interpretation. In addition to eye movements, there is attention, automaticity, recognition of numbers, phonological coding, visual-verbal integration time, articulation rate, the ability to recover from error, and continuous workload capacity. If a child exhibits increased time to complete a naming test, then any of these factors may be contributing to that performance.

The visual, cognitive, and language processes required for rapid naming are quite similar to those needed to identify and recognize words during silent reading.[63,64] An assessment of naming speed is important, because recent evidence[65,66] suggests that a majority of the readingdisabled, regardless of the presence of other types of processing dysfunctions, have a phonological coding deficit. Slow naming is a reflection of this basic phonological deficiency. The subprocesses involved in retrieval of a verbal label in the naming process are similar to those necessary for word recognition. Reading and naming both require lexical access and retrieval in the context of rapid scanning, sequencing, and processing of serially presented material. Naming speed is also an index of automaticity (i.e., fast and obligatory processing), which requires only a limited use of cognitive resources. With intact and automatized lower-level processing, attentional allocation can be reserved for higher-level processing. There is substantial evidence[65,66] that a significant inverse relationship exists between naming speed and reading achievement.

CLINICAL PEARL

The visual, cognitive, and language processes required for rapid naming are quite similar to those needed to identify and recognize words during silent reading. An assessment of naming speed is important because recent evidence suggests that a majority of the reading disabled, regardless of the presence of other types of processing dysfunctions, have a phonological coding deficit.

For naming tests to be valid and clinically useful measures, they must be designed to separate the effects of eye movement function from these other variables. The Developmental Eye Movement (DEM)

Test[67] was developed to address these concerns. The DEM incorporates a subtest of rapid continuous naming of numbers presented in a vertical array. This arrangement represents naming speed in the absence of horizontal eye movements. Vertical naming performance is then compared with the ability to name an equal set of numbers displayed in a horizontal array. The ratio of horizontal time to vertical time represents the change induced by incorporation of eye movements.

This method differentially isolates the influence of eye movements from phonological or automaticity problems as potential causes of diminished performance. Even though the DEM does not provide direct information on eye movement parameters (like fixation duration or regressions), it does provide an indirect normative measure, based on time, of potential delays in reading-related eye movement control. When used in conjunction with other visual information processing tests, the DEM can assist you with the differential diagnosis of eye movement dysfunction in reading disability.

Similarities and contrasts

A comment is required about the relationship between chairside tests of saccadic function and visual-verbal naming performance like the DEM. Although both have been shown to be related to reading disability individually, their interrelationship is unknown at this time. They are considered to test the same function but are quite different in the following way: Naming tests simulate the requirements for saccadic programming involved in reading. The next-in-sequence number must be found accurately among an array of distractors. Few if any distractors exist with chairside tests. Two targets held 6 to 12 inches apart are easily visible against the background of the examiner.

This does not mean that chairside tests are unimportant. On the contrary, both types of tests are meaningful in assessing eye movement function. A naming test evaluates eye movement function in the context of visual-spatial awareness in a reading-like phonological environment and not necessarily eye movement programming per se. Chairside tests may be considered as providing information about basic saccadic programming, in the absence of higher visual-spatial and phonological demands. Knowledge of this difference has important implications for vision therapy or, at a minimum, the sequences of and emphases for therapy.

Diagnosis and Therapy

Solan and others have provided some evidence that eye movement parameters and reading efficiency can be improved with appropriate therapeutic intervention in achieving young adults whose only complaints are of inefficient reading (slow and laborious).

Solan's reported therapy[68-70] used a tachistoscope to promote speed of processing and controlled reading instruments to promote a directional attack. After therapy the number of fixations and regressions decreased while perceptual span, reading rate, and comprehension all increased. Reading efficiency indeed improved. These subjects also received instruction in reading strategy, which makes any conclusion as to the efficacy of vision therapy alone questionable. However, the results do suggest that a complete remedial program, including both reading and vision therapy, is important. The subjects in these studies did show significant improvements, not only in eye movement parameters but also in reading efficiency.

Another study[71] divided a group of optometry students who scored lowest on a standardized reading test into an experimental group that received 4 weeks of vision therapy with no reading instruction and a no-therapy control group. Reading efficiency (as determined by reduced number of fixations, fewer regressions, and greater perceptual span) was enhanced. However, there were no concomitant improvements in reading comprehension.

The clearest indications of the need for therapy in eye movement disorders are the concordance of presenting signs and symptoms, chairside performance, and DEM results. Ratio scores on the DEM at least 1.5 standard deviations below age or grade means should be considered inadequate. We do not recommend therapy unless there is a consistency between the nature of the reported reading disturbance and the criterion level of eye-movement performance. The objective of therapy is to reduce or eliminate symptoms, with accompanying improvement in eye-movement performance. Reading performance may or may not improve immediately. Clinicians should also consider the impact of such therapy on other school-related activities, for example, visual-motor integration and playground skills. Another overlooked effect of therapy is on attention. As described earlier, there are clear physiological and anatomical associations between eye-movement control and attentional processes. Therapy programs implemented primarily for eye-movement dysfunctions can have a secondary impact on attention. Therefore the success of therapy may be sought in changes in "off-task" behavior, distractability, and impulsivity. This effect of changes in eye movements becomes more evident when we critically examine and review many of the vision-therapy procedures and programs employed today[59,72-74] for eye-movement dysfunctions. In fact, attentional deficits are largely contributory to the manifestations of faulty eye movements, particularly fixation maintenance and smooth pursuit. It is quite likely that eye-movement therapy is, in reality, visual-attention therapy reflected through changes in oculomotor behavior. In other words, as visual attentional processes are enhanced eye-movement control becomes more automatic and efficient, providing a sounder and more consistent basis for information processing.

CLINICAL PEARL

It is quite likely that eye-movement therapy is, in reality, visual-attention therapy reflected through changes in oculomotor behavior.

References

1. Tinker MA: Eye movements in reading, *J Educ Res* 30:241-277, 1936.
2. Tinker MA: The study of eye movements in reading, *Psychol Bull* 43:93-120, 1946.
3. Rayner K: The perceptual span and eye movement control during reading. In Rayner K (ed): *Eye movements in reading,* New York, 1983, Academic Press.
4. Rayner K: Eye guidance in reading: fixation locations within words, *Perception* 8:21-30, 1979.
5. O'Regan JK, Jacobs AM: Optimal viewing position effect on word recognition: a challenge to the current theory, *J Exp Psychol Hum Percept Perform* 18:185-197, 1992.
6. Taylor SE: Eye movements while reading: facts and fallacies, *Am Educ Res J* 2:187-202, 1965.
7. McConkie GW, Zola D, Grimes J, et al: Children's eye movements during reading. In Stein JF (ed): *Vision and dyslexia,* Boca Raton, Fla, 1991, CRC Press.
8. Epelboim J, Booth JR, Steinman RM: Reading unspaced text: implications for theories of reading eye movements, *Vision Res* 34:1735-1766, 1994.
9. Taylor EA: *The fundamental reading skill,* ed 2, Springfield, Ill, 1966, Charles C Thomas.
10. Taylor EA, Solan HA: *Functional readiness and school adjustment,* New York, 1956, Reading & Study Skills Center.
11. McConkie GW: Eye movements and perception during reading. In Rayner K (ed): *Eye movements in reading,* New York, 1983, Academic Press.
12. Zangwill OL, Blakemore C: Dyslexia: reversal of eye-movements during reading, *Neuropsychologia* 10:371-373, 1972.
13. Elterman RD, Abel LA, Daroff RB, et al: Eye movement patterns in dyslexic children, *J Learn Disabil* 13:16-21, 1980.
14. Ciuffreda KJ, Bahill AT, Kenyon RV, Stark L: Eye movements during reading: case reports, *Am J Optom Physiol Opt* 53:389-395, 1976.
15. Ciuffreda KJ, Kenyon RV, Stark L: Saccadic intrusions contributing to reading disability: a case report, *Am J Optom Physiol Opt* 60:242-249, 1983.
16. Ciuffreda KJ, Kenyon RV, Stark L: Eye movements during reading: further case reports, *Am J Optom Physiol Opt* 62:844-852, 1985.
17. Pavlidis GT: Eye movement differences between dyslexics, normal, and retarded readers while sequentially fixating digits, *Am J Optom Physiol Opt* 62:820-832, 1985.
18. Olson RK, Kliegl R, Davidson BJ: Dyslexic and normal readers' eye movements, *J Exp Psychol Hum Percept Perform* 9:816-825, 1983.
19. Black JL, Collins DWK, DeRoach JN, Zubrick S: A detailed study of sequential saccadic eye movements for normal- and poor-reading children, *Percept Mot Skills* 59:423-434, 1984.
20. Stanley G, Smith GA, Howell EA: Eye-movements and sequential tracking in dyslexic and control children, *Br J Psychol* 74:181-187, 1983.
21. Garzia RP, Peck CK: Vision and reading. II. Eye movements, *J Optom Vis Dev* 25:4-37, 1993.
22. Eden GF, Stein JF, Wood HM, Wood FB: Differences in eye movements and reading problems in dyslexic and normal children, *Vision Res* 34:1345-1358, 1994.
23. Conte R: Attention disorders. In Wong BYL (ed): *Learning about learning disabilities,* New York, 1991, Academic Press.

24. Silver LB: The relationship between learning disabilities, hyperactivity, distractability and behavioral problems: a clinical analysis, *J Am Acad Child Adolesc Psychiatry* 20:385-397, 1981.

25. Goldstein S, Goldstein M: *Managing attention disorders in children,* New York, 1990, John Wiley & Sons.

26. Morrison RE: Manipulation of stimulus onset delay in reading: evidence for parallel programming of saccades, *J Exp Psychol Hum Percept Perform* 10:667-682, 1984.

27. Steinman BA, Steinman SB, Garzia RP: Reading with an M neuron: how a defective magnocellular (M) pathway interferes with normal reading. In Garzia RP (ed): *Vision and reading,* St Louis, 1996, Mosby.

28. Fischer B, Weber H: Saccadic reaction times of dyslexic and age-matched normal subjects, *Perception* 19:805-818, 1990.

29. Fischer B, Biscaldi M, Otto P: Saccadic eye movements of dyslexic subjects, *Neuropsychologia* 31:887-906, 1993.

30. Fischer B, Boch R: Saccadic eye movements after extremely short reaction times in the monkey, *Brain Res* 260:21-26, 1983.

31. Fischer B, Ramsberger E: Human express saccades; extremely short reaction times of goal directed eye movements, *Exp Brain Res* 57:191-195, 1984.

32. Fischer B, Breitmeyer B: Mechanisms of visual attention revealed by saccadic eye movements, *Neuropsychologia* 25:73-83, 1987.

33. Rayner K: Eye movements in reading and information processing, *Psychol Bull* 85:618-660, 1978.

34. Buswell GT: *Fundamental reading habits: a study of their development,* Chicago, 1922, Chicago University Press.

35. Rayner K: Eye movements and the perceptual span in beginning and skilled readers, *J Exp Child Psychol* 41:211-236, 1986.

36. LaBerge D, Samuels SJ: Toward a theory of automatic information processing in reading, *Cogn Psychol* 6:293-323, 1974.

37. Nicolson RI, Fawcett AJ: Automaticity: a new framework for dyslexia research? *Cognition* 35:159-182, 1990.

38. Richman JE, Walker AJ, Garzia RP: The impact of automatic digit naming on a clinical test of eye movement functioning, *J Am Optom Assoc* 54:617-622, 1983.

39. Newsome WT, Wurtz RH, Dursteler MR, Mikami A: Disturbances in motion processing following ibotenic acid lesions of the middle temporal visual area of the macaque monkey, *J Neurophysiol* 5:825-840, 1985.

40. Lynch JC, Mountcastle VB, Talbot WH, Yin TCT: Parietal lobe mechanisms for directed visual attention, *J Neurophysiol* 40:362-389, 1977.

41. Leigh RJ, Zee DS: *The neurology of eye movements,* ed 2, Philadelphia, 1991, FA Davis.

42. Petersen SE, Robinson DL, Currie JN: Influences of lesions of parietal cortex on visual spatial attention in humans, *Exp Brain Res* 76:267-280, 1989.

43. Posner MI, Walker JA, Friedrich FJ, Rafal RD: How do the parietal lobes direct covert attention? *Neuropsychologia* 25:135-145, 1987.

44. Duhamel JR, Colby CL, Goldberg ME: The updating of the representation of visual space in parietal cortex by intended eye movements, *Science* 255:90-92, 1992.

45. Lehmkuhle S, Garzia RP, Turner L, et al: A defective visual pathway in reading disabled children, *N Engl J Med* 328:989-996, 1993.

46. Lovegrove WJ, Garzia RP, Nicholson SB: Experimental evidence for a transient system deficit in specific reading disability, *J Am Optom Assoc* 61:137-146, 1990.

47. Williams MC, Molinet K, LeCluyse K: Visual masking as a measure of temporal processing in normal and disabled readers, *Clin Vis Sci* 4:137-144, 1989.

48. Garzia RP, Sesma M: Vision and reading. I. Neuroanatomy and electrophysiology, *J Optom Vis Dev* 24:4-53, 1993.

49. Pelham WE: Attention deficits in hypreactive children and learning disabled children, *Except Educ Q* 2:13-23, 1981.

50. Douglas VI, Peters KG: Toward a clearer definition of attentional deficit of hyperactive children. In Hale GA, Lewis M (eds): *Attention and cognitive development,* New York, 1973, Plenum Press.

51. Douglas VI: Stop, look, and listen: the problem of sustained attention and impulse control in hyperactive and normal children, *Can J Behav Sci* 4:259-282, 1972.

52. Kupietz SS, Richardson E: Children's vigilance performance and inattentiveness in the classroom, *J Child Psychol Psychiatry* 19:145-154, 1978.

53. Richman JE: Use of a sustained visual attention task to determine children at risk for learning problems, *J Am Optom Assoc* 57:20-26, 1986.

54. Maples WC, Atchley J, Ficklin T: Northeast State University College of Optometry's oculomotor norms, *J Behav Optom* 3:143-150, 1992.

55. Gordon M: *The Gordon Diagnostic System,* Dewitt, NY, 1983, Gordon Systems.

56. Conners CK: *Continuous Performance Test (CPT),* Los Angeles, 1993, Western Psychological Services.

57. Vogel G, Shearer C: *Computer therapy for visual skills,* South Bend, Ind, 1994, Bernell.

58. Ciuffreda K, Tannen B: *Eye movement basics for the clinician,* St Louis, 1995, Mosby.

59. Griffin JR: *Binocular anomalies: procedures for vision therapy,* ed 2, Chicago, 1982, Professional Press.

60. Pierce J: *Pierce Saccade Test,* Bloomington, Ind, 1972, Cook.

61. King AT, Devick S: *The proposed King-Devick test and its relation to the Pierce Saccade Test and reading levels,* Senior research project, 1976, Illinois College of Optometry.

62. Lieberman S, Cohen AH, Rubin J: NYSOA K-D test, *J Am Optom Assoc* 54:631-637, 1983.

63. Murphy LA, Pollatsek A, Well AD: Developmental dyslexia and word retrieval deficits, *Brain Lang* 35:1-23, 1988.

64. Wolf M: Naming, reading, and the dyslexias: a longitudinal overview, *Ann Dyslexia* 34:87-115, 1984.

65. Denckla MB, Rudel RG: Rapid "automatized" naming (R.A.N.): dyslexia differentiated from other learning disabilities, *Neuropsychologia* 14:471-479, 1976.

66. Fawcett AJ, Nicolson, RI: Naming speed in children with dyslexia, *J Learn Disabil* 27:641-646, 1994.

67. Garzia RP, Richman JE, Nicholson SB, Gaines CS: A new visual-verbal saccade test: the Developmental Eye Movement test (DEM), *J Am Optom Assoc* 61:124-135, 1990.

68. Solan HA: The improvement of reading efficiency: a study of sixty-three achieving high school students, *J Read Spec* 7:8-13, 1967.

69. Solan HA: Deficient eye-movement patterns in achieving high school students: three case histories, *J Learn Disabil* 18:66-70, 1985.

70. Solan HA: Eye movement problems in achieving readers: an update, *Am J Optom Physiol Opt* 62:812-819, 1985.

71. Rounds BB, Manley CW, Norris RH: The effect of oculomotor training on reading efficiency, *J Am Optom Assoc* 62:92-99, 1991.

72. Richman JE, Cron MT: *Guide to vision therapy,* South Bend, Ind, 1994, Bernell.

73. Scheiman M, Wick B: *Clinical management of binocular vision,* Philadelphia, 1994, JB Lippincott.

74. Birnbaum MH: *Optometric management of near point vision problems,* Boston, 1993, Butterworth-Heinemann.

8

Visual Perception and Reading

Eric Borsting

Key Terms

visual perception	visual spatial	vision development
visual information	visual analysis	management
processing	visual motor	vision therapy

Optometrists have managed individuals with vision perception and reading problems for more than 30 years. This role originally grew out of a necessity to address these unique and atypical presenting problems. Parents or educators working with children readily identified mistakes in reading (e.g., reversals of *b*s & *d*s) that were judged to be caused by faulty vision perception. To address these problems, management strategies were developed that attempted to reduce the frequency of the observed behaviors. Research done in a parallel time frame supported the link between vision perception and reading. However, the exact nature of this relationship, in individual patients, proved to be quite complex and elusive. Many patients with reading disability have both a visual-perceptual and a language deficit, whereas others have a more predominantly visual-perceptual or more predominantly language deficit. Thus the role of the clinician is to determine how the perceptual problem interferes with the reading process for such a diverse group of patients. This task forces an understanding of the literature that links vision perception and reading, and the need to have a clinical model that accounts for significant individual variations.

CLINICAL PEARL

Many patients with reading disability have both a visual-perceptual and a language deficit, whereas others have a more predominatly visual-perceptual or more predominantly language deficit.

What Is Vision Perception?

When a child performs school-based activities (such as writing letters or numbers, remembering spelling words, or copying), visual information-processing skills are required. *Vision perception* or *visual information processing* refers to a group of visual skills used to extract and organize visual information from the environment and to integrate it with information from other sensory modalities and higher cognitive functions.[1] This information can be retained, stored, and recalled to assist in new learning situations. Current opinion in cognitive psychology indicates that visual memory, visual figure ground, and visual closure can be considered forms of visual information processing.[2]

CLINICAL PEARL

Visual perception *or* visual information processing *refers to a group of visual skills used to extract and organize visual information from the environment and to integrate it with information from other sensory modalities and higher congitive functions.*

Relationship Between Vision Perception and Reading

The relationship between vision perception and reading has been controversial. Some researchers[3-6] have found a positive relationship between the two skills, while others[7-9] have found that disabled readers do not differ from normal readers on measures of vision perception. Despite the controversy, the literature taken as a whole indicates that vision perception is one of the multiple factors that contribute to reading performance. Kavale[3] used a metanalytical statistical technique to compile results from 161 studies. He looked at the relationship between reading and several visual processing skills (visual discrimination, visual memory, visual closure, visual-spatial relationship, visual-motor integration, visual figure ground, visual association, and visual-auditory integration). Each of the visual-perceptual skills was related to reading ability. Within this group, visual discrimination and visual memory showed the strongest association with reading ability. Kavale concluded that visual-perceptual skills appear sufficiently associated with reading to be considered among the complex factors that predict reading ability. This conclusion is supported by the work of Solan and Mozlin[4] and Solan[5], who found correlations between several perceptual skills (visual-motor integration, form perception, visual memory, and visual-auditory integration) and reading in the primary and later grades.

Supportive evidence also comes from studies that categorize reading-disabled children according to subtypes.[10,11] Children with reading disabilities are not a homogeneous group but consist of heterogeneous groups with differing cognitive deficits. To determine distinct subtypes, researchers have evaluated reading-disabled children in many processing areas and used statistical analysis to define different homogeneous groupings within the population. The exact definition of the subtypes depends on the methods of testing used,[10] but there is general agreement that approximately 20% of poor readers have a predominantly visual-perception deficit and another 20% have a visual deficit that exists in combination with a dysfunction in another aspect of cognitive processing.[12]

Much of the information about the relationship between visual perception and reading is based on correlational studies. These do not provide causal mechanisms for determining how a visual-perceptual deficit interferes with the reading process. The difficulty in finding a cause-and-effect relationship is largely due to the complex nature of both vision perception and reading. It is difficult in a research paradigm to isolate an individual factor while keeping all other factors equal across the two groups. For example, two children with deficits in visual memory may have very different levels of success in compensation. One child could have excellent auditory memory and rely on verbal information, whereas another child may not have adequate compensation mechanisms available and may avoid school-work altogether.

Despite difficulties in finding a cause-and-effect relationship between vision perception and reading, there are many common errors that children with reading problems make that have origins in visual processing deficits. Identifying such distinctive behaviors can help determine the contribution of vision perception problems to poor reading. Willows and Terepocki[13] summarize such behavioral characteristics based on case reports, interviews with clinicians, and their own clinical experiences. In the earliest stages of learning how to read, the poor reader will have great difficulty with recognizing letters and numbers. Mistaken identifications are frequently based on visual similarities between the letters (e.g., a/o, b/d, or u/n). After recognition is mastered, recalling numbers and letters also is difficult. Again many mistakes are based on the visual characteristics of the symbols. For example, poor readers tend to confuse upper and lower case letters that differ by minor visual features (e.g., K/k or P/p) or substitute upper case letters for lower case forms when the letters are easily reversed (e.g., b or d). Recognition of sight words, the next stage in the reading process, is a serious problem for the poor reader. One commonly seen problem is that the child has difficulty recalling simple sight recognition words from week to week. That is, reading-disabled children appear to have mastered the word, but, when they encounter the same word in a few weeks, they act as if they have never seen the word before. Finally, after poor readers can recognize words, they have difficulty recalling the words from memory. This results in spelling difficulties and such children frequently resort to using a phonetic strategy (e.g., "laf" for laugh). Willows and Terepocki[13] argue that these types of errors cannot be accounted for by a verbal/linguistic explanation alone. Instead, there appears to be a difficulty with visual processing that contributes to the errors made by many poor readers.

CLINICAL PEARL

There are many common errors that children with reading problems make that have origins in visual processing deficits. Identifying such distinctive behaviors can help you determine the contribution of vision perception problems to poor reading.

Identifying behaviors indicative of a visual processing difficulty serve as the foundation for a clinical model that addresses the interaction between vision perception and reading. However, such distinctive behaviors alone are not sufficient to diagnose a visual processing problem. The deficit in visual processing must be substantiated by finding corresponding deficits correlated with standardized tests of vision perception. For example, a child who tends to make transposition errors should have a corresponding deficit in visual sequential memory. If test results do not confirm the behaviors, then the problem probably does not have a visual origin. A child may tend to make transposition errors because of difficulties in processing language. For example, a child may write "sak" for "ask" because of a deficient understanding of the rules of phonics.

Developing a Diagnostic Strategy

There are two major models for the diagnosis of vision perception dysfunction—the visual-motor model and the visual information-processing model.[14] The central theme of the *visual-motor model*[15-16] is that motor development serves as a foundation for later emerging vision perception skills. In other words, as the child grows older, performance is characterized by a shift to more visual and less motoric gathering of information. The child moves through four basic stages— motor, motor-visual, visual-motor, and finally visual. This has also been referred to as the visual-motor hierarchy. The visual-motor model has been criticized[17] because the assumption that motor development precedes visual perceptual development is inconsistent with current models of visual development. Another difficulty with the motor-based model is its reliance on the clinician's skill to make critical observations to arrive at a diagnosis.[14]

CLINICAL PEARL

Two major models for the diagnosis of vision perception dysfunction are the visual-motor model and the visual information-processing model.

In the *visual information-processing model*, the visual system analyzes sensory information to derive meaning, puts items into memory, and integrates information with other sensory modalities. Specific elements of visual processing are defined (e.g., visual memory or visual closure), and standardized testing procedures are used to quantify the functioning within each skill.

There are some overlaps between the visual-motor and visual information-processing models, and the best approach is a synthesis of the two. The approach outlined in this chapter is based on the visual information-processing model, but components of the visual-motor model are incorporated as well.

The test battery for evaluating developmental visual information-processing (DVIP) skills should use standardized tests in which administration procedures and scoring are uniform. To identify anomalies within an individual component skill (e.g., visual discrimination), I recommend using percentile ranks and then grading the performance on a 1 to 5 scale (see Table 8-1). Performance that is one standard deviation below the mean (16th percentile) or worse is abnormal and, in most cases, should be managed with an appropriate intervention program. Performance that is between the 16th and 35th percentiles is considered weak or suspect and may represent a problem for the child. A confirmation with signs and symptoms in the

TABLE 8-1

Scale For Evaluating DVIP Test Scores

1	2	3	4	5
Very weak 0 to 16th	Weak 17th to 35th	Average 36th to 65th	Strong 66th to 83rd	Very strong 84th to 99.9th

history will indicate if an anomaly is present. Performance above the mean is usually considered normal or above average. For a more detailed description of test interpretation of vision information processing skills, refer to other sources.[14,18]

Observations are another important, but often overlooked, component of the testing process. You need to identify where breakdowns in performance occur. For example, a child may be very impulsive in a test of visual memory but not visual discrimination. This may indicate that the child does not apply the appropriate strategy for solving a visual memory problem and may start guessing. However, on visual discrimination the child is able to use the appropriate strategy and, as a result, works through all the problems without guessing. This child's responses are very different from those of the child who is impulsive on all tests administered and may represent a primary attention deficit that would have to be treated by medication or educational intervention. Thus, observations help confirm diagnoses. Observations are also essential for arriving at the appropriate management plan. For example, a child with a problem in visual-motor integration may have a poor pencil grip, and development of adequate visual-motor ergonomic skills would need to occur during the therapy program.

The approach for analyzing the effects of vision-perception or DVIP deficiencies on reading is based on systems analysis. In systems analysis the clinician assembles a case history, performs tests, and makes observations to evaluate the integrity of all major components of DVIP. When applying systems analysis approach to DVIP, three components can be defined: visual spatial, visual analysis, and visual motor. A brief description of each component will be presented. Behaviors associated with deficient DVIP are illustrated along with recommended testing sequences.

Visual-Spatial System

The visual-spatial system consists of a set of abilities used to understand directional concepts that organize external visual space. These skills relate to understanding the difference between the concepts of up and down, front and back, and right and left. The individual develops an awareness of his or her body position in space and the relationship of objects to self.[19] Spatial abilities are important for many skills, including navigating through the world (e.g., right and left turns), understanding directions ("Put your name on the top right hand side of the page"), recognizing the orientation and sequence of linguistic symbols (*b* vs *d*), and further manipulating this information.

The visual-spatial system is subdivided into three abilities—bilateral integration, laterality, and directionality. Bilateral integration is the ability to be aware of and to use the two sides of the body separately and simultaneously.[20] This serves as a motor foundation for understanding the difference between the right and left sides of the body. Laterality is the ability to be internally aware of and to identify right and left on oneself.[1] Directionality is the ability to interpret right and left directions in external space and itself consists of three skills.[1] First is the ability to identify the directional position of objects in space (e.g., "Is the window to my right or left"). Second is the ability to identify right and left positions on another person. This is dependent on understanding that right and left positions on another person change depending on the person's orientation. Third is the ability to apply directional concepts to the spatial orientation of linguistic symbols (such as *b* and *d*).

> **CLINICAL PEARL**
>
> *The visual-spatial system consists of a set of abilities used to understand directional concepts that organize external visual space. It is subdivided into three abilities—bilateral integration, laterality, and directionality.*

A variety of behaviors, including poor motor coordination and difficulty with right and left knowledge, are associated with visual-spatial dysfunction (see the box on p. 156). The primary effect on reading attributed to deficiencies in visual-spatial skills is reversal errors. Many children with visual-spatial problems (poor knowledge of right and left) are easily confused by letters that are mirror images of each other (*b* and *d*).[21,22] Additionally, poor spatial skills result in a tendency to rotate letters or numbers around the vertical axis (rotations around the horizontal axis are less common, such as *b* and *p*).[23] Remember that reversal errors are considered normal when the child enters school. A steady decline in the number of reversal errors occurs as the child proceeds through kindergarten and first grade, but by 8 years of age most children have ceased making reversal errors.[23,24] Persistent reversals beyond this age are abnormal and frequently associated with reading disability.[22,25] However, reversal errors alone do not always lead to a reading disability.

The testing sequence for the visual spatial system consists of three tests (see the box below):

1. The Standing Angels in the Snow Test[19] evaluates bilateral integration (Figure 8-1). The patient is asked to make specific movements with the arms and legs. The movement patterns are homologous (both arms or legs moving at the same time), monolateral (isolated movement of the arm or leg), homolateral (simultaneous movement of the arm and leg on the same side of the body), and contralateral (simultaneous movement of the arm and leg on opposite sides of the body). The ability of the patient to make smooth and coordinated movements with the right and left arms indicates bilateral integration ability.

2. The Piaget Right-Left Awareness Test[26] evaluates laterality and two aspects of directionality. A series of questions is asked about the right and left of the patient, the examiner, and objects (see the box on p. 158). The ability of the patient to identify right and left on himself measures laterality. The ability to identify right and left positions on the examiner and of objects in space assesses directionality. Observations are very important when administering this test because the child has a 50% chance of guessing the correct answer. Occasionally a child is able to respond correctly but the knowledge of right and left is inconsistent[27] (i.e., if the child was asked similar questions 2 weeks later, he or she might not respond correctly). Therefore, it is often helpful to question the child's right and left knowledge in a variety of contexts. For example, when assessing visual acuity, ask the child to place the occluder over his or her right eye.

═══◉ Diagnostic/Therapeutic Strategies for the Visual-Spatial System

Behaviors that are representative of a visual-spatial dysfunction

Clumsy, falls and bumps into things
Poor athletic performance
Difficulty learning right and left
Reverses letters and words
Confuses right and left directions

Testing sequence by component ability

1. Bilateral integration: Standing Angels in the Snow Test
2. Laterality: Piaget Right-Left Awareness Test
3. Directionality: Piaget Right-Left Awareness Test
   Gardner Reversal Frequency Test

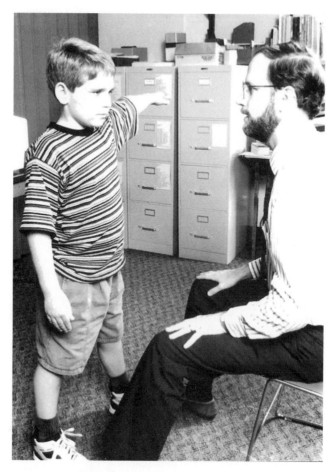

FIGURE 8-1 The Standing Angels in the Snow Test. The child is performing a homolateral movement.

3. The Gardner Reversal Frequency Test[28] evaluates the patient's ability to use directionality concepts when identifying the correct orientation of single letters and numbers. It is important to use isolated letters and numbers when evaluating reversal errors because language components are minimized. For example, a child might say "bab" for "bad" because of poor phonetic knowledge. Using isolated letters minimizes phonological influences since most children can easily identify single letters and numbers by name and phonetic knowledge is minimally involved. I recommend using the first two subtests on the Gardner Reversal Frequency Test—execution and recognition. The execution subtest evaluates the occurrence of reversal errors when the child writes individual letters and numbers (Figure 8-2). The recognition subtest evaluates the child's ability to recognize letters and numbers that are rotated around the vertical axis (Figure 8-3).

Piaget Right-Left Awareness Test

Show me your right hand
Show me your left leg
Show me your right leg
Touch your left ear
Show me your right leg
Show me your left hand
Point to your right eye

(Sit opposite the child)
Show me my right hand
Now show me my left hand
Show me my right leg
Now my left leg

(Place a coin on the table left of a pencil in relation to the child)
Is the pencil to the right or to the left?
And the penny, is it to the right or to the left?
(Have the child go around to the opposite side of the table)
Is the pencil to the right or to the left?
And the penny, is it to the right or to the left?

(Sit opposite the child with a coin in your right hand and a bracelet or watch on your left arm)
You see this coin. Have I got it in my right hand or my left?
And the bracelet, is it on my right arm or my left?

(Place three objects in front of the child: a pencil to the left, a key in the middle, and a coin to the right)
Is the pencil to the left or to the right of the key?
Is the pencil to the left or to the right of the penny?
Is the key to the left or to the right of the penny?
Is the key to the left or to the right of the pencil?
Is the penny to the left or to the right of the pencil?
Is the penny to the left or to the right of the key?

Visual Analysis System

The visual analysis system consists of a group of abilities used to recognize, recall, and manipulate visual information.[1] These skills are an important part of many activities, including judging similarities or differences among forms and symbols, remembering forms and symbols, and visualizing. The visual analysis system is subdivided into four component skills: form perception, visual attention, perceptual speed, and visual memory.

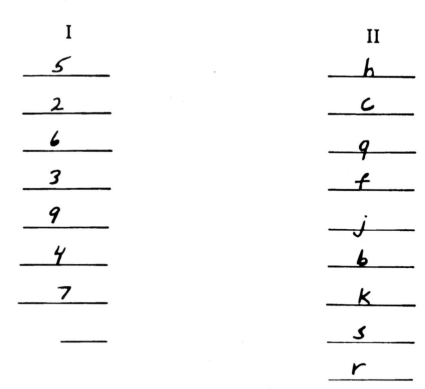

FIGURE 8-2 The Gardner Reversal Frequency Test—Execution Subtest.

CLINICAL PEARL

The visual analysis system consists of a group of abilities used to recognize, recall, and manipulate visual information. These skills are an important part of many activities—including judging similarities or differences among forms and symbols, remembering forms and symbols, and visualizing.

Form perception

Form perception is the ability to discriminate, recognize, and identify forms and objects and is usually subdivided into four categories: (1) *visual discrimination* is the ability to be aware of the distinctive features of forms, including size, shape, color, and orientation, to determine similarities and differences between them[29]; (2) *visual figure ground* is the ability to attend to a specific feature or form, while maintaining an awareness of the relationship of the form to background information[29]; (3) *visual closure* is the ability to be aware of clues in the visual array that allow the individual to determine the final percept without the necessity of all the details being present[29];

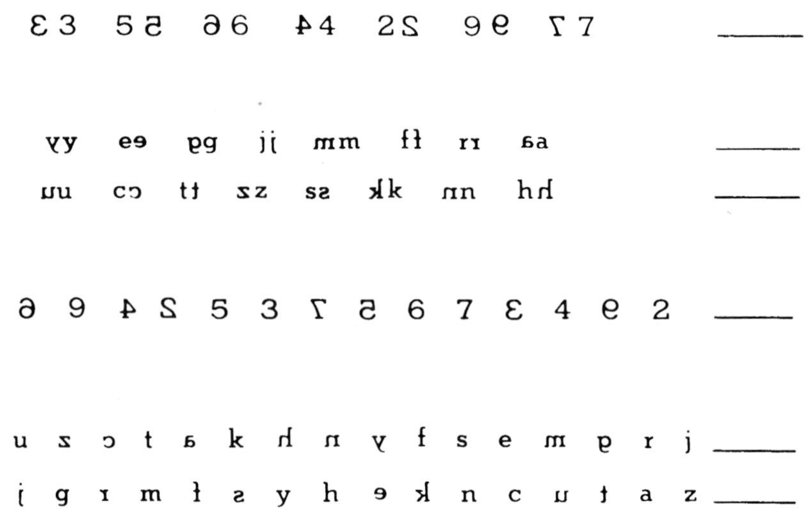

Ɛ3   5Ƨ   ә6   Ꞁ4   2Ƨ   9ҽ   Ɛ7   _____

γy   eә   ᖩg   jᵢ   ɱm   fꞁ   ɪɪ   ɓa   _____

ɹu   cɔ   tꞁ   ƨz   sƨ   ʞk   ɳn   hꞁ   _____

ә 9 Ꞁ Ƨ 5 3 Ꞁ ƨ 6 7 Ɛ 4 ҽ 2   _____

u ƨ ɔ t ᖷ k ꓶ ɳ γ f s e ɱ ᖱ r j _____

ᵢ g ɪ m ꞁ ƨ y h ә ʞ n c ɹ ꞁ a z _____

FIGURE 8-3 The Gardner Reversal Frequency Test—Recognition Subtest.

and (4) *visual form constancy* is the ability to identify the invariant features of a form when a transformation has altered the size, rotation, or orientation.[30]

Visual attention

Visual attention is included in the visual analysis system because many of the clinical methods used to evaluate attention are similar to tests of form perception. When a child performs a visual processing task, certain parts of the form will be attended to and others ignored.[31] How the child approaches such tasks relates to visual attention.

There are several clinical and theoretical models of attention. One model will be highlighted because it represents the aspects of attention that would be of most concern to you in managing a child with vision perception deficiencies.[32]

In this model, originally developed by Keogh and Margolis,[33] attention consists of three separate but interrelated components: coming to attention, decision making, and sustaining attention. *Coming to attention* is the ability to analyze, organize, and determine salient features of a visual target. In other words, it is the ability to focus attention on the requirements of the task, allowing the child to get appropriately involved in the activity. *Decision making* refers to visual cognitive style. There is a continuum of decision making, from the child who is impulsive (a fast and inaccurate decision maker) to the one who is reflective (a thoughtful problem solver). Finally, *sustaining attention* is the ability to maintain attention once the task is engaged.

All three components of attention can be evaluated by observations during the testing sequence.[34] Typically, a direct assessment of these skills is not performed because of time constraints. By observing performance on all tests, it is possible to assess the components of visual attention. Another reason for not directly assessing the three components of attention is that attentional skills can be task dependent. For example, a child may be impulsive on a visual-motor task but not on a visual figure ground task. This often results when a child has a deficit that is specific to a certain visual processing skill.

Perceptual speed

Perceptual speed assesses the ability to perform visual processing tasks rapidly with little cognitive effort. In my experience a significant number of children perform adequately on perceptual tests when given sufficient time, but when asked to perform the same skill quickly, their performance breaks down. Inferior processing speed is one of the commonly observed characteristics of the learning-disabled child.[12] Slow processing speed is a significant problem because a majority of the information processing and attentional resources are allocated for lower-level visual perceptual analysis instead of for higher-order cognition. As an example, when writing, the teacher assumes that the child is able to remember the whole word or several items at a time. However, a child with poor visual memory may have to glance at the word several times because he can remember only small segments.

Visual memory

Visual memory is the ability to recall visually presented material.[1] Usually two types of memory are evaluated: spatial and sequential. The spatial component of memory refers to the ability to recall the spatial location of an object (e.g., its orientation about the y axis). Visual sequential memory refers to the ability to remember the exact order of items in a left-to-right sequence.

Deficiencies in the visual analysis system can affect the acquisition of reading skills (see the box on p. 162 for the list of behaviors). These abilities may be thought of as readiness skills necessary for the child to respond to educational instruction. Poor form perception affects the ability to recognize letters, numbers, and simple words in the beginning stages of learning to read. Mistakes based on the visual characteristics of the form (e.g., *a* and *o* or *m* and *n*) should occur instead of errors based on poor phonetic awareness. Problems with visual memory affect the ability to recall individual letters or numbers in the early stages of reading and the ability to recall words in the later stages. Again, mistakes with individual letters and numbers are based on the visual characteristics of the symbols. Poor visual memory can affect the child's ability to recall whole word gestalt, forcing him or her to spell phonetically.

Diagnostic/Therapeutic Strategies for the Visual Analysis System

Behaviors indicative of dysfunction

Confuses similar letters and numbers (such as *a* and *o*)
Difficulty learning the alphabet
Tends to spell phonetically
Poor recall of letter, numbers, and simple words
Difficulty visualizing what is read
Difficulty retaining spelling words from week to week
Difficulty tuning into the important part of a task
Easily distracted
Works slowly compared to peers

Testing sequence by component ability

1. Form perception: Test of Visual Perceptual Skills: Visual Discrimination, Visual-Spatial Relationship, Visual Form Constancy, Visual Figure Ground, Visual Closure
2. Visual memory: Test of Visual-Perceptual Skills: Visual Memory, Visual Sequential Memory
3. Perceptual speed and visual memory: Tachistoscope Test

Perceptual speed can affect reading through automaticity or the ability to process visual information fast and effortlessly. If the information is processed slowly, then understanding the material will be impaired. For example, LaBarge and Samuels[35] described a model of automatic information processing to explain some aspects of reading disorders. They argued that beginning readers may not be able to learn to read for meaning until they have learned to identify words and letters automatically.

Finally, poor attention probably affects reading indirectly by influencing the time on task. Children with poor attention will spend less time on task and as a result may develop reading skills at a slower rate.

The testing sequence of visual analysis skills can be performed with two tests. The Test of Visual Perceptual Skills is a nonmotor test of vision perception and has seven subtests.[30] It evaluates five components of form perception (visual discrimination, visual-spatial relationship, visual form constancy, visual figure ground, and visual closure) (Figure 8-4) and two components of memory (spatial and sequential) (Figure 8-5). The Tachistoscope Test evaluates perceptual speed and visual memory under dynamic conditions. In this test a series of numbers are flashed at one tenth of a second and the child is asked to write down the numbers. The battery of tests for evaluating visual analysis are heavily weighted toward visual memory because this skill appears most associated with reading.[3,6]

Visual-Motor System

Visual-motor integration is the general ability to coordinate visual information-processing skills with motor skills. One component of visual- motor integration is the ability to integrate form perception with the fine-motor system in order to reproduce complex visual patterns.[36] This component is most important for academic achievement. In the school-age years, children suffering from a visual-motor dysfunction often have difficulty copying written work accurately and efficiently (see the box on p. 164).

CLINICAL PEARL

Visual-motor integration is the general ability to coordinate visual information-processing skills with motor skills. One component is the ability to integrate form perception with the fine-motor system in order to reproduce complex visual patterns.

Three component skills are necessary to reproduce complex forms[1,37]—visual form perception, fine motor coordination, and integration of visual and motor systems. *Visual form perception* is evaluated as part of the visual analysis system. *Fine motor coordination* is the ability to manipulate small objects (e.g., a pencil). *Integration of the visual and motor systems* depends upon the ability to coordinate an internally generated spatial program with the fine motor system in order to copy letters and numbers.[29]

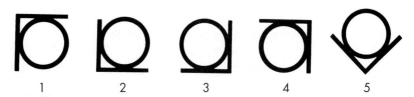

1   2   3   4   5

FIGURE 8-4 The Test of Visual Perceptual Skills—Visual Discrimination Subtest.

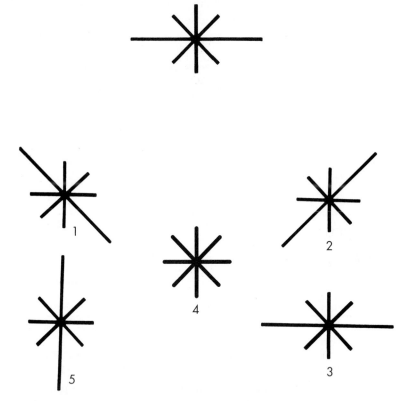

FIGURE 8-5   The Test of Visual Perceptual Skills—Visual Memory Subtest.

Diagnostic Strategy for the Visual-Motor System

Behaviors representative of a visual-motor problem

Poor handwriting
Poor drawing skills
Difficulty coloring, cutting, or pasting
Poor spacing and inability to stay on lines when writing
Difficulty completing written work in the time allotted

Testing sequence by component ability

1. Visual fine motor ability: Grooved Pegboard
2. Visual-motor integration: Developmental Test of Visual-Motor Integration
3. Qualitative aspects of writing: Wold Sentence Copying Test

CLINICAL PEARL

Three component skills are necessary to reproduce complex forms—visual form perception, fine motor coordination, and integration of visual and motor systems.

Poor visual-motor skills probably do not affect decoding skills or reading for comprehension directly. However, to enhance vocabulary development, many reading programs require the child to write letters and numbers in the beginning stages and words in the later stages of reading. Children with poor visual-motor integration have difficulty writing quickly and accurately. Thus, a child with a visual-motor dysfunction may not learn as well using writing to reinforce the recognition and recall of letters and words.

Visual-motor skills can be evaluated by three tests. The ability to integrate the visual and motor systems is evaluated with the Developmental Test of Visual-Motor Integration[38] (Figure 8-6). Visual fine motor skills are evaluated with the Grooved Pegboard[39] (Figure 8-7). The Wold Sentence Copying Test[40] has the child copy a paragraph (Figure 8-8) and measures the quality of the child's writing skills, allowing the practitioner to directly observe handwriting errors that are reported by the teacher or parent (e.g., writing up- or downhill or inconsistent spacing between words).

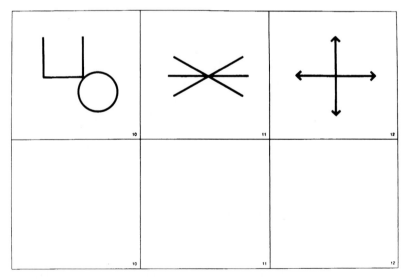

FIGURE 8-6 The Developmental Test of Visual-Motor Integration.

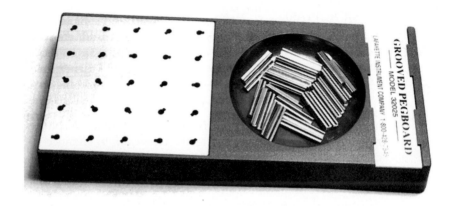

FIGURE 8-7 The Grooved Pegboard Test.

While testing visual-motor skills, it is important to evaluate the child's posture, the presence of a lead-support system, and the pencil grip. This is also referred to as visual-motor ergonomics.[29]

Posture looks at the relationship between the visual axis and the writing surface. The optimal posture is when the visual axis forms a 90-degree angle with the writing surface.[41,42] The appropriate working distance is approximated by the distance between the middle knuckle and the elbow, which is also referred to as the Harmon distance.[41,42] Many children with visual-motor problems work very close to the writing surface and have postural asymmetries.

A *lead-support system* occurs when the nondominant hand holds the paper and the dominant hand is used for writing. A minority of children with visual-motor problems do not use the dominant hand to hold the writing surface.

Finally, many children with visual-motor problems hold the writing tool rigidly, using the wrist and forearm for control. The optimal *pencil grip* is the tripod grip,[23] in which the thumb and index finger grasp the pencil while resting on the middle finger. With the tripod grip the child should be able to manipulate the writing tool with his or her fingers instead of using the wrist or forearm.

Determining the Diagnosis

The diagnosis of a developmental visual information-processing deficit is determined by matching behavioral signs and symptoms with results of the testing sequence. When a match occurs, a DVIP or vision perception problem exists. For example, if a parent reports that the child is reversing letters when reading and writing and the results of the Gardner Reversal Frequency Test indicate an abnormally high rate of reversal errors, this child has a problem in the visual-spatial system, and a vision therapy program is one treatment option. The decision on when to intervene is complex and depends on the degree of the visual deficit (along with other variables). Before arriving at a treatment decision, you should obtain information from previous evaluations (e.g., psychological, educational). Such reports will provide a global picture of the child's difficulties and allow for a more informed decision about the goal of therapy. In my experience the intervention decision depends mainly on the degree to which the visual problem is interfering with child's performance. For example, a fourth grader who has borderline low visual-motor integration (30th percentile) with no corresponding signs and symptoms will probably not benefit from treatment of the visual processing problem; however, a second grader with many deficits (e.g., reversals, visual memory, and visual-motor integration) and corresponding symptoms may.

Four men and a jolly boy came out of the black and pink house quickly to see the bright violet sun, but the sun was hidden behind a cloud.

Name _____ Age _____ Time _____

FIGURE 8-8 The Wold Sentence Copying Test.

When discrepancies exist between behavioral signs and symptoms and test results, the patient's problem may not have a visual perception origin. For example, a parent may report that the child is reversing letters when reading and writing but performance is adequate on all tests of visual-spatial skills. In this case the reversal errors may be caused by a language problem and not a visual-spatial problem. Occasionally, the case history is negative but test results are poor. In this situation the case history must be reviewed to ensure that no school-related difficulties have been overlooked. Another possibility is that the child was malingering during testing.

CLINICAL PEARL

When discrepancies exist between behavioral signs and symptoms and test results, the patient's problem may not have a visual perception origin.

Managing Visual Perception Deficiencies

The treatment of DVIP deficiencies is based on a sequential management strategy. First, significant refractive anomalies should be corrected before anything else is done. Second, remediation of visual efficiency (binocular vision, ocular motility) problems should also precede specific therapy for DVIP problems. Treatment of deficient visual efficiency skills has resulted in concurrent improvement of visual perceptual skills.[43,44] Finally, vision therapy is the optimal treatment to improve or abate the remaining DVIP anomalies.

Vision therapy for DVIP deficits is an interactive process that results in learning new strategies or methods to solve visual processing problems in certain domains. For example, the child with poor visual memory cannot simply be told to remember visual items more efficiently. Rather, a vision therapy technique must be implemented to help him learn a strategy or method to solve a problem (e.g., "Form an image in your head"). The therapist, through an interactive process, must help with the learning of new skills. It is essential that you interact with the patient by asking questions, providing feedback, and helping the patient to develop alternative problem-solving strategies.

Efficacy of DVIP/Perceptual Therapy

The efficacy of therapy for improving perceptual-motor skills and associated learning problems has met with considerable controversy. Kavale and Matson,[45] using a metanalytical technique, found that perceptual-motor therapy had little impact on a child's learning problems. There was also little evidence to support the claim that perceptual therapy improves specific perceptual-motor skills. This has led some authorities[46] to discourage perceptual-motor therapy for children with learning disabilities.

Evaluating studies taken from a variety of sources creates several difficulties. First, many studies that assessed visual perceptual therapy did not ensure that significant refractive errors and visual efficiency problems had been remedied before starting therapy. Second, many studies done in the 1950s and 1960s performed perceptual therapy either on all children with learning problems or as part of broad-based readiness programs. As discussed earlier, only a minority of children with learning problems have a predominant visual perception deficit. The efficacy of visual perception therapy for this subgroup of reading-disabled children has not been adequately addressed. Third, newer approaches for addressing vision perception problems[29] have emphasized the development of visual cognitive strategies in order to improve visual processing skills and have deemphasized motor-based therapy in favor of specific visual information-processing deficits. Similar approaches that emphasize cognitive strategy development[47] have been advocated for working with learning-disabled children. Finally, therapy programs need to be individualized for the patient's visual deficits, developmental level, visual style, and auditory skills. The experienced clinician knows that a successful therapy program depends upon the ability to adjust the program to meet the individual needs of the patient. It is very difficult to make adjustments without contaminating a research paradigm in which treatment is the same across all subjects in the experimental group.

In reviewing the literature that addresses therapy for visual perceptual skills, Solan and Ciner[48] cited several factors that are important for a successful therapy program. First, the patient should have a documented perceptual deficit that is associated with the reading or learning disorder. Broad-based therapy programs to improve readiness skills in normal patients may not be effective. Second, therapy programs should be individualized to address the specific deficits that the patient manifests. Finally, therapy should complement and not replace reading and other educational instruction. The goal of the treatment of DVIP deficits is to improve visual-spatial, visual analysis, and visual-motor skills in children who manifest these problems. This should result in more effective participation in the classroom and receptive benefit from other educational therapies.

Despite the controversy in the literature, there are several well-designed studies that support the efficacy of therapy for DVIP anomalies. When investigating the effectiveness of visual perception therapy, you should be addressing two issues: First, how effective is therapy at improving DVIP skills? For example, in a therapy program for visual-motor skills, is it likely that these skills will improve? Second, if there are improvements in DVIP skills, is the child more available or responsive to educational instruction? In other words, after remediation of specific visual deficits, will the child respond more appropriately to academic intervention for specific educational deficits?

CLINICAL PEARL

Broad-based therapy programs to improve readiness skills in normal patients may not be effective. Therapy programs should be individualized to address the specific deficits that the patient manifests. The therapy should complement and not replace reading and other educational instruction.

In addressing the first issue, most studies evaluating the effectiveness of visual therapy have used a broad variety of training procedures in all three areas of visual information processing (visual spatial, visual analysis, and visual motor) at the same time. Academic performance was then reevaluated following the treatment. Several of these studies[49,50] have found significant improvements in DVIP skills following therapy. Studies that have concentrated on the treatment of isolated visual perceptual skills have also supported the effectiveness of therapy for visual-spatial,[51,52] visual analysis,[53,54] and visual-motor skills.[55] Improving the ability of the child to benefit from academic instruction has been supported by similar research.[50,53,56-58] These studies demonstrate statistically significant improvements in standardized tests of academic skills compared with improvements in a control group.

Designing a Vision Therapy Program

It is beyond the scope of this chapter to provide a detailed description of the possible vision therapy programs for all patients with DVIP deficits. Instead, I will review a more recent approach to DVIP therapy that was outlined by Rouse and Borsting.[29] They argue that a successful visual perception therapy program depends on understanding individual therapy goals and their appropriate sequencing. The central theme of a therapy program is to help develop more appropriate strategies for visual information processing. In this approach a therapy goal is defined for each component skill in the DVIP profile (e.g., visual discrimination), and then a sequence of subgoals is delineated. Successful completion of the subgoals leads to attainment of the therapy goal. The advantage of this system is that individual therapy procedures can be organized into an overall treatment strategy.

Another important component of the Rouse and Borsting[29] approach is that the vision therapy program is designed to remedy only those skills that are deficient in the three general systems—visual spatial, visual analysis, and visual motor. The diagnostic evaluation reveals specific component abilities that are deficient within each system. For example, if visual discrimination is adequate but figure ground is deficient, then therapy will address figure ground and not visual discrimination. Additionally, within an individual component ability (e.g., visual memory) the therapy program may begin at a different subgoal depending on the degree of deficiency in that skill.

As an illustration of the use of a system of goals and subgoals for therapy, I will review a therapy sequence for visual memory. The overall goal and the sequence of four subgoals for developing adequate visual memory are listed in the box below.

Goals, Subgoals, and Techniques for Visual Memory

Therapy goal: Develop the patient's short-term memory abilities

Subgoal 1: Develop the ability to form an image of the visual input using multisensory input
Therapy techniques
Winterhaven templates
Parquetry blocks

Subgoal 2: Develop the ability to recall spatial characteristics of figures using only visual information
Therapy techniques
Winterhaven templates
Parquetry blocks
Concentration

Subgoal 3: Develop the ability to recall the sequential characteristics of figures using only visual information
Therapy techniques
Three-in-a-row
Sequential beads

Subgoal 4: Develop the patient's ability to recall information as the amount of information is increased and the viewing time is decreased
Therapy techniques
Tachistoscope

Before starting therapy, it should be determined whether the patient has a deficit in spatial (poor performance on TVPS subtest visual memory) or sequential (poor performance on TVPS subtest sequential memory) memory. When a patient has more difficulty with spatial aspects of memory storage, therapy should begin with subgoal 1. In contrast, if the patient has only sequential memory problems therapy should start with subgoal 3.

The third subgoal for visual memory is designed to have the patient reproduce the sequential characteristics of figures or displays using only visual information. The first step in therapy is to leave a sequential pattern design in view while the patient copies the design. The patient needs to understand that it is necessary to remember or code the exact left-to-right sequence. In the next step the design is hidden from view and the patient constructs it based on the mental image of it (Figure 8-9). The therapist should start with two or three items and emphasize that the patient needs to form an image of the left-to-right sequence. The patient should be able to reproduce a pattern of four to six items.

The final subgoal in the development of visual memory is to increase both the speed and the span of visual memory. This phase of therapy is designed to improve the automaticity of visual response. In it the target is presented rapidly (e.g., less than 1 second). In contrast to the previous stage, the patient cannot rely on memory strategies while directly viewing the target. Instead he or she must form an image of the visual stimulus and then use memory strategies for short-term recall. The goal is to remember the grade-appropriate number of digits at 0.1 second.

Similar goals and subgoals have been delineated for all the component abilities within the three major systems (visual spatial, visual analysis, and visual motor) that were defined in the diagnostic section. A wide variety of therapy procedures can be used to manage DVIP anomalies. However, the most important aspect of therapy is for the patient to develop more efficient strategies for solving visual information-processing problems.

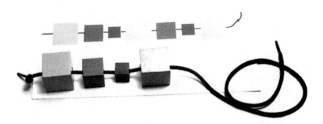

FIGURE 8-9 Sequential beads technique for addressing deficits in visual sequential memory deficits.

Conclusion

The relationship between vision perception and reading is complex. The clinician who works with children with vision perception deficits needs to understand the literature that links perception and reading problems. Such information guides the diagnostic strategy for identifying anomalies in visual-spatial, visual-analysis, and visual-motor skills. Once identified, significant vision perception anomalies should be remedied with the appropriate vision therapy program. The intervention program should be individualized to account for patient factors and specific anomalies in vision perception. Finally, vision therapy should not replace educational therapy but should supplement it when specific vision anomalies are identified.

CLINICAL PEARL

Once identified, significant vision perception anomalies should be remedied with the appropriate vision therapy program. The intervention program should be individualized.

References

1. Borsting E: Overview of visual and visual processing development. In Scheiman MM, Rouse MW (eds): *Optometric management of learning related visual problems,* St Louis, 1989, Mosby.
2. Rogow SM, Rathwell D: Seeing and knowing: an investigation of visual perception among children with severe visual impairments, *J Vis Rehabil* 3:55-66, 1989.
3. Kavale K: Meta-analysis of the relationship between visual perceptual skills and reading achievement, *J Learn Disabil* 5:142-151, 1982.
4. Solan HA, Mozlin R: The correlations of perceptual-motor maturation to readiness and reading in kindergarten and the primary grades, *J Am Optom Assoc* 57:28-35, 1986.
5. Solan HA: A comparison of the influences of verbal-successive and spatial-simultaneous factors on achieving readers in fourth and fifth grade: a multivariate correlational study, *J Learn Disabil* 20:237-242, 1987.
6. Willows DM, Kruk R, Corcos E: Are there differences between disabled and normal readers in their processing of visual information? In Willows DM, Kruk R, Corcos E (eds): *Visual processes in reading and reading disabilities,* Hillsdale, NJ, 1993, Lawrence Erlbaum.
7. Stanovich KE: Explaining the variance in reading ability in terms of psychological processes: What have we learned? *Ann Dyslexia,* 1987.
8. Vellutino FR: *Dyslexia, theory and research,* Cambridge, Mass, 1979, MIT Press.
9. Vellutino FR: Dyslexia, *Sci Am* 256:34-41, 1987.
10. Flynn JM, Boder E: Clinical and electrophysiological correlates of dysphonetic and dyseidetic dyslexia. In Stein JF (ed): *Vision and visual dyslexia,* Boca Raton, Fla, 1991, CRC Press.
11. Hooper SR, Willis WG: *Learning disability subtyping: neuropsychological foundations, conceptual models, and issues in clinical differentiation,* New York, 1989, Springer-Verlag.

12. Groffman S. The relationship between visual perception and learning. In Scheiman MW, Rouse MW (eds): *Optometric management of learning related visual problems,* St Louis, 1989, Mosby.

13. Willows DM, Terepocki M: The relation of reversal errors to reading disabilities. In Willows DM, Kruk R, Corcos E (eds): *Visual processes in reading and reading disabilities,* Hillsdale, NJ, 1993, Lawrence Erlbaum.

14. Scheiman MM, Gallaway M: Visual information processing: assessment and diagnosis. In Scheiman MM, Rouse MW (eds): *Optometric management of learning related visual problems,* St Louis, 1994, Mosby.

15. Getman GN: The visuomotor complex in the acquisition of learning skills. In Helmuth J (ed): *Learning disorders,* Seattle, 1965, Special Child Publications.

16. Kephart NC: *The slow learner in the classroom,* Columbus, Ohio, 1971, Charles E Merrill.

17. Cratty BJ: Sensory-motor and perceptual-motor theories and practice: an overview and evaluation. In Walk RD, Pick HL (eds): *Intermemory perception and sensory integration,* New York, 1981, Plenum Press.

18. Solan HA, Suchoff IB: *Tests and measurements for the behavioral optometrist,* Santa Ana, Calif, 1991, Optometric Extension Program Foundation.

19. Suchoff IB: *The visual-spatial development in the child,* New York, 1981, State University of New York.

20. Hoffman LG: An optometric learning disability evaluation, *Optom Month* 70:78-81, 1979.

21. Ginsburg GP, Hartwick A: Directional confusion as a sign of dyslexia, *Percept Mot Skills* 32:535-543, 1971.

22. Kaufman NL: Review of research on reversal errors, *Percept Mot Skills* 51:55-79, 1980.

23. Gardner RA: *The objective diagnosis of minimal brain dysfunction,* Cresshill, NJ, 1979, Creative Therapeutics.

24. Davidson HP: A study of confusing letters b, d, p, and q, *J Genet Psychol* 47:458-468, 1935.

25. Boone HC: Relationship of left-right reversals to academic achievement, *Percept Mot Skills* 62:27-33, 1986.

26. Piaget J: *Judgement and reasoning in the child,* London, 1928, Routledge & Kegan Paul.

27. Laurendeau M, Pinard A: *The development of the concept of space in the child,* New York, 1970, International Universities Press.

28. Gardner RA: *The Reversal Frequency Test,* Cresshill, NJ, 1979, Creative Therapeutics.

29. Rouse MW, Borsting E: Management of visual information processing problems. In Scheiman MM, Rouse MW (eds): *Optometric management of learning related visual problems,* St Louis, 1994, Mosby.

30. Gardner MF: *The test of visual perceptual skill,* Burlingame, Calif, 1988, Health Publishing.

31. Brown RT, Wynne ME: An analysis of attentional components in hyperactive and normal boys, *J Learn Disabil* 17:162-166, 1984.

32. Borsting E: Measures of visual attention in children with and without visual efficiency problems, *J Behav Optometry* 6:151-156, 1991.

33. Keogh BK, Margolis J: Learn to labor and to wait: attentional problems of children with learning disorders, *J Learn Disabil* 9:276-286, 1976.

34. Richman JE: Use of sustained attention task to determine children at risk for learning problems, *J Am Optom Assoc* 57:20-26, 1986.

35. LaBarge D, Samuels SJ: Toward a theory of automatic information processing in reading, *Cogn Psychol* 6:293-323, 1974.

36. Solan HA, Groffman S: Understanding and treating developmental and perceptual motor disabilities. In Solan HA (ed): *Treatment and management of children with learning disabilities,* Springfield, Ill, 1982, Charles C Thomas.

37. Leonard P, Foxcroft C, Kroukamp T: Are visual-perceptual and visual-motor skills separate abilities? *Percept Mot Skills* 67:423-426, 1988.

38. Beery KE: *The developmental test of visual motor integration,* Cleveland, 1982, Modern Curriculum Press.
39. *Grooved Pegboard Test,* Lafayette, Ind, 1991, Lafayette Instruments.
40. Wold RM: *Screening tests to be used by the classroom teacher,* New York, 1970, Academic Therapy Publications.
41. Harmon DB: *Notes on a dynamic theory of vision,* ed 3, Austin, Texas, 1958, DB Harmon.
42. Harmon DB: *The coordinated classroom,* Grand Rapids, Mich, 1949, American Seating.
43. Hoffman LG: The effect of accommodative deficiencies on the developmental level of perceptual skills, *Am J Optom Physiol Opt* 59:254-262, 1982.
44. Weisz CL: Clinical therapy for accommodative responses: transfer effects upon performance, *J Am Optom Assoc* 50:209-215, 1980.
45. Kavale K, Mattson PD: One jumped off the balance beam: meta-analysis of perceptual-motor training, *J Learn Disabil* 16:165-173, 1983.
46. American Academy of Ophthalmology: *Learning disabilities, dyslexia, and vision,* Position statement, 1984.
47. Myers PI, Hammill DD: *Learning disabilities: basic concepts, assessment practices, and instructional strategies,* Austin, Texas, 1990, Pro-ed.
48. Solan HA, Ciner EB: Visual perception and learning: issues and answers, *J Am Optom Assoc* 60:457-460, 1989.
49. Farr J, Leibowitz HW: An experimental study of the efficacy of perceptual-motor training, *Am J Optom Physiol Opt* 53:451-455, 1976.
50. Halliwell JW, Solan HA: The effects of a supplemental perceptual training program on reading achievement, *Except Child* 38:613-2, 1972.
51. Hendrickson LN, Muehl S: The effect of attention and motor response pretraining on learning to discriminate b and d in kindergarten children, *J Educ Psychol* 53:236-241, 1962.
52. Greenspan SB: Effectiveness of therapy for children's reversal confusions, *Acad Ther* 11:169-178, 1975-76.
53. Brown RT, Alford N: Ameliorating attentional deficits and concomitant academic deficiencies in learning disabled children through cognitive training, *J Learn Disabil* 17:20-26, 1984.
54. Walsh JF, D'Angelo R: Effectiveness of the Frostig program for visual perceptual training with Head Start children, *Percept Mot Skills* 32:944-946, 1971.
55. Rosner J: The development of a perceptual skills program, *J Am Optom Assoc* 44:698-707, 1973.
56. Getz DJ: Learning enhancement through visual training, *Acad Ther* 15:457-466, 1980.
57. Seiderman AS: Optometric vision therapy—results of a demonstration project with a learning disabled population, *J Am Optom Assoc* 51:489-493, 1980.
58. Rowell RB: *The effect of tachistoscope and visual tracking program on the improvement of reading at the second grade level,* Ann Arbor, Mich, 1976, University Microfilms.

9

Could a Transient Visual System Deficit Play a Causal Role in Reading Disability?

William Lovegrove

Key Terms

transient system	flicker masking	phonological
visible persistence	visual evoked	processing
contrast sensitivity	potential (VEP)	temporal processing
		temporal order

This chapter is concerned with the nature of visual processing in reading-disabled and normal-reading children. The central issue for our research for some time was whether these children differ from normal readers in basic visual processes. The emphasis of the research has now changed a little to ask what are the implications for the reading process of the visual processing differences between disabled readers and controls that we and others have now demonstrated. Both questions will be considered here.

For many years the commonly accepted view within the reading-disability literature has been that reading disability is not attributable to visual deficits and that normal readers and disabled readers do not differ systematically in terms of visual processing.[1,2] Extensive work over the last 10 years in a number of laboratories, however, has clearly demonstrated that the two groups do differ in terms of visual processing. Despite this, we still know little about the possible implications of these findings. Much of this recent research has resulted in part from developments in theoretical vision that have been applied to reading, thus providing a more suitable theoretical framework in which to consider reading and vision. The following section briefly outlines one approach to vision that has been usefully applied. A more detailed discussion of this framework can be found elsewhere.[3]

The Sustained and Transient Subsystems

The spatial frequency approach to vision research[4,5] indicates that information is transmitted from the eye to the brain via a number of separate parallel pathways. The separate pathways are frequently referred to as channels. Each channel is specialized to process information about particular features of visual stimuli. A large amount of research has identified a number of channels, each sensitive to a narrow range of spatial frequencies (or stimulus widths) and orientations in cats, monkeys, and humans.

Spatial frequency or size-sensitive channels may be relevant to reading because when we read we process both general (low spatial frequency) and detailed (high spatial frequency) information in each fixation. We extract detailed information from an area approximately 5 or 6 letter spaces to the right of fixation. Beyond this we also extract visual information but only of a general nature such as word shape.[6] These two types of information must in some way be combined.

It has also been shown that the different channels transmit their information at different rates and respond differently to different rates of temporal change. Some are sensitive to very rapidly changing stimuli, and others to stationary or slowly moving stimuli. Similarly, some channels respond primarily at stimulus onset and offset, whereas others respond throughout stimulus presentation. Such results have led to the proposal of two subsystems within the visual system. Many of the properties of these subsystems have been identified (see Table 9-1). An extended discussion of the properties of the systems, how they are identified, and the evidence indicating their physiological basis can be found elsewhere.[7] The magnocellular system and the parvocellular system, respectively, are often equated with the transient and sustained subsystems.

CLINICAL PEARL

Different channels transmit their information at different rates and respond differently to different rates of temporal change. Some are sensitive to very rapidly changing stimuli, and others to stationary or slowly moving stimuli. Similarly, some channels respond primarily at stimulus onset and offset, whereas others respond throughout stimulus presentation. Such results have led to the proposal of two subsystems within the visual system, transient and sustained.

Table 9-1
General Properties of the Transient and Sustained Subsystems

Transient system	Sustained system
High sensitivity to contrast	Low sensitivity to contrast
Most sensitive to low spatial frequencies	Most sensitive to high spatial frequencies
Most sensitive to high temporal frequencies	Most sensitive to low temporal frequencies
Fast transmission times	Slow transmission times
Responds at stimulus onset and offset	Responds throughout stimulus presentation
Predominates in peripheral vision	Predominates in central vision
The transient system may inhibit the sustained system	The sustained system may inhibit the transient system

It has been demonstrated physiologically and psychophysically[8,9] that the two systems may inhibit each other. In particular, if the sustained system is responding when the transient system is stimulated, the transient will terminate the sustained activity. Breitmeyer[9] and Matin[10] have argued that such transient-on-sustained inhibition is important in metacontrast. Metacontrast, in turn, is important in saccadic suppression. These two subsystems and the interactions between them may serve a number of functions essential to reading.

Because the transient system is predominantly a flicker- or motion-detecting system that transmits information about stimulus change and general shape, it is well suited for transmitting peripheral information in reading. The sustained system, being predominantly a detailed-pattern system, should be most important for extracting detailed information during fixations. Below we shall see that the two systems interact in important ways.

CLINICAL PEARL

Because the transient system is predominantly a flicker- or motion-detecting system that transmits information about stimulus change and general shape, it is well suited for transmitting peripheral information in reading. The sustained system, being predominantly a detailed-pattern system, should be most important for extracting detailed information during fixations.

Sustained and Transient Subsystems and Reading

When reading, the eyes move through a series of rapid eye movements called saccades. These are separated by fixation intervals when the eyes are stationary. The average fixation duration is approximately 200 to 250 msec for skilled readers, and it is during these stationary periods that information from the printed page is seen. The average saccade length is 6 to 8 characters or about 2° of visual angle.[6] Saccadic eye movements function to bring unidentified regions of text into foveal vision for detailed analysis during fixations. Foveal vision is the area of high acuity in the center of vision extending approximately 2° (6 to 8 letters) around the fixation point on a line of text. Beyond the fovea, acuity drops off rather dramatically.

The role of transient and sustained subsystems in reading has been considered by Breitmeyer.[7,9] Breitmeyer[9] has implicated transient and sustained system interactions in reading via saccadic suppression. He has argued that two forms of transient-sustained interactions are involved in saccadic suppression—metacontrast and the peripheral shift effect. Metacontrast, in particular, is argued to reflect transient-on-sustained inhibition. For this reason much of the work to be reported here has been done within the framework of transient-sustained interactions. The following is a selective review of some recent research done in a number of laboratories, including ours.

Transient and Sustained Processing in Disabled Readers and Controls

Even though we have used a range of measures to identify transient and sustained system processing, I will focus primarily on those involving flicker sensitivity. Some of our earliest studies concentrated on measuring visible persistence. *Visible persistence* is a measure of temporal processing and refers to the continued perception of a stimulus after it has been physically removed. This is assumed to reflect ongoing neural activity initiated by the stimulus presentation. In adults the duration of visible persistence increases monotonically with increasing spatial frequency.[11] Several studies[12] have compared disabled readers and controls on measures of visible persistence and have shown that disabled readers experience a significantly smaller increase in persistence duration with increasing spatial frequency than do controls.

In an attempt to understand further the nature of these differences between disabled readers and controls in visible persistence as a function of spatial frequency, Slaghuis and Lovegrove[13] used uniform-field masking to reduce transient system involvement in the persistence task. (See Breitmeyer, Levi, and Harwerth[14] for a full discussion of the rationale of this procedure.) In brief, they argued that uniform-field masking should reduce transient system involvement without any significant effect on sustained system processing. When visible persistence is measured in both groups under these conditions, differences between the groups disappear.[13] This is precisely what would be expected if the transient system in disabled readers is already weak.

A number of groups have measured sensitivity of disabled readers and controls to flicker. This is because of the evidence that the transient system is what processes flicker under a wide range of conditions. In the first studies of this sort,[15,16] sensitivity to counterphasing gratings, with stimuli varying in spatial and temporal frequency, were measured. Martin and Lovegrove[15,16] showed that disabled readers were less sensitive to flicker than controls and that this difference increased as temporal frequency increased. Brannan and Williams[17] showed similar results with whole field flicker. In addition they showed that this effect was present in children aged 8, 10, and 12 years. Importantly, this finding has been replicated with chronological-age-matched controls and with reading-age-matched controls.[18,19] This is important in establishing that flicker differences are not the result of reading-disabled children failing to learn to read. Livingstone et al.[20] have reported data consistent with these psychophysical findings measuring visual evoked potentials (VEPs) to flickering stimuli. They found disabled readers and controls to differ at high, but not low, flicker rates. Consequently, flicker differences between controls and disabled readers have been reported by a number of groups using different procedures and with both reading-age- and chronological-age-matched controls.

It has also been demonstrated[18,19] that flicker sensitivity differences between disabled readers and reading-age controls are luminance dependent. Differences have been found at 10 cd/m^2 but not at 30 cd/m^2. This result may be explained in terms of the differences in the gain of M and P cells as a function of luminance.[21] At low luminance levels flicker is processed primarily in M cells, but at higher luminance levels M and P cells have similar sensitivity to flicker.[21] To the extent that the M and P pathways correspond to the transient and sustained systems, the findings concerning disabled readers and flicker sensitivity as a function of luminance are consistent with the transient deficit hypothesis.

Further supporting evidence has recently been provided by Lehmkuhle et al.[22] They recorded visual evoked potentials (VEPs) from controls and disabled readers with and without uniform-field flicker. Under nonflicker conditions, they showed that the latency of early VEP components was longer for disabled readers at low spatial frequencies but not at high spatial frequencies. Uniform-field flicker significantly increased the latency and reduced the amplitude of the early VEP components in normal readers. In disabled readers the uniform-field flicker reduced the amplitude only of the same components. The net outcome was that the results for the two groups did not differ as much under uniform-field flicker masking conditions. This strongly reinforces the visible persistence data, but under conditions where it is essentially impossible to interpret the results in terms of criterion differences between the two groups.

Additional support for differences in transient system activity between the groups has been found in other VEP[20,23] and anatomical studies.[20] The data collected by May et al.[23] will be discussed in more detail later.

Lovegrove and colleagues[24,25] have also conducted a series of experiments comparing sustained system processing in controls and disabled readers. These studies measured orientation and spatial frequency tuning and the magnitude of the oblique effect.[25] Using similar procedures, equipment, and subjects as the experiments outlined previously, they failed to show any significant differences between the two groups. This implies that either there are no differences between the groups in the functioning of their sustained systems or such differences are smaller than the transient differences demonstrated.

It should be noted that both Williams and Bologna[26] and Ruddock[27] have demonstrated differences between the two groups on a visual search task. This task should have involved some sustained system activity. Furthermore, Williams, Molinet, and LeCluyse[28] have shown some interesting facilitation effects in a metacontrast experiment (this experiment will be discussed in more detail later). While the precise interpretation of these data is not clear, they do suggest some differences between normal and disabled readers in the sustained system. The exact nature of the differences requires further research, but it is likely that many tasks involving transient-sustained interactions are likely to show differences between the groups.

In summary: A number of measures of low-level visual processing suggest a transient deficit in disabled readers. The differences between the groups are quite large on some measures and discriminate well between individuals in the different groups, with approximately 75% of disabled readers showing reduced transient system sensitivity.[29] At the same time, evidence to date suggests that the two groups do not differ as clearly in sustained system functioning.

CLINICAL PEARL

A number of measures of low-level visual processing suggest a transient deficit in disabled readers. The differences between the groups are quite large on some measures and discriminate well between individuals in the different groups, with approximately 75% of disabled readers showing reduced transient system sensitivity.

In terms of the conflict on the issue of reading disability and vision in the literature, there are a number of questions that follow from the data outlined previously. The first is how many disabled readers differ from controls on these measures, and the second concerns the reliability of these measures. Each of these will be considered in turn.

Do the Measures Discriminate Between Individuals?

In an attempt to answer this question, Slaghuis and Lovegrove[29] combined data from a number of studies measuring duration of visible persistence as a function of spatial frequency in disabled and normal readers. They calculated a regression coefficient for the slope of this function for each subject in each group. To permit combining of the scores from different experiments, all regression coefficients were converted to z scores. A discriminant analysis was then performed on the z scores for 61 disabled readers and 61 controls. This showed that 75% of the disabled readers differed from the controls on this measure. Five percent of controls had functions as in the majority of the disabled readers. It is not clear why this is so, but it possibly relates to measurement error.

A second approach to this problem has been to use the latency scores from visual evoked potential data. In the May et al.[23] study, subjects were presented with sine-wave gratings ranging in spatial frequency from 0.5 to 8.0 cycles per degree flickering at a rate of 2 Hertz (Hz). Stimulus duration was 200 msec. This allowed analysis of two components of the VEP elicited by both stimulus onset and stimulus offset. The major findings indicated that poor readers had significantly lower amplitudes and significantly shorter latencies for components produced by stimulus offsets when low-spatial frequency stimuli were used.

Factor analyses of these data revealed two factors for both the low-spatial frequency and the high-spatial frequency stimuli.[30] With a low-spatial frequency stimulus, factor II was associated with latencies on the first onset component and factor I with latencies on all components. These scores were subject to a discriminant analysis, based on the differential scores on the two factors, that showed good and poor readers to be well differentiated by the factor scores on the low-spatial frequency but not the high-spatial frequency factor. Thus, this measure also differentiates well between individuals in the two groups.

Are These Measures Reliable?

Lovegrove et al.[12] have addressed the question of reliability of the measures within subjects by measuring the consistency of the regression coefficients for the spatial frequency by duration of visible persistence function referred to above. Slaghuis and Lovegrove[29] measured this function a number of times in the same children in a series of studies separated by 3 to 6 months. This issue is important in light of the claim by Georgeson and Georgeson[31] that this is an extremely unreliable measure. Our analyses showed that in the children we tested there were significant correlations on these measures over the three testing occasions.[32] Consequently our measures appear to be more reliable than those reported by Georgeson and Georgeson.[31]

Vision, Reading Disability, and Causality?

Hulme[33] has argued that it is most unlikely that there is a causal link between transient system processing and reading disability. Lovegrove[34] has countered that this question still should be regarded as open. I will consider this issue in two ways. The first will look at possible relationships between visual deficits and phonological processing. The second will take up the question of whether it is possible to make predictions about conditions that may improve reading in disabled readers from what we know about transient system processing in disabled readers.

Is There Any Link Between Transient System and Phonological Processing?

It is well documented that disabled readers experience major difficulties in phonological awareness[35] and phonological recoding.[36] Less is known, however, about possible relationships between transient processing and phonological processing. This issue was considered in a study of approximately 60 disabled readers and 60 controls.[37] Lovegrove et al.[37] took measures of transient system processing (flicker sensitivity), phonological awareness (segment comparison[38]), and phonological recoding (nonsense words and sentence verification[39]) in each child. These measures were subjected to a factor analysis that showed the phonological recoding measures and the phonological awareness measure loaded on the same factor as the measure of transient processing used. This shows some relation between the two processing areas without revealing the precise nature of that relationship.

Further information on this issue has been provided by Stein and his colleagues. Cornelissen et al.[40] measured the number of nonword errors made by groups of disabled readers and controls. They divided the subjects into two groups depending on whether they passed the Dunlop test of stability of ocular dominance.[41] Subjects were required to recognize words printed in different sizes. Cornelissen et al.[40] argued that nonword errors generally may be attributed to phonological awareness abilities. On the other hand, if errors varied with print size, they would more likely reflect visual problems. The results of these workers showed that children who passed the Dunlop test made more nonword errors than children who failed the Dunlop test when reading large print but they made fewer nonword errors with medium and small print. This group-by-print-size interaction indicates a causal role for the visual problems.

Eden, Stein, and Wood[42] measured the contribution made by measures of visual processing (a binocular fixation index) and phonological recoding (pig Latin completion time) to reading scores in a large group of disabled readers and controls. Their data showed that chronological age and IQ accounted for 38% of the variance. When phonological recoding data were added in, the accounted-for variance rose to 50%. And with the addition of visual measures, the variance rose to 65%.

It should be noted that Stein[43] has argued that the visual anomalies his group have identified in disabled readers reflect transient system processing. In particular, his group's work implicates the posterior parietal cortex, which receives primary magnocellular input.[44]

Evidence also is found in work[45] showing that there are disabled readers who have no phonological recoding problems but do have visual problems as measured by a visual segmentation task. This suggests that, although phonological awareness is an important part of the explanation of reading disability, it is not the full explanation in all cases.

In a recent study, Neville et al.[46] measured auditory and visual event-related potentials (ERPs) as well as ERPs to sentences in language-impaired children who also had reading disabilities. The most surprising aspect of their data was that the groups differed more on the visual ERPs than on the auditory ERPs. Subgroups of disabled readers differed on the auditory tasks, but the disabled readers as a whole differed from the controls only on the visual measures. These results show strongly that children whose major difficulties are in language and reading have clear differences from controls in visual processing. The differences were not found on all visual measures but were restricted to conditions in which stimuli were presented in rapid succession rather than presented at a slower rate, which is consistent with earlier psychophysical results of Tallal's group.[47] An interpretation of these results is discussed following.

Common Underlying Mechanisms?

Another possibility is that the deficits in both vision and phonological processing reflect some common underlying process or processes. Indirect support for this hypothesis comes from a number of sources. For example, it is possible that some of these deficits are related by virtue of the fact that some disabled readers have a problem processing rapidly presented stimuli in more than one sensory modality. Tallal,[48] for example, has shown disabled readers to have problems in audition that are similar to those we have measured in vision. She has shown that disabled readers perform as well as control readers on an auditory temporal order judgment task or an auditory fusion task when the two stimuli are separated by an interval of 428 msec. When this interval was reduced to 8 to 305 msec, disabled readers performed clearly worse than controls. Furthermore, Tallal[48] showed a highly significant positive correlation between her auditory temporal measures and nonsense word performance.

There is evidence, then, showing a relationship between rapid visual processing (as measured by transient system processing) and measures of both phonological awareness and phonological recoding. Similarly, a strong relationship has been demonstrated between rapid auditory processing and nonsense word performance. It has not been easy to integrate these various findings in previously available theoretical frameworks. Lovegrove[49] suggested the possibility of a general sensory timing problem in disabled readers. More recently this tentative suggestion has received further support. Livingstone et al.[20] have noted that, like the visual system, the auditory and somatosensory systems also may be subdivided into fast and slow components. They speculated further that problems may occur in disabled readers in the fast system of more than one modality. Their speculation was based in part on finding smaller magnocellular cells in disabled readers than in controls.

CLINICAL PEARL

There is evidence showing a relationship between rapid visual processing (as measured by transient system processing) and measures of both phonological awareness and phonological recoding.

The study by Neville et al.[46] discussed previously provides further support for this hypothesis. It is difficult to see why children with language deficits would have visual processing deficits. The proposal that these different deficits may be linked via a common sensory perceptual temporal processing deficit is one way of reconciling the different sets of data.

The relationship between temporal processing across modalities and reading has recently been investigated in normal adult readers.[50] We used a number of measures in vision and audition. Following on from Tallal, Stark, and Mellits[47] and from May, Williams, and Dunlap,[51] we measured temporal order judgment thresholds in vision and audition. We also found fusion thresholds with both auditory and visual stimuli. In addition, we measured intelligence using the Raven *Standard Progressive Matrices*[52] and nonsense word accuracy in 49 university students with normal reading ability. The data were subject to a hierarchical multiple regression analysis, with nonword accuracy being the dependent variable. The only variables that significantly contributed to the variance in nonword ability were visual and auditory temporal order judgment thresholds, which accounted for 17% of the variance in nonsense word recognition ability. Furthermore, the Raven *Progressive Matrices* scores of intelligence did not contribute significantly to this analysis.

Temporal order judgments in vision and audition did not, however, significantly correlate with each other. This is not consistent with a common temporal processing deficit found in both vision and audition.

This study, therefore, shows that there is a significant correlation between measures of rapid visual and auditory processing, on the one hand, and nonword reading, on the other, with intelligence partialed out. While not establishing causality, it further strengthens the links suggested by Cornellissen et al.[40] and Eden et al.[42] discussed previously. At the same time, the data show that, although some measures of rapid temporal processing in vision and audition are correlated with each other, not all are. Further work is required to reveal the complete picture.

Although this hypothesis requires further direct testing with disabled readers, it is an exciting prospect that may help integrate a large amount of apparently discrepant data. It is currently being investigated in our laboratory, among others.

What Can We Predict from a Transient Deficit?

The issue of causality may also be considered by predicting conditions that would lead to different levels of performance in normal readers and disabled readers based on transient system deficits. In terms of Breitmeyer's theory,[9] outlined earlier, a transient deficit should lead to more errors for disabled readers when reading continuous text than when reading isolated words, because the reading of continuous text requires integration of peripheral information from one fixation with central information from the next. Breitmeyer has argued that this task would largely involve the transient system. We have recently tested this by varying the mode of visual presentation when reading.[18] The general aim of our work was to vary the mode of visual presentation while holding semantic context constant.

CLINICAL PEARL

A transient deficit should lead to more errors for disabled readers when reading continous text than when reading isolated words, because the reading of continuous text requires integration of peripheral information from one fixation with central information from the next.

Three conditions of visual presentation on a computer monitor were used while holding the semantic context constant. This was done by presenting stories in three different ways. In the first condition one word at a time was presented in the middle of the screen; the subjects never had to move their eyes and never had information presented to the right of fixation. In the second condition one word was presented at a time but its position was moved across the screen; the subjects were required to move their eyes across the screen but still were never presented with information to the right of fixation. The final condition was a whole-line presentation, which most closely approximated normal reading. The rate of word presentation was held constant in all three conditions.

The results in Figure 9-1 showed that normal readers were most accurate in the two eye-movement conditions and made slightly more errors in the one-word-at-a-time condition. The reverse was true for the disabled readers, who read significantly more accurately in both one-word conditions than in the whole-line condition. The mode of presentation of written material that maximized reading accuracy in controls, therefore, produced the most errors in disabled readers. These findings have both theoretical and practical implications. Theoretically, they support the prediction, based on Breitmeyer's theory,[9] that disabled readers with a transient deficit should have difficulties

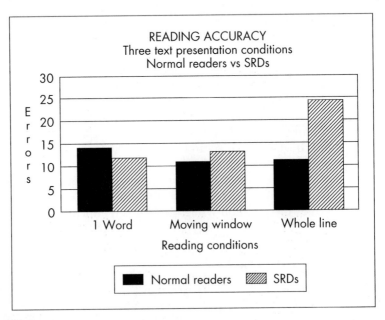

FIGURE 9-1 Mean number of errors for dyslexics and controls as a function of type of text presentation.

integrating peripheral and central information. Practically, they offer a means of presenting written text to beginning readers that may facilitate attempts at learning to read.

Conclusions

Although none of the previous discussion constitutes conclusive evidence that there is a causal link between transient system processing and reading disability, the data do show this to be a more open question than has been the case for some time. Some of the data from several types of studies indicate that visual factors make an independent contribution to reading disability. They also indicate that the issue warrants further investigation, which may lead to a fuller understanding of the problem of reading disability. Finally, the possibility of a general sensory timing deficit provides a convenient hypothesis that allows the possible integration of a large amount of existing data; in addition, the preliminary data available offer some support for this hypothesis.

References

1. Benton AL: Dyslexia in relation to form perception and directional sense. In Money J (ed): *Reading disability: progress and research needs in dyslexia*, Baltimore, 1962, Johns Hopkins Press, pp 81-102.
2. Vellutino FR: *Dyslexia: theory and research*, Cambridge, Mass, 1979, MIT Press.
3. Breitmeyer BG: Sustained (P) and transient (M) channels in vision: a review and implications for reading. In Willows DM, Kruk RS, Corcos E (eds): *Visual processes in reading and reading disabilities*, Hillsdale, NJ, 1993, Lawrence Erlbaum.
4. Campbell FW: The transmission of spatial information through the visual system. In Schmidt FO, Worden FS (eds): *The neurosciences third study program*, Cambridge, Mass, 1974, MIT Press.
5. Graham N: Spatial frequency channels in human vision: detecting edges without edges detectors. In Harris CS (ed): *Visual coding and adaptability*, Hillsdale, NJ, 1980, Lawrence Erlbaum.
6. Rayner K: The perceptual span and peripheral cues in reading, *Cogn Psychol* 7:65-81, 1975.
7. Lehmkuhle S: Neurological basis of visual processes in reading. In Willows DM, Kruk RS, Corcos E (eds): *Visual processes in reading and reading disabilities*, Hillsdale, NJ, 1993, Lawrence Erlbaum.
8. Singer W, Bedworth N: Inhibitory interaction between X and Y units in the cat lateral geniculate nucleus, *Brain Res* 49:291-307, 1973.
9. Breitmeyer BG: Unmasking visual masking: a look at the "why" behind the veil of "how," *Psychol Rev* 87:52-69, 1980.
10. Martin E: Saccadic suppression: a review and an analysis, *Psychol Bull* 81:899-915, 1974.
11. Meyer GE, Maguire WM: Spatial frequency and the mediation of short-term visual storage, *Science* 198:524-525, 1977.
12. Lovegrove W, Heddle M, Slaghuis W: Reading disability: spatial frequency specific deficits in visual information store, *Neuropsychologia* 18:111-115, 1980.

13. Slaghuis W, Lovegrove WJ: Flicker masking of spatial frequency dependent visible persistence and specific reading disability, *Perception* 13:527-534, 1984.
14. Breitmeyer B, Levi D, Harwerth RS: Flicker masking in spatial vision, *Vision Res* 21:1377-1385, 1981.
15. Martin F, Lovegrove W: Flicker contrast sensitivity in normal and specifically disabled readers, *Perception* 16:215-221, 1987.
16. Martin F, Lovegrove W: Uniform field flicker in control and specifically-disabled readers, *Perception* 17:203-214, 1988.
17. Brannan J, Williams M: The effects of age and reading ability on flicker threshold, *Clin Vis Sci* 3:137-142, 1988.
18. Hill R, Lovegrove W: One word at a time: a solution to the visual deficit in the specific reading disabled. In Wright SF, Groner R (eds): *Facets of dyslexia and its remediation,* Amsterdam, 1993, North Holland.
19. Cornelissen P: Fixation, contrast sensitivity and children's reading. In Wright SF, Groner R (eds): *Facets of dyslexia and its remediation,* Amsterdam, 1993, North Holland.
20. Livingstone MS, Rosen G, Drislane F, Galaburda A: Physiological and anatomical evidence for a magnocellular defect in developmental dyslexia, *Proc Natl Acad Sci USA* 88:7943-7947, 1991.
21. Kaplan E, Lee BB, Shapley RM: New views of primate retinal function, *Prog Ret Res* 9:273-336, 1990.
22. Lehmkuhle S, Garzia RP, Turner L et al: A defective visual pathway in reading disabled children, *N Engl J Med* 328:989-996, 1993.
23. May J, Lovegrove W, Martin F et al: Pattern-elicited visual evoked potentials in good and poor readers, *Clin Vis Sci* 2:131-136, 1991.
24. Lovegrove W, Martin F, Slaghuis W: A theoretical and experimental case for a visual deficit in specific reading disability, *Cogn Neuropsychol* 3:225-267, 1986.
25. Lovegrove W, Martin F, Bowling A et al: Contrast sensitivity functions and specific reading disability, *Neuropsychologia* 20:309-315, 1982.
26. Williams M, Bologna N: Perceptual grouping in good and poor readers, *Percept Psychophys* 38:367-374, 1985.
27. Ruddock K: Visual search in dyslexia. In Stein J (ed): *Vision and visual dyslexia,* London, 1991, Macmillan.
28. Williams M, Molinet K, LeCluyse K: Visual masking as a measure of temporal processing in normal and disabled readers, *Clin Vis Sci* 4:137-144, 1989.
29. Slaghuis W, Lovegrove WJ: Spatial-frequency mediated visible persistence and specific reading disability, *Brain Cogn* 4:219-240, 1985.
30. May J, Dunlap W, Lovegrove W: Factor scores derived from visual evoked potential latencies, *Clin Vis Sci* 7:67-70, 1992.
31. Georgeson MA, Georgeson JM: On seeing temporal gaps between gratings: a criterion problem for measurement of visible persistence, *Vision Res* 25:1729-1733, 1985.
32. Lovegrove W, Slaghuis W: How reliably are visual differences found in dyslexics? *Irish J Psychol* 10:542-550, 1989.
33. Hulme C: The implausibility of low-level visual deficits as a cause of children's reading difficulties, *Cogn Neuropsychol* 5:369-374, 1988.
34. Lovegrove W: Is the question of the role of visual deficits as a cause of disabilities a closed one? Comments on Hulme, *Cogn Neuropsychol* 8:435-441, 1991.
35. Bradley L, Bryant P: Categorising sounds and learning to read: a causal connection, *Nature* 301:419-421, 1983.
36. Snowling M: Phonemic deficits in developmental dyslexia, *Psychol Res* 43:219-234, 1981.
37. Lovegrove W, McNicol D, Martin F et al: Phonological recoding, memory processing and memory deficits in specific reading disability. In Vickers D, Smith P (eds): *Human information processing: measures, mechanisms, and models,* Amsterdam, 1988, North Holland.

38. Trieman R, Baron J: Segmental analysis ability: development and relation to reading. In Waller TG, Mackinnon GE (eds): *Reading research: advances in theory and practice,* New York, 1978, Academic Press.

39. Baron J: Phonemic stage not necessary for reading, *Q J Exp Psychol* 25:241-246, 1973.

40. Cornelissen P, Bradley L, Fowler MS, Stein JF: What children see affects how they read, *Dev Med Child Neurol* 33:755-762, 1991.

41. Dunlop P: Dyslexia: an orthoptic approach, *Aust J Orthopt* 12:16-20, 1972.

42. Eden G, Stein JF, Wood FB: Visuospatial ability and language processing in reading disabled and normal children. In Wright SF, Groner R (eds): *Facets of dyslexia and its remediation,* Amsterdam, 1993, North Holland.

43. Stein JF: Visuospatial sense, hemispheric asymmetry, and dyslexia. In Stein JF (ed): *Vision and visual dyslexia,* Boca Raton, Fla, 1991, CRC Press.

44. Livingstone MS, Hubel DH: Psychophysical evidence for separate channels for the perception of form, color, movement, and depth, *J Neurosci* 7:3416-3468, 1987.

45. Johnstone R, Anderson M, Duncan L: Phonological and visual segmentation problems in poor readers. In Snowling M, Thomson M (eds): *Dyslexia: integrating theory and practice,* London, 1991, Whurr Publishers.

46. Neville HJ, Coffey SA, Holcomb PJ et al: The neurobiology of sensory and language processing in language-impaired children, *J Cogn Neurosci* 5:235-253, 1993.

47. Tallal P, Stark RE, Mellits D: The relationship between auditory temporal analysis and receptive language development: evidence from studies of developmental language disorder, *Neuropsychologia* 23:527-534, 1985.

48. Tallal P: Auditory temporal perception, phonics, and reading disabilities in children, *Brain Lang* 9:182-198, 1980.

49. Lovegrove W: Do dyslexics have a visual deficit? In Wright S, Groner R (eds): *Facets of dyslexia and its remediation,* Amsterdam, 1993, North Holland.

50. Lovegrove W, Pepper K, Campbell T et al: The role of rapid visual and auditory processing in nonword reading. (In preparation.)

51. May J, Williams M, Dunlap W: Temporal order judgments in good and poor readers, *Neuropsychologia* 26:917-924, 1988.

52. Raven JC: *Standard progressive matrices,* Hawthorne, Victoria, 1989, ACER.

C H A P T E R

10

Visual Evoked Potentials in Reading Disability

John A. Baro
Ralph P. Garzia
Stephen Lehmkuhle

Key Terms

visual evoked potential (VEP)	parvocellular pathway	electrophysiology VEP latency
magnocellular pathway		

As technology evolved to record brain responses from the scalp to specific visual stimuli and to distinguish visual evoked potentials (VEPs) from concurrent background activity of the brain, it was soon applied to the study of reading disability. This new technology provided one of the first opportunities to differentiate the neurophysiology of normal readers from those of disabled readers.

There have been continuous attempts to examine the physiological status of the brains of disabled readers; but over the 30 years of electrophysiological research, the early research efforts have been confusing and contradictory and have yielded equivocal results. Stimuli and recording procedures in many instances were more suitable for generating event-related potentials (ERPs) than sensory-evoked potentials.

ERPs are endogenous responses that depend more on the particular characteristics of the subject and less on the physical attributes of the stimulus. VEPs are stimulus driven, and their properties depend more upon the characteristics of the stimulus, such as spatial and temporal frequency, and contrast.

Conners[1] was the first to report that differences between normal and disabled readers can be demonstrated electrophysiologically. He used interspersed bright and dim flashes presented at a rate of 45 Hz. Potentials were recorded only for the bright flashes as the subjects depressed a response button each time a bright flash was presented. A significant correlation was found between the amplitude of a positive wave occurring at approximately 140 msec recorded from parietal electrodes and reading achievement.

Preston, Gutherie, and Childs[2] studied a reading-disabled and two control groups, one age matched and the other reading level matched. Among an array of four different stimuli were a 50 msec light flash and a 50 msec exposure of the word "cat." A smaller-amplitude wave occurring about 200 msec after stimulus onset was found in the reading-disabled group compared with the two control groups. Similar results were noted for the nonlinguistic (light flash) and linguistic (word) stimuli. The differences found between the reading-disabled and the control groups suggested that the results could be attributed neither to age nor to reading level effects.

Sobotka and May[3] used an experimental paradigm similar to those of Conners.[1] Stimuli were short-duration dim and bright light flashes. The subjects were instructed to attend to the dim flashes by depressing a response key; however, potentials were recorded only from the bright flashes. Sobotka and May found larger amplitudes in a reading-disabled group compared with a control group. They attributed these results to a selective attention deficit, because the disabled readers developed a stronger response to the experimentally unattended bright light flashes.

Symann-Louett et al.[4] investigated waveform differences related to reading ability. They used as stimuli simple words—either the names of animals or the names of body parts—three or four letters in length and counted the total number of "peaks" and "troughs" of a certain threshold amplitude in the averaged waveforms. The reading-disabled were noted to have fewer waveforms than the controls. Although potentials were purportedly elicited by word stimuli, a distinct luminance-generated response was likely present.

Not all research results within this time frame were in agreement. Three large families with multiple reading-disabled members were studied by Weber and Omenn[5] using light flashes. They found no significant differences between family members with and family members without reading disability. These results were extended in a subsequent expanded study of a larger sample of unrelated disabled readers.

Two more recent investigations used pattern-elicited VEPs to study vision and reading disability. Mecacci, Sechi, and Levi[6] recorded from two occipital locations to study hemispheric symmetry. Checkerboard-elicited transient evoked potentials were recorded for patterns from 0.5 to 12.0 c/deg. Larger VEP amplitudes for all check sizes were found for the control group compared with the reading-disabled group. In addition, controls exhibited a very high correlation between the two hemispheres for VEP amplitude whereas reading-disabled subjects had significant hemispheric asymmetry.

Solan et al.[7] were primarily interested in the question of binocular summation in reading-disabled people, but other relevant information can be extracted from their data. Pattern-reversal VEPs were elicited by high-contrast checkerboards of 2 and 4 c/deg, reversing at 1 and 4 Hz. The control group exhibited larger monocular and binocular VEP amplitudes than the reading-disabled group did, by as much as a factor of 2.

These last two reports are somewhat troubling. There are no intuitive reasons why VEP amplitudes should have been reduced in the reading-disabled groups. Slowly reversing or transiently presented high-contrast checkerboards should have provided a strong visual stimulus. There have been no published reports suggesting that disabled readers have organic visual pathway dysfunction of the kind that would produce such dramatic VEP abnormalities. Perhaps the reading-disabled group had poor accommodation that produced stimulus blur, reducing VEP amplitude.

In contrast to earlier work, recent electrophysiological studies[8-10] have been guided by the results of recent psychophysical investigations. These studies, in which differences between reading-disabled and normal observers have been obtained, were based on the wealth of psychophysical evidence suggesting differences in spatial and temporal response characteristics between two of the primary visual pathways, parvocellular (P) and magnocellular (M). The P pathway is predominant in central vision and is responsive principally to high-spatial frequency stimuli. It responds relatively slowly and exhibits low temporal resolution. The M pathway predominates in peripheral vision and responds well to low spatial frequencies, lower contrasts, and higher temporal rates. The next sections will consider in more detail the response characteristics of these two pathways and how their functionality can be assessed through the use of evoked potential techniques.

CLINICAL PEARL

Recent electrophysiological studies in which differences between reading-disabled and normal observers have been obtained were based on the wealth of psychophysical evidence suggesting differences in spatial and temporal response characteristics between two of the primary visual pathways, the parvocellular (P) and magnocellular (M).

M- and P-Pathway Response Characteristics

The M and P pathways differ with respect to contrast sensitivity (i.e., the minimum amount of contrast necessary to detect a pattern), spatial-frequency tuning (the range of spatial frequencies that elicits a maximum response), and temporal-frequency tuning (the range of temporal frequencies that elicits a maximum response).[11-13] Generally speaking, the M pathway has greater contrast sensitivity than the P pathway. Low-contrast patterns are more likely to be detected by the M pathway, whereas the response of the P pathway is less likely to saturate at higher contrasts. This overall difference in contrast sensitivity is complicated by the difference in spatial-tuning characteristics between the two pathways. The M pathway tends to respond best to lower spatial frequencies, which typically convey information about the global characteristics—shape and form—of an image. The P pathway tends to respond best to higher spatial frequencies, which typically convey information about the local characteristics—fine detail—of an image.

These response profiles of the two pathways are further delineated by their difference in temporal tuning characteristics. The M pathway responds best to images that are changing or moving rapidly, while the P pathway responds best to images that are changing very little or moving slowly. Because the response of the M pathway can follow higher temporal rates, it is not surprising that the M pathway also responds quickly to a stimulus. With optimal stimulation, the response latency of the M pathway is shorter than the latency of the P pathway (see Table 10-1 for a summary of the differences in response characteristics of the M and P pathways).

Given this information about the response characteristics of the two pathways, we can determine the optimum combination of stimulus characteristics for separating the responses of the two pathways as well as predict how each pathway will respond to less-than-optimal stimuli. The optimal stimulus for the M pathway has low contrast, low spatial frequency, and high temporal frequency (e.g., the overall form of moving objects). On the other hand, the optimal stimulus for

TABLE 10-1
Characteristics of Parallel Pathways

	M pathway	P pathway
Sensitivity	Low	High
Temporal frequency	High	Low
Contrast	Low	High
Response speed	Fast	Slow

the P pathway has relatively high contrast, high spatial frequency, and low temporal frequency (e.g., the fine detail in stationary objects). It should be noted, however, that virtually all stimuli elicit *some* response from each pathway—the extent to which a stimulus conforms to the "optimal" configuration determining the relative strength of the response in each pathway. In other words, the overall response of the visual system can be dominated by contributions from the M pathway, the P pathway, or (typically) some combination of the two.

CLINICAL PEARL

The optimal stimulus for the M pathway has low contrast, low spatial frequency, and high temporal frequency (e.g., the overall form of moving objects). On the other hand, the optimal stimulus for the P pathway has relatively high contrast, high spatial frequency, and low temporal frequency (e.g., the fine detail in stationary objects).

Psychophysical Evidence For An M-Pathway Deficit In Reading Disability

Lovegrove et al.[8,9] reported that the contrast sensitivity to low-spatial frequency patterns (1 to 4 c/deg) is lower in reading-disabled children than in normal readers, the difference tending to be greatest with briefly presented stimuli (150 to 500 msec). Contrast sensitivity to higher spatial frequency stimuli was typically the same for the two groups but was sometimes higher in reading-disabled children. Because contrast sensitivity, particularly to low spatial frequencies, is determined by sensitivity of the M pathway, decreased sensitivity in reading-disabled children is consistent with an M-pathway deficit. The finding that the difference in sensitivity between the two groups was more pronounced with brief stimulus presentation also points to an M-pathway deficit, because of the M pathway's higher sensitivity to high temporal frequencies. The increase in sensitivity to high spatial frequencies obtained in some reading-disabled observers is also consistent with this interpretation, if we assume that a reduced M-pathway contribution reveals the P pathway's higher sensitivity to high spatial frequencies.

Martin and Lovegrove[14] measured the effects of uniform-field flicker masking on contrast sensitivity in normal and reading-disabled children. Contrast sensitivity to sinewave gratings was determined with a steady uniform background and a uniform background modulated in luminance at a high temporal frequency. They found that a high-frequency flickering background reduced contrast sensitivity to low spatial frequencies in normal readers while having no effect on reading-disabled observers. This finding can also be accounted for in the context of an M-pathway deficit. The uniform flickering field, which has a low spatial frequency and high temporal frequency, provides an optimal stimulus for the M pathway, eliciting a maximal response. The addition of a target stimulus therefore produces little or no additional response from the saturated M pathway, while the P pathway, which does not respond well to the flickering background, responds normally to the target. This effect is most prominent with low spatial frequency targets because the low frequency response is normally dominated by the M pathway. The response to high frequency targets is normally dominated by the P pathway, so a reduced M-pathway contribution has negligible effect. The absence of this flicker-masking effect in reading-disabled observers indicates that the M-pathway contribution to contrast sensitivity is either reduced or more like the normal P-pathway response.

Brannan and Williams[15] measured flicker-detection thresholds in normal and reading-disabled children at three age levels and in normally reading adults. They found that poor readers had higher flicker-detection thresholds than both good readers and adults. Although the flicker thresholds of poor readers decreased with age, the differences between good and poor readers did not change—which suggests the presence of a temporal visual processing deficit as opposed to a maturational delay. Brannan and Williams[15] suggested that this deficit represents a loss in temporal resolution, thus implicating an M-pathway deficit.

Taken together, the psychophysical studies discussed previously (and the majority of other recent psychophysical studies) suggest the presence of an M-pathway deficit in reading-disabled children that appears to involve both spatial and temporal response characteristics of the M pathway and can be demonstrated with a variety of psychophysical techniques. Because of the nature of these deficits revealed psychophysically, recent electrophysiological studies of reading disability have focused their efforts on measuring M-pathway activity. Stimulus parameters and viewing conditions have been selected to isolate and compare activity in the M and P pathways. The results of these electrophysiological studies are generally consistent with those of psychophysical studies.

Electrophysiological Assessment of the M and P Pathways

The rationale behind electrophysiological studies of reading disability is based on the assumption that the VEP, especially its early components, represents the combined contributions of the M and P pathways. Because these pathways differ in their spatial and temporal response characteristics, stimuli can be selected that preferentially activate one or the other. The result is that the relative contributions of the two pathways to the VEP are altered, which can be manifested by changes in VEP latency, VEP amplitude, or both (Figure 10-1). For example, if a stimulus is selected that is optimal for the M pathway, the VEP will be dominated by an M-pathway contribution and will change in a predictable way. In this example, because the M pathway generally responds more quickly than the P pathway, the latency of a transient VEP will be reduced because the contribution of the relatively slow P pathway has been reduced relative to the contribution of the quicker M pathway. It is thus possible to segregate and measure activity in the M and P pathways electrophysiologically in much the same way as has been done psychophysically.

CLINICAL PEARL

If a stimulus is selected that is optimal for the M pathway, the VEP will be dominated by an M-pathway contribution and will change in a predictable way.

Three psychophysical methods used to isolate responses of the M and P pathway have been described. If similar approaches are applied to electrophysiological paradigms, particular results would be anticipated in normal and reading-disabled observers. First, M and P pathways can be distinguished by their spatial frequency response function. The M pathway responds more quickly and better to low spatial frequencies, while the P pathway responds more slowly and better to higher spatial frequencies. We would therefore expect VEP latency (i.e., a measure of the speed at which information is processed) to increase with increasing spatial frequencies in normal observers. Baro and Lehmkuhle[16] have shown that, although VEP amplitude peaks at middle spatial frequencies, latency of the transient VEP does increase with spatial frequency. If the M-pathway contribution were reduced or slowed, an increase in VEP latency, primarily at low spatial frequencies, would be expected.

A second psychophysical technique used to isolate the M-pathway response is flicker masking. High-frequency uniform-field flicker provides an optimal M-pathway stimulus, saturating its response and therefore masking its contribution to the target-evoked response. Psychophysically this effect can be manifested by decreased contrast sensitivity at low spatial frequencies. Masking of the M-pathway response can also be revealed in a task that measures temporal processing. For example, it has been shown[17-19] that reaction times to low spatial frequency targets are increased by a flickering mask, while reaction times to high spatial frequency targets are not affected. It follows that a similar temporal effect of flicker masking would be observed in the latency of the VEP. This prediction has been confirmed in normal observers by Baro and Lehmkuhle,[16] who demonstrated that uniform-field flicker increases transient VEP latency at

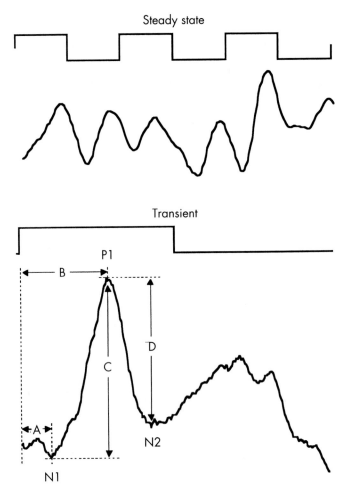

FIGURE 10-1 A comparison of steady state and transient VEPs. *Top,* Steady-state stimulus (e.g., a counterphasing sinewave grating) above the steady-state waveform. In this 1-second record the stimulus counterphases three times (i.e., switches light and dark regions and then switches back again), evoking a response that alternates at twice the frequency of the stimulus (i.e., at each light/dark transition). *Bottom,* Transient stimulus (e.g., a sinewave grating turned on and then off) above the transient waveform. In this example, the stimulus is on for 250 msec and the duration of the record is 500 msec. The major positive and negative deflections have been labeled *N1, P1,* and *N2.* The measures typically obtained from a transient VEP are (*A*) N1 latency (i.e., the time from stimulus onset or offset to N1), (*B*) P1 latency, (*C*) N1-P1 amplitude, and (*D*) P1-N2 amplitude.

low spatial frequencies. If the M pathway were slowed relative to the P pathway, the P pathway–dominated VEP should be affected much less by flicker masking.

A third means of assessing M-pathway activity is the flicker-detection threshold. Because the M pathway has higher temporal resolution than the P pathway, psychophysical studies have demonstrated reduced temporal resolution in reading-disabled observers. The task used to measure the flicker-detection threshold is similar to the paradigm used to record steady-state VEPs. In contrast to the transient VEP, in which the stimulus is turned on and off once during discrete trials, when recording steady-state VEPs the stimulus is always on and is continuously counterphasing (i.e., alternating light and dark regions) throughout the recording (Figure 10-1). In a system with reduced temporal resolution, it could be predicted that VEPs would not be obtained at temporal frequencies as high as those in normal observers.

Thus, a number of psychophysical techniques used to isolate and measure M-pathway activity can be adapted to electrophysiological techniques. Based on psychophysical results, specific predictions can be made about how an M-pathway deficit should be manifested electrophysiologically. A reduced or slowed M-pathway response should result in VEPs with smaller amplitudes and/or longer latencies primarily at lower spatial frequencies. An M-pathway deficit should be revealed in a flicker-masking paradigm in a variety of ways (e.g., by a failure to observe a reduction in the amplitude of the VEP at low spatial frequencies or by failure to observe an increase in the latency of the VEP produced by low spatial frequency targets). With respect to temporal resolution, an M-pathway deficit would produce reduced-amplitude steady-state VEPs at high temporal frequencies.

CLINICAL PEARL

A reduced or slowed M-pathway response should result in VEPs with smaller amplitudes and/or longer latencies primarily at lower spatial frequencies. An M-pathway deficit should produce reduced-amplitude steady-state VEPs at high temporal frequencies.

Electrophysiological Evidence For An M-Pathway Deficit in Reading Disability

Electrophysiological techniques offer many advantages over psychophysical procedures with respect to the identification of children who experience reading problems due to visual processing deficits. Psychophysical measures typically require a large number of trials, during which the observer must attend to stimuli and make responses over an extended time. With training and practice, the observer's participation is often spread over several testing sessions, and it is therefore often difficult to obtain reliable measures from the young child usually tested in studies of reading disability. Electrophysiological measures are especially well suited to this application because, in contrast to psychophysical tasks, the recording of evoked potentials is fast and requires no training of the observers, nor does it require sustained attention or active participation. Thus, not only can electrophysiological techniques provide support for conclusions based on psychophysical studies, they also offer advantages in the collection of reliable data from a large population in a timely manner.

Livingstone et al.[20] recorded both transient and steady-state VEPs in adults who were normal readers and those who had been diagnosed as reading disabled. Their stimuli were checkerboard patterns. In the transient VEP conditions, low- versus high-contrast stimuli (0.02 vs 0.2) were compared. In the high-contrast conditions VEPs were similar in both groups of observers. However, in the low-contrast conditions the N1 components of the VEPs were later, by 20 to 40 msec, in the disabled readers as compared with the controls. For some reading-disabled observers the N1 component was missing and the P1 component was also delayed. In the steady-state VEP conditions both stimulus contrast and counterphase frequency were varied. In the high-contrast and low-frequency (1 Hz) condition, VEPs were similar in both groups of observers. However, in the low-contrast conditions (0.01 and 0.02) at a frequency of 15 Hz, while VEP amplitude in the normal observers was slightly reduced, VEP responses in the reading-disabled almost disappeared.

However, Victor et al.[21] failed to observe differences in VEP latency and temporal resolution between normal and reading-disabled observers. These authors also used low- and high-contrast checkerboard stimuli reversed at low and high temporal rates. Their failure to replicate this effect is difficult to reconcile in terms of the differences in stimuli, procedures, and subject selection. One possible difference is in the rate used to sample the EEG activity to average a potential. The sampling rate was 135 Hz (every 7 msec) in the Victor et al. study[21] but was 100 KHz (every 10 μsec) in the Livingstone et al. study.[20] The higher sampling rate used in the Livingstone et al. study would provide a more sensitive procedure to detect small temporal differences in the potential.

May et al.[22] also recorded transient VEPs. However, their stimuli were sinewave grating patterns, and they were recorded from reading-disabled and normal high school students. In addition to recording onset VEPs (i.e., elicited by stimulus onset), they recorded offset VEPs. With respect to onset VEP amplitude, they found no differences between the two groups for stimuli at any spatial frequency. Offset

VEP amplitudes were smaller in the reading-disabled group for 0.5 c/deg stimuli but similar in both groups at higher spatial frequencies. This difference in amplitude was obtained only for early VEP components (N1 and P1); later components were similar in both groups at all spatial frequencies tested. Offset latencies of later VEP components (N2 and P2) were shorter in the reading-disabled group for the 1 c/deg stimuli. At other spatial frequencies, latencies of early and late VEP components were similar in both groups.

Recently May et al.[23] reanalyzed their results discussed previously. They examined correlations among amplitudes and latencies of VEP components and used factor analysis to differentiate between the two groups according to factor score. Although VEPs were the same in both disabled and normal readers with high-spatial frequency stimuli (8 c/deg), the factor analysis revealed differences with low-spatial frequency stimuli (1 c/deg). The factor analysis indicated longer latencies for early-onset VEP components (N1, P1) in the reading-disabled group. Shorter latencies were obtained for later-onset VEP components (N2, P2) and both early- and late-offset VEP components in the reading disabled group.

Lehmkuhle et al.[24] employed a technique that enabled both within-subject and between-subject comparisons of transient VEPs to be obtained in reading-disabled children and normal readers. Stimuli were low-contrast, low and high spatial frequency sinewave gratings (0.5 and 4.5 c/deg) that were surrounded by either a steady background with the same mean luminance as the target or a uniform flickering field mask—a homogeneous field that was flickered at 12 Hz at a modulation of 0.70. Latencies and amplitudes were determined for early VEP components (N1, P1). Overall, steady background VEP latencies were slightly longer for the reading-disabled observers in the low spatial frequency condition (< 7 msec), but there were no differences in latency or amplitude in the high spatial frequency condition. Given the small difference in latency observed in this study, it is not surprising that Victor et al.,[21] using a 7 msec sampling rate, failed to detect any latency differences between normal and reading-disabled observers with low spatial frequency stimuli. Moreover, although the low spatial frequency difference was statistically significant in the Lehmkuhle et al. study,[24] the large amount of within-group variability makes conclusions based on their between-group comparison uncertain.

Assessing the effects of flicker masking provides for a within-group comparison, which is a comparison more immune to the inter-subject variability often observed in evoked potential experiments. At high spatial frequencies the flickering field had no effect in either group of observers. In normal readers the presence of the flickering field produced VEP components, which were generally slower and smaller in amplitude at low spatial frequencies. In contrast, the effects of the flickering field at low spatial frequencies were only partial in the reading-disabled observers. There was a significant reduction in the amplitude of the VEP, but latency did not shift (Figure 10-2).

This finding extends previous results beyond what is possible to infer from psychophysics alone. The reduction in VEP amplitude with flicker masking in reading-disabled observers suggests the presence of an intact functioning M pathway. If there were little or no M-pathway contribution to the VEP, the flickering mask should have no effect. The reduction in amplitude indicates a reduced M-pathway contribution to the VEP. The absence of a shift in latency, however, points to a deficit that is primarily temporal in nature. Therefore the effect of flicker masking on amplitude without a corresponding effect on latency provides evidence that the M pathway is intact in reading-disabled observers but sluggish in its response. In other words, the M pathway in reading-disabled observers behaves more like the P pathway, thus disrupting the normal temporal flow of information.

TABLE 10-2
Effects Obtained in Reading-Disabled Observers

Stimulus	Study	M pathway			P pathway	
		Low SF	High TF	Low Con	High SF	Low TF
Checkerboard	Transient VEP (Solan et al.[7])	X	-	-	-	-
Checkerboard	Steady-state VEP (Solan et al.[7])	X	X	-	-	-
Checkerboard	Transient VEP (Mecacci et al.[8])	X	-	-	X	-
Checkerboard	Transient VEP (Livingstone et al[20])	-	-	X	-	-
Checkerboard	Steady-state VEP (Livingstone et al.[20]) (but see Victor et al.[21])	-	X	X	-	-
Grating	Transient onset VEP (May et al.[22])	-	-	-	-	-
Grating	Transient offset VEP (May et al.[22])	X	-	-	-	-
Grating	Transient onset VEP (May et al.[23])	X	-	-	-	-
Grating	Transient offset VEP (May et al.[23])	X	-	-	-	-
Grating	Transient VEP (Lehmkuhle et al.[24])	X	-	-	-	-

SF, Spatial frequency; TF, temporal frequency; Con, contrast.

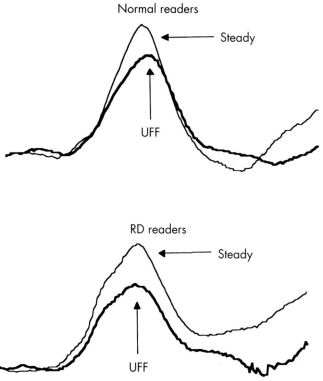

FIGURE 10-2 Difference between the transient VEP of normal and reading-disabled observers in a flicker masking paradigm. These waveforms are composites; that is, they are the sum of normalized waveforms from many observers. Although this technique serves to illustrate some basic differences between groups, it also tends to make the VEP components less distinct (e.g., as compared with Figure 10-1, which shows the waveform obtained from a single observer). All comparisons and statistical analyses were performed on individual waveforms. *Top,* Flicker masking effect in normal observers. *Steady* indicates that the grating stimulus was presented on a steady uniform background; *UFF,* uniform field flickering background. Note the increased latency of the N1 and P1 components and the decreased amplitude of N1-P1. *Bottom,* Flicker masking effect in reading-disabled observers. Note the decrease in N1-P1 amplitude, similar to that in the normal observers, but the absence of a corresponding increase in latencies. (Modified from Lehmkuhle S et al: A defective visual pathway in reading disabled children, *N Engl J Med* 328:989-996, 1993.)

CLINICAL PEARL

The effect of flicker masking on amplitude without a corresponding effect on latency provides evidence that the M pathway is intact in reading-disabled observers but sluggish in its response. In other words, the M pathway in reading-disabled observers behaves more like the P pathway, thus disrupting the normal temporal flow of information.

Based on the recent psychophysical studies of reading disability, three predictions were made regarding VEPs recorded from normal and reading-disabled observers. An M-pathway deficit in reading disability should be revealed by (1) a slowed response to low-spatial frequency stimuli, (2) a reduced effect of flicker masking at low spatial frequencies, and (3) a reduced response to high temporal rates. Although different stimuli, recording procedures, and analysis techniques were employed in these studies, the studies tend to support each prediction (see Table 10-2 for a summary of the results of VEP studies that found deficits in reading-disabled subjects).

References

1. Connors CK: Cortical visual evoked response in children with learning disorders, *Psychophysiology* 7:418-428, 1970.
2. Preston MS, Guthrie JT, Childs B: Visual evoked responses (VERs) in normal and disabled readers, *Psychophysiology* 11:452-457, 1974.
3. Sobotka KR, May JG: Visual evoked potentials and reaction time in normal and dyslexic children, *Psychophysiology* 14:18-24, 1977.
4. Symann-Lovett N, Gascon GG, Matsumiya Y, Lombroso CT: Waveform differences in visual evoked responses between normal and reading disabled children, *Neurology* 27:156-159, 1977.
5. Weber BA, Omenn GS: Auditory and visual evoked responses in children with familial reading disabilities, *J Learn Disabil* 10:153-158, 1977.
6. Mecacci L, Sechi E, Levi G: Abnormalities of visual evoked potentials by checkerboards in children with specific reading disability, *Brain Cogn* 2:135-143, 1983.
7. Solan HA, Sutija VG, Ficarra AP, Wurst SA: Binocular advantage and visual processing in dyslexic and control children as measured by evoked potentials, *Optom Vis Sci* 67:105-110, 1990.
8. Lovegrove WJ, Heddle M, Slaghuis W: Reading disability: spatial frequency specific deficits in information store, *Neuropsychologia* 18:111-115, 1980.
9. Lovegrove WJ, Martin F, Bowling A et al: Contrast sensitivity functions and specific reading disability, *Neuropsychologia* 20:309-315, 1982.
10. Lovegrove W, Martin G, Slaghuis W: A theoretical and experimental case for a transient system deficit in specific reading disability, *Cogn Neuropsychol* 3:225-267, 1986.
11. Van Essen DC: Visual areas of the mammalian cerebral cortex, *Ann Rev Neurosci* 2:227-263, 1979.
12. Bassi CJ, Lehmkuhle S: Clinical implications of parallel visual pathways, *J Am Optom Assoc* 61:98-110, 1990.

13. Livingstone MS, Hubel DH: Segregation of form, color, movement and depth: anatomy, physiology, and perception, *Science* 240:740-749, 1988.
14. Martin F, Lovegrove WJ: Uniform-field flicker masking in control and specifically-disabled readers, *Perception* 17:203-214, 1988.
15. Brannan J, Williams M: The effects of age and reading ability on flicker thresholds, *Clin Vis Sci* 3:137-142, 1988.
16. Baro JA, Lehmkuhle S: The effects of a luminance-modulated background on human grating-evoked cortical potentials, *Clin Vis Sci* 5:265-270, 1990.
17. Baro JA, Brzezicki LJ, Lehmkuhle S, Hughes HC: The perceived duration of gratings, *Perception* 21:161-166, 1992.
18. Bowling A: The effects of peripheral movement and flicker on the detection thresholds of sinusoidal gratings, *Percept Psychophys* 37:181-188, 1985.
19. Breitmeyer B, Levi DM, Harwerth RS: Flicker masking in spatial vision, *Vision Res* 21:1377-1385.
20. Livingstone MS, Rosen GD, Drislane FW, Galaburda AM: Physiological and anatomical evidence for a magnocellular defect in developmental dyslexia, *Proc Natl Acad Sci USA* 88:7943-7947, 1991.
21. Victor JD, Conte MM, Burton L, Nass RD: Visual evoked potentials in dyslexics and normals: failure to find a difference in transient or steady-state responses, *Vis Neurosci* 10:939-946, 1993.
22. May JG, Lovegrove WJ, Martin F, Nelson P: Pattern-elicited visual evoked potentials in good and poor readers, *Clin Vis Sci* 6:131-136, 1991.
23. May JG, Dunlop WP, Lovegrove WJ: Factor scores derived from visual evoked potential latencies differentiate good and poor readers, *Clin Vis Sci* 7:67-70, 1992.
24. Lehmkuhle S, Garzia RP, Turner L et al: A defective visual pathway in reading disabled children, *N Engl J Med* 328:989-996, 1993.

11

Reading with an M Neuron: How a Defective Magnocellular Pathway Interferes with Normal Reading

Barbara A. Steinman
Scott B. Steinman
Ralph P. Garzia

Key Terms

visual attention	psychophysics	line-motion illusion
magnocellular	transient attention	attention index
pathway	attentional focus	

The visual system comprises two specialized pathways, the magnocellular (M) and the parvocellular (P). The M pathway preferentially processes rapid-motion, fast-flicker, and gross (low spatial frequency) shapes and can respond even at very low luminance contrasts. The P pathway, on the other hand, best responds to fine details, edges, and isoluminant (color-defined) targets, but it requires higher luminance contrast to be activated. The M pathway has been referred to[1] as the "where" system, and the P pathway the "what" system—that is, the

M pathway helps orient targets in the visual field, while the P pathway helps identify and recognize them.

Recently it has been shown[2-7] that a deficient M pathway is associated with reading disabilities. There are four convergent lines of psychophysical evidence that an M-pathway deficit is associated with reading disability. First, visual persistence for stimuli is prolonged in disabled readers as compared with age-matched normal readers. The duration of this persistence is significantly longer for stimuli of low spatial frequency.[2] A second measure on which the two groups differ is contrast sensitivity. Reading-disabled children are less sensitive to contrast at low spatial frequencies.[3] The third, more direct, measurement of M-pathway function is flicker sensitivity, which has been shown to be reduced in disabled readers compared with normal readers.[4,5] In fact, the differences between the two groups are greater as temporal frequency increases. Deficient temporal resolution among reading-disabled has also been found by a masking-by-light paradigm.[6] The fourth line of evidence comes from studies of metacontrast masking.[7] In metacontrast, a target is briefly presented and is followed at various delays by a spatially adjacent masking stimulus. The accuracy of target identification is determined by the time course of the interaction between the P-pathway (sustained) and M-pathway (transient) components of the visual response. Metacontrast functions in disabled readers have shown the M-pathway response to be weaker and slower.

CLINICAL PEARL

It has been shown that a deficient M pathway is associated with reading disabilities. There are four convergent lines of psychophysical evidence for this.

In this chapter we will present arguments for a fifth line of evidence for the involvement of the M pathway in reading disability—abnormalities in reflexive (stimulus-induced) visual attention.

A number of the psychophysical techniques used to isolate and measure M-pathway activity have been adapted to electrophysiological recordings. The diminished or slowed M-pathway response of disabled readers is reflected in visual evoked potentials (VEPs) with smaller amplitudes[8] and/or longer latencies, primarily with lower spatial frequency stimuli.[9] An M-pathway deficit has also been revealed with a flicker masking paradigm, in which there is a failure to observe a VEP latency increase produced by low spatial frequency targets.[9] With respect to temporal resolution, an M-pathway deficit produces reduced amplitude steady-state VEPs at high temporal frequencies.[10]

The psychophysical and electrophysiological data clearly point to an M-pathway deficit in reading-disabled subjects. Precisely how the deficit affects reading is poorly understood at this time. Thus far, three hypotheses have been advanced. The first of these, Breitmeyer's visual masking model,[11,12] has been discussed most frequently. This model is based on the presence of increased visible persistence in disabled readers due to a reduced inhibition of sustained P-pathway responses by transient M-pathway responses.[13] In normal reading, each fixation-saccade sequence requires integration of information across saccades. M-pathway neurons, stimulated by the saccadic eye movement, inhibit the sustained P response from the previous fixation. Thus information extracted during each fixation is separated from, and not confused with, information seen during the preceding fixation. There is no perceptual overlap but rather a clear temporal segregation of information flow. With a defective M pathway this inhibition is reduced, allowing information from the previous fixation to persist and merge into the current fixation. Increased fixation durations would be required to compensate for sluggish M function to produce clear fixation intervals. Complaints of words running together or overlapping portions of the text with reading may be manifestations of increased visible persistence.

CLINICAL PEARL

The psychophysical and electrophysiological data clearly point to an M-pathway deficit in reading-disabled subjects. Precisely how the deficit affects reading is poorly understood at this time.

The second hypothesis relating M-pathway deficiency and reading disability can be called the saccadic suppression-visual localization hypothesis. Saccadic suppression refers to the fact that vision is impaired during saccades and for a short time before and after the actual eye movement. Readers normally do not see movement or smearing of the text when making saccadic eye movements. The same can be said for any perceived movement in the environment associated with saccades. Although eye movements cause retinal image displacement, the central nervous system can differentiate object movement from eye movement. The mechanism that accounts for this perceptual stability is probably a signal of the intention to move the eyes, also known as corollary discharge or efference copy.[14] This mechanism is probably one of the processes responsible for saccadic suppression.

M-pathway inhibitory processes on the P pathway are thought[12,15] to be responsible for the phenomenon of saccadic suppression. Matin[16] related the maintenance of visual localization to visible persistence. The compensations or adjustments that must occur during saccades to maintain constancy of visual direction occur only after the persistence of visual image from the preceding fixation is eliminated. Decreased M-pathway activation or its delayed activation will also disrupt this mechanism. A defect in these mechanisms might cause visual objects—or words during reading—to appear to move when the eyes move. Even during steady fixation we make miniature eye movements. Some of the sensations of movement reported during reading may be due either to a defect in registration of the changes in eye position per se or to alterations in the processes of combining visual and eye position information.

A third possible mechanism of M-pathway involvement in reading disability involves the disruption of temporal precedence of information flow during the fixation phase of reading.[17] If we accept a global-to-local mode of visual processing (global precedence) mediated by M and P pathways respectively, then at the beginning of a fixation, information is available for processing sooner from the normally faster M pathway than information is from the relatively slower P pathway. The M-pathway processes lower spatial frequency components of text (word shape or length information, or visual gestalts), followed by an analysis of higher spatial frequency content by the P pathway (letter shapes). If this normal order or timing differential is disrupted, then visual difficulties during reading can result that will slow word identification.[17] Both lesion studies of the lateral geniculate nucleus[18] and measurements of average response latencies in the striate cortex[19,20] suggest that the M-derived responses of striate cortex occur 10 to 20 msec before P-derived responses.

There is evidence that the normally faster M pathway is slowed in reading-disabled subjects. Livingstone et al.[10] found that low-contrast N1 components of the VEP were later by 20 to 40 msec in reading-disabled compared with normal readers. Lehmkuhle et al.[9] reported VEPs in the absence of a flickering background to be slightly longer (7 msec) in reading-disabled observers for low spatial frequency targets.

Reports of clinical success using compensatory filters or overlays may be explained by the restoration of temporal precedence of the M pathway by slowing transmission times of the P pathway.[21]

Although there is ample evidence that deficits in the M pathway may be implicated in reading disability, none of the current theories provides a complete explanation of the neurophysiological mechanisms by which this deficit contributes to reading disability. We would like to propose that this neurophysiological mechanism is a deficit in reflexive visual attentional processes, and that it must be differentiated from the disorders of attention observed by teachers in the classroom. Such children are diagnosed with attention deficit disorder

(ADD) and are described as impulsive, lacking sustained attention, unable to selectively attend to relevant stimuli, and hyperactive. ADD is frequently included among the presumed causes of reading and learning disability. There can be little doubt that defects in higher level cognitive and motor attentional control mechanisms delay reading development. However, we will present evidence that deficient low-level visual attentional processes also may disrupt the reading process. To read effectively, a person must move visual attention facilely from word to word, from fovea to parafovea to fovea. These rapid attentional shifts, ostensibly dominated by the M pathway, must operate efficiently to permit effortless reading.

CLINICAL PEARL

Although there is ample evidence that deficits in the M pathway may be implicated in reading disability, none of the current theories provides a complete explanation of the neurophysiological mechanisms by which this deficit contributes to reading disability.

CLINICAL PEARL

Deficient low-level visual attentional processes also may disrupt the reading process. To read effectively, a person must move visual attention facilely from word to word, from fovea to parafovea to fovea. These rapid attentional shifts, ostensibly dominated by the M pathway, must operate efficiently to permit effortless reading.

What Is Visual Attention?

The visual system is continuously bombarded by a steady supply of constantly changing visual stimuli. It is beyond the limits of the visual system to process all of these stimuli simultaneously. To avoid an overload, visual information must be prioritized so the most important stimuli can be detected and identified while others are effectively ignored. This task is accomplished by a neural mechanism called visual attention. When attention is paid to one particular location in the visual field, response times (as measured by reaction speed) for detection and discrimination of visual stimuli in that area are faster.[22-26] Concurrently, response times are slower for stimuli falling in the remaining portions of the visual field.[22,24,27-29] These changes in visual processing speed and accuracy are produced directly by visual attention mechanisms.

CLINICAL PEARL

When attention is paid to one particular location in the visual field, response times (as measured by reaction speed) for detection and discrimination of visual stimuli in that area are faster.

The portion of the visual field in which processing is enhanced is the attentional focus. The attentional focus can be moved independently of eye movement, producing the ability to fixate on one location while attending to another.[12,30] However, when the two are coincident, visual tasks are performed more efficiently. When attentional focus and fixation are at different locations, visual tasks can still be performed but with greater difficulty. Visual attention may be focused by consciously attending to a desired spatial location. This is called voluntary[31] or sustained[32] attention. Attention may also be focused involuntarily as a reflexive response to the onset of a new stimulus within the visual field. The sudden onset of any stimulus is a compelling cue to direct attention.[33] Attention focused by the onset of a cue is called transient[32] stimulus-induced,[31] or reflexive[34] attention. This type of attention allows for quick localization, identification, and response to new and potentially life-threatening stimuli. Unlike voluntary attention, which remains present as long as one can concentrate, reflexive visual attention has a temporary or transient nature. It lasts for only a few hundred milliseconds and then fades.[32,34] Any subsequent stimuli appearing at the same location will be inhibited from producing a strong attentional response for at least 1500 msec. This prevents attention from becoming "stuck" on repeating stimuli such as a blinking light, allowing attention to move on to new and novel stimuli.[35]

CLINICAL PEARL

The portion of the visual field in which processing is enhanced is the attentional focus. The attentional focus can be moved independently of eye movement, producing the ability to fixate on one location while attending to another.

CLINICAL PEARL

Attention focused by the onset of a cue is called transient attention, stimulus-induced attention, or reflexive attention. It allows for quick localization, identification, and response to new and potentially life-threatening stimuli.

Regardless of whether the focus of attention is moved reflexively or voluntarily, it has the same effect on visual processing speed and accuracy—enhancement within the attentional focus and inhibition in the remaining visual field.

Measuring Visual Attention

It is possible to observe and measure these attentionally induced changes in visual processing speed with a visual illusion.[36] The illusion is as follows: immediately after the sudden onset of a cue (e.g., a small dot), a line is displayed adjacent to the cue (Figure 11-1). Even though the entire line is displayed at one time, it does not appear to have been presented in its entirety. Instead, the portion of the line closest to the cue appears first; then, each successively more distal portion of the line is perceived. In other words, the line seems to "grow," with its leading edge moving away from the cue. The induced motion in the line occurs because the cue onset activates visual attention, which then accelerates visual processing speed in the zone adjacent to the cue and then radiates outward. The differential processing speed, faster for portions of the line closest to the cue relative to those portions more distant from the cue, induces the illusion of motion.[31,36]

This illusion has been referred to in the literature as the line-motion illusion.[36-39] When viewed, the illusion of line motion appears to the observer as identical to apparent motion (phi motion), which is produced by actually presenting a line as a series of small line segments in sequence from one end to the other. Both induce the perception of motion from one end of the line to the other. Because of this, it has been hypothesized that the line-motion illusion is simply an extension of the phi motion effect between the cue and line. However, this is not the case—the two types of motion are independent. The line-motion illusion differs from phi motion in several important ways:[31] (1) the line-motion illusion occurs within a single object rather than between two or more objects as in apparent motion; (2) the line-motion illusion can be observed under conditions in which apparent motion between the cue and the line is not seen; (3) apparent motion always moves in a direction from the offset of one stimulus to the onset of another, whereas the line-motion illusion moves away from the cue regardless of whether the cue is onset or offset.

The line-motion illusion is an exciting new tool, not just for demonstrating visual attention but also for quantifying it. Initially, the problem of finding a sensitive and accurate method to measure this illusion presented a stumbling block to scientists who wanted to measure the strength of attention. This has been overcome recently by using the strong resemblance between line-motion illusion and apparent motion. When apparent motion is produced in a line by breaking

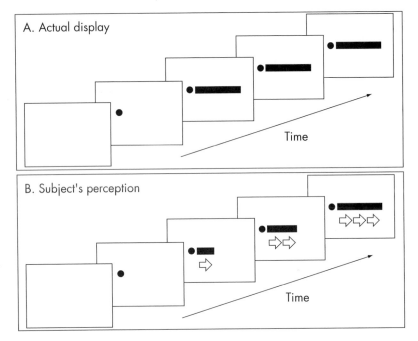

FIGURE 11-1 The line-motion illusion. **A,** A line displayed alone is perceived to appear all at once, not "growing" in either direction. **B,** A line displayed near a visual cue that has recently appeared seems to grow away from the cue. *Open arrows* indicate the direction of the observer's percept of line motion or growth. (From Steinman BA, Steinman SB, Lehmkuhle S: Visual attention mechanisms show a center-surround organization, *Vision Res* 35:1859-1869, 1995.)

the line into a series of small segments and then displaying each in consecutive order from one end of the line to the other, it is indistinguishable from the line-motion illusion (Figure 11-2).

The velocity of the apparent motion in the line can be varied by altering the number of segments and the time between presentations of each segment. The attentionally induced line-motion illusion's velocity can be measured by canceling the illusory motion with the apparent motion. Following presentation of the cue, instead of presenting the target line all at once, the line is presented with apparent motion toward the cue in the opposite direction from the illusory motion.[37] When the velocity of the apparent motion in the line exactly matches that of the illusory line motion, both motions will cancel each other and no motion will be observed in the line.

This motion-nulling technique has been used to determine that the increased speed of visual processing produced by an attentional cue is not uniform across the entire attentional focus. When visual processing speed is plotted as a function of the separation between cue and

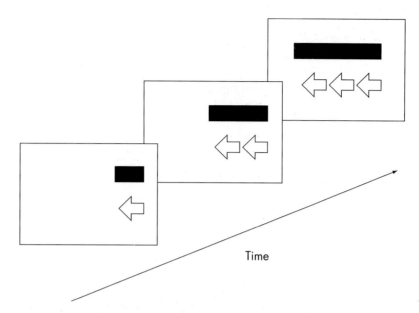

FIGURE 11-2 Apparent motion. The line is broken down into a number of segments. Each segment is displayed in sequence from the right end of the line to the left. As each section of the line is added, the line appears to grow from right to left. *Open arrows* indicate the direction of the observer's percept of line motion or growth.

line, a sharp peak occurs at close cue-line separations that initially drops off rapidly as the separation between cue and probe line enlarges and then more gently until no further increase in processing speed occurs (at about a 3° radius).[37]

Cues are followed by lines that have apparent motion presented at random velocities as well as lines that have no apparent motion. Subjects' perceptions of the motion in these lines are compared with those for similar lines that are not preceded by a cue. The differences in strength and direction of the perceived motion in the presence versus in the absence of a cue are used to calculate an Attention Index score.[40] The trials with apparent motion are used as distracter trials to prevent a subject from anticipating motion in any one direction relative to the cue. These distracter trials help determine the subject's accuracy in correctly reporting the direction of the line motion.

As an example of how the Attention Index is calculated, consider the hypothetical case in which a subject reports that a line not preceded by a cue appears to grow to the left 48% of the time and to the right 52% of the time. When no cue is presented, the subject should guess the direction of line motion and report seeing motion to the left and to the right about equally as often. On the other hand, when the target line is preceded by a cue on its right side, the line now is reported to grow in a leftward direction 87% of the time and when preceded by a cue on its left to grow rightward 94% of the time. Therefore, the effect of using a cue on the right side is to increase the percept of leftward line growth by 39% (87–48). Likewise, the effect of a cue on the left is to increase the percept of rightward line growth by 42% (94–52). The calculated Attention Index scores are therefore +39 for a rightward cue and +42 for a leftward.

The Attention Index score provides a measure of the strength of the attentional percept—the higher the Attention Index score, the stronger the percept and therefore the stronger the attentional effect—and allows for measurement of the direction of a line-motion illusion by its sign. When a cue produces accelerated processing speed, the line motion is away from the cue and a positive Attention Index score is generated. Conversely, slowed visual processing produces line motion toward the cue and results in negative Attention Index scores.

Spatial Distribution of Attention across the Visual Field

Figure 11-3 is the plot of visual Attention Index scores across the visual field at an optimal time interval between the cue and line (50 msec) for three subjects. In all subjects the direction of the illusory line motion reversed at cue-line separations larger than the limits of the attentional focus, indicating a slowing of visual processing outside the focus.[34] The curve resembles a typical "Mexican hat" difference-of-gaussians (DOG) shape of on-center/off-surround receptive fields found throughout the visual system.[41] The final panel of Figure 11-3 shows a DOG curve fitted to the data. The close approximation of the data with the DOG curve suggests that the visual attention mechanisms, like other neural substrates of the visual system, have an on-center/off-surround nature. The center of the attentional "receptive field" would correspond to the attentional focus—the central excitatory zone in which visual processing speed is enhanced as demonstrated by positive Attention Index scores. The large surround region would encompass the entire remaining visual field. In this inhibitory zone, visual processing speed is slowed down, resulting in negative Attention Index scores.

CLINICAL PEARL

The visual attention mechanisms, like other neural substrates of the visual system, have an on-center/off-surround nature. The center of the attentional "receptive field" would correspond to the attentional focus—the central excitatory zone in which visual processing speed is enhanced.

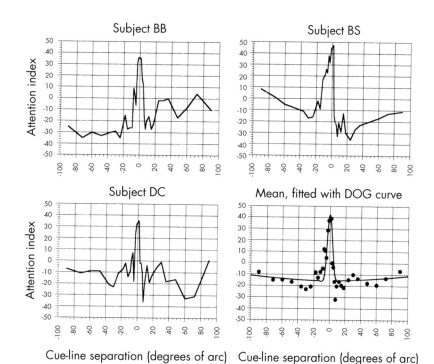

FIGURE 11-3 Attention index measurements across the visual field. Measurements for three subjects at a 50 msec cue lead time reveal an attentional function with an on-center/off-surround shape similar to that of numerous visual receptive fields. Positive cue-line separations indicate cues displayed on the right side of the line, and negative cue-line separations indicate results for cues to the left of the line. The positive central peak denotes a zone of accelerated visual processing speed, the attentional focus. The surrounding negative scores indicate that visual processing is slowed or inhibited. The *final panel* shows mean scores for all three subjects. *Closed circles* indicate the subjects' mean scores, while the *line* denotes the best-fitting DOG curve. (From Steinman BA, Steinman SB, Lehmkuhle S: Visual attention mechanisms show a center-surround organization, *Vision Res* 35:1859-1869, 1995.)

Parallel Processing and Visual Attention

In addition to revealing the shape of the visual attention response, the line motion illusion provides a tool to examine which properties of visual cues best "catch" our attention, which in turn invites speculation about the involvement of the magnocellular (M) and parvocellular (P) pathways.

As the pathway that provides localization information and has the more rapid transmission speeds, the M pathway is a logical candidate to initiate the attentional response by providing information necessary to rapidly move the attentional focus to the correct location. The M pathway provides a conduit through which visually significant objects can rapidly attract attention and be subsequently fixated.[42] It also has previously been suggested[13] to be the source of information about cue location for the voluntary visual attention mechanism. If the conscious direction of attention relies on M-pathway information, the reflexive attentional mechanisms must rely upon it even more heavily, because they require even faster transmission times and respond most strongly to sudden changes of stimuli. The "where" information provided by the M pathway may provide a powerful trigger to generate this response as quickly as possible so it has benefits for the survival of the viewer.

CLINICAL PEARL

The M pathway is a logical candidate to initiate the attentional response. It conducts the information necessary for rapid movement of the attentional focus to the correct location.

Indirect evidence supporting M-pathway involvement in visual attention includes the fact that cues of various modalities (color, luminance, stereopsis, and motion) can produce attentional effects, but the effects are subjectively stronger for luminance-defined cues than for color-defined cues.[38] Additionally, deficits in attention have been linked[43] to the posterior parietal cortex, a target of M-pathway projections.

A recent study using the line motion illusion[44] directly explored the possibility that the M pathway mediates reflexive visual attention. Cues were used that selectively biased the responses of the visual system to either the M or the P pathway. Attention Index scores were measured for each type of stimulus individually.

Because the M pathway is most sensitive to low-contrast and low spatial frequencies and is relatively color blind,[45,46] low-contrast gray cues of ample size were used to preferentially activate it. The P pathway is most sensitive to high spatial frequencies and colors, so finely detailed isoluminant chromatic cues were used to preferentially activate it. High-contrast black cues were used as a control stimulus to activate both pathways. Although manipulation of cue properties cannot exclusively activate either the M or the P pathway, it can bias responses so that one pathway will be favored over the other. Differential activation of visual attention by these pathways would be expected to produce different line motion percepts that vary according to cue type.

Figure 11-4 shows the Attention Index scores for five subjects in whom individual high-contrast (M and P), low-contrast (M), and isoluminant (P) cues were plotted against cue lead times (the delay between the cue and the line) and cue-line separation. The strength of attention produced by low-contrast cues was not significantly different from that produced by high-contrast cues. However, the attentional response to an isoluminant cue was much weaker. Surprisingly, the low-contrast cues were much less visible than the isoluminant cues. This is highly significant, because it shows that even barely visible stimuli that activate the M pathway elicit stronger attentional responses than very visible cues do that preferentially stimulate the P system.

Not only do these two pathways differ in terms of the magnitude of an attentional response that they can elicit, they also differ in terms of the spatial extent of their attentional responses. High-contrast cues produced a robust attentional response extending to cue-line separations of 5.5° ± 0.5°. Conversely, the greatest cue-line separation over which isoluminant cues produced line motion was smaller, only 3.2° ± 0.51°.

However, it might be argued that, because the M pathway always processes faster than the P pathway, attention would be dominated by the pathway that reaches the cortical attention pathways first. To test this, the same experiment was repeated at the cue-line separation that produced the strongest attentional response (1.5°), but the isoluminant cue was given a "head start" of 17 or 33 msec to allow information from the P pathway to reach the cortex first. However, regardless of this head start, the dominant percept of line motion remained in a direction away from the low-contrast cue, although the strength of the percept was somewhat degraded.

Visual Attention and Reading Disability

Because M-pathway deficits have been implicated in reading disability, the link between visual attention and the M pathway leads to the conjecture that compromised visual attention may be a factor in reading disability. Early results in our laboratory suggest that it probably is.

CLINICAL PEARL

Because M-pathway deficits have been implicated in reading disability, the link between visual attention and the M pathway leads to the conjecture that compromised visual attention may be a factor in reading disability.

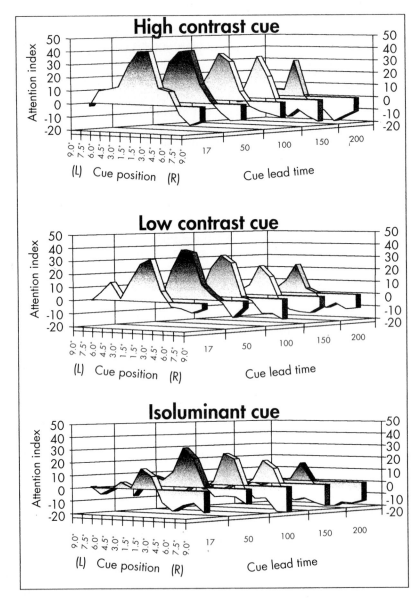

FIGURE 11-4 High-contrast, low-contrast, and isoluminant Attention Index plots. At all cue lead times and cue line separations, responses to low-contrast cues were only slightly less than those for high-contrast cues. Responses to isoluminant cues were significantly weaker and were elicited over a smaller radius than either high- or low-contrast cues. Positive cue-line separations indicate cues displayed on the right side of the line, and negative cue-line separations cues to the left of the line. (From Steinman BA, Steinman BS, Lehmkuhle S: Visual attention is dominated by the M stream, *Vision Res* [In press].)

We measured visual attention in a 30-year-old woman with a lifelong history of reading problems.[47] A standard optometric examination indicated no evidence of past or present refractive error, binocular vision anomalies, or ocular health problem that could account for her reading difficulty. The presence of a reading disability was confirmed with the Nelson-Denny reading test, which showed a reading comprehension 2 years below her vocabulary. In addition, scores on the vertical subtest of the Developmental Eye Movement test were more than four standard deviations below normal. The Boder Test of Reading-Spelling Patterns indicated a mixed dysphonetic and dyseidectic dyslexia, but with more phonetic spelling errors. A visual evoked potential recording showed the absence of flicker masking, an indication of a deficit in the M pathway.

The Attention Index scores for this patient are shown in Figures 11-5 and 11-6, along with the mean scores for five normal adult readers. Figure 11-5 shows the progression of peak values of the attention function (averaging together the two maximum points) for cue-line separations between −1.5° and +1.5° as a function of cue lead time from 17 to 200 msec before the target line presentation. Initially

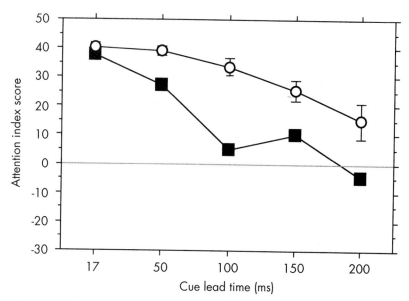

FIGURE 11-5 The temporal course of attention in a reading disabled subject. *Open circles* represent the average attention index scores for five normal readers. *Closed squares* denote scores for a reading-disabled 30-year-old woman. Initially, following the cue, there is no difference in the amount of attention produced. However, attention deteriorates much faster in the reading-disabled subject.

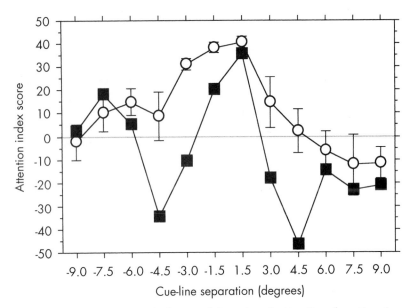

FIGURE 11-6 The spatial shape of the visual attention function in a reading-disabled subject. *Open circles* represent the average attention index scores for five normal readers. *Closed squares* denote scores for the same reading-disabled 30-year-old woman as in Figure 11-5. The attentional focus is significantly narrowed and surrounded by a zone of strong suppression in the reading-disabled subject. However, at separations of greater than 6.0° the attentional surround is not significantly different from that in normal readers.

(at the 17 msec cue lead time), the reading-disabled subject demonstrates the same strength of attentional response as the normal readers. However, attention quickly deteriorated in this subject so that little attention response can be measured at 100 msec. In normal readers the strength of visual attention does not deteriorate to the same degree, even at delays as long as 200 msec, which suggests that in reading disability the attentional focus cannot be maintained as long as in normal subjects.

Figure 11-6 is a plot of Attention Index scores as a function of cue-line separations from −9.0% to +9.0% for the same subjects at the optimal 50 msec cue lead time. The reading-disabled subject differs significantly from normal subjects in two fundamental ways: (1) the attentional focus is much narrower in extent and (2) the degree of suppression in the surround region outside the attentional focus is much stronger over a range of 4.5° cue-line separation. At greater separations, the differences between normal and reading-disabled subjects diminish. The restriction of the zone of abnormal visual attention to the center of the attentional receptive field suggests that it is primarily the central excitatory attentional processes that are affected in reading-disabled subjects, with little to no deficit of the surrounding inhibitory attentional processes. In other words, the reading disabled may be unable to activate a strong positive attentional response at the cued location. This has the effect of unmasking negative attention that is also present at that location but normally overridden by the stronger attentional focus. The result is that reading-disabled subjects are left with a weak attentional focus and more pronounced inhibition just outside the focus. Such a dissociation between the effects of visual processing disorders on excitatory and inhibitory processes has been demonstrated previously[48] in other visual defects such as amblyopia.

The strong zone of suppressed attention flanking the attentional focus could explain the finding[49] that severely reading-disabled subjects have better performance on letter identification tasks for letters at least 5° from fixation compared to letters 2.5° from fixation. It might also help explain the erratic eye movements of reading-disabled subjects in shifting fixation from one word of text to the next.

These data provide the first evidence that visual attention may be the mechanism through which M-pathway deficits exert their influence on reading. In reading, the eyes and attentional focus fixate on a word. Attentional mechanisms then must locate and move the attentional focus to a new point a short distance to the right of fixation to pick up the next word. Once attention has moved to the new point, a saccade is made moving the eyes to the new location.[50,51] Recent evidence[52] has shown that the M pathway is suppressed during saccadic eye movements. When the saccade is completed, the M pathway is again activated and the visual system can take in words or portions of words falling within the new attentional focus.

CLINICAL PEARL

Visual attention may be the mechanism through which M-pathway deficits exert their influence on reading.

A narrowing of the spatial extent of attentional focus and the strong inhibitory surround in disabled readers would make parafoveal words difficult to process and direct saccades too, causing difficulty in keeping place when reading. It might also be possible that these inhibitory effects make the formerly fixated word relatively more salient, resulting in the "smearing" together of words. This effect may explain the patient of Rayner et al.[53] with selective attentional dyslexia. These authors described an adult who had had a reported history of reading difficulties from childhood. Reading rate was substantially improved when parafoveal vision was restricted with a mask. This was interpreted to mean that letters from words in the parafovea interfered with processing of the foveally fixated word.

The release from suppression of the M pathway after a saccadic eye movement would produce the same stimulation of attentional mechanisms as the sudden onset of a visual cue, generating a reflexive attentional response. Because this reflexive response lasts for a shorter time, as seen in our reading-disabled subject, there would be less time during which words within the attentional focus could be processed. If the time provided by reflexive attention is not sufficient to process the word, the reader is forced to invoke conscious attention to read any remaining characters. This would require greater effort and concentration from the reader to keep the attentional focus in the correct location, making reading that much more difficult.

References

1. Ungerleider LG, Mishkin M: Two cortical visual systems. In Ingle DJ, Goodale MA, Mansfield RJW (eds): *Analysis of visual behavior,* Cambridge, Mass, 1982, MIT Press.
2. Lovegrove WJ, Heddle M, Slaghuis W: Reading disability: spatial frequency specific deficits in information store, *Neuropsychologia* 18:111-115, 1980.
3. Lovegrove WJ, Martin F, Bowling A et al: Contrast sensitivity functions and specific reading disability, *Neuropsychologia* 20:309-315, 1982.
4. Martin F, Lovegrove WJ: Flicker contrast sensitivity in normal and specifically disabled readers, *Perception* 16:215-221, 1987.
5. Martin F, Lovegrove WJ: Uniform-field flicker masking in control and specifically-disabled readers, *Perception* 17:203-214, 1988.
6. Williams M, LeCluyse K, Bologna N: Masking by light as a measure of visual integration time and persistence in normal and disabled readers, *Clin Vis Sci* 5:335-343, 1990.
7. Williams MC, Molinet K, LeCluyse K: Visual masking as a measure of temporal processing in normal and disabled readers, *Clin Vis Sci* 4:137-144, 1989.
8. May JG, Lovegrove WJ, Martin F, Nelson P: Pattern-elicited visual evoked potentials in good and poor readers, *Clin Vis Sci* 6:131-136, 1991.
9. Lehmkuhle S, Garzia RP, Turner L et al: A defective visual pathway in reading disabled children, *N Engl J Med* 328:989-996, 1993.
10. Livingston MS, Rosen GD, Drislane FW, Galaburda AM: Physiological and anatomical evidence for a magnocellular defect in developmental dyslexia, *Proc Nat Acad Sci USA* 88:7943-7947, 1991.
11. Breitmeyer BG: *Visual masking: an integrated approach,* New York, 1984, Oxford University Press.
12. Breitmeyer BG: Reality and relevance of sustained and transient channels in reading and reading disability. In Schmid R, Zambarbieri D (eds): *Oculomotor control and cognitive processes,* Amsterdam, 1991, Elsevier/North-Holland.
13. Breitmeyer BG, Ganz L: Implications of sustained and transient channels for theories of visual pattern masking, saccadic suppression, and information processing, *Psychol Rev* 83:1-36, 1976.
14. von Holst E: Relations between the central nervous system and the peripheral organs, *Br J Anim Behav,* pp 89-94, 1954.
15. Matin E: Saccadic suppression: a review and analysis, *Psychol Bull* 81:899-917, 1974.

16. Matin L: Visual localization and eye movements. In Boff KR, Kaufman L, Thomas JP (eds): *Handbook of perception and human performance. Vol 1, Sensory processes and perception,* New York, 1986, John Wiley.
17. Lehmkuhle S: Neurological basis of visual processes in reading. In Willows DM, Kruk R, Corcos E (eds): *Visual processes in reading and reading disabilities,* Hillsdale, NJ, 1993, Lawrence Erlbaum.
18. Maunsell JHR, Gibson JR: Visual response latencies in striate cortex of the macaque monkey, *J Neurophysiol* 68:1332-1344, 1992.
19. Marrocco RT: Sustained and transient cells in monkey lateral geniculate nucleus: conduction velocities and response properties, *J Neurophysiol* 39:340-353, 1976.
20. Novak LG, Munk MJH, Girard P, Bullier J: Visual latencies in areas V1 and V2 of the macaque monkey, *Vis Neurosci* 12:371-384, 1995.
21. Williams MC, May JG, Solman R, Zhou H: The effects of spatial filtering and contrast reduction on visual search times in good and poor readers, *Vision Res* 35:285-291, 1995.
22. Posner MI, Cohen Y, Rafal RD: Neural systems control of spatial orienting, *Phil Trans R Soc Lond* B298:187-198, 1982.
23. Eriksen CW, Collins JF: Temporal course of selective attention, *J Exp Psychol* 80:254-261, 1969.
24. Downing CJ, Pinker S (eds): *The spatial structure of visual attention,* Hillsdale, NJ, 1985, Lawrence Erlbaum.
25. Tsal Y: Movements of attention across the visual field, *J Exp Psychol* 9:523-530, 1983.
26. Eriksen CW, St. James JD: Visual attention within and around the field of focal attention: a zoom lens model, *Percept Psychophys* 40:225-240, 1986.
27. Posner MI, Boies SJ: Components of attention, *Psychol Rev* 78:391-408, 1971.
28. Posner MI: *Psychobiology of attention,* New York, 1975, Academic Press.
29. Posner MI, Snyder CRR (eds): *Facilitation and inhibition in the processing of signals,* New York, 1976, Academic Press.
30. James W: *The principles of psychology,* New York, 1890, Holt.
31. Hikosaka O, Miyauchi S, Shimojo S: Voluntary and stimulus-induced attention detected as motion sensation, *Perception* 22:517-526, 1993.
32. Nakayama K, Mackeben M: Sustained and transient components of focal visual attention, *Vision Res* 29:1631-1647, 1989.
33. Yantis S, Jonides J: Abrupt visual onsets and selective attention: evidence from visual search, *J Exp Psychol Hum Percept Perform* 10:601-621, 1984.
34. Steinman BA, Steinman SB, Lehmkuhle S: Visual attention mechanisms show a center-surround organization, *Vision Res* 35:1859-1869, 1995.
35. Posner MI, Cohen Y (eds): *Components of visual orienting,* Hillsdale, NJ, 1984, Lawrence Erlbaum.
36. Hikosaka O, Miyauchi S, Shimojo S: Focal visual attention produces motion sensation in lines, *Invest Ophthalmol Vis Sci Suppl* 32:716, 1991.
37. Miyauchi S, Hikosaka O, Shimojo S: Visual attention field can be assessed by illusory line motion sensation, *Invest Ophthalmol Vis Sci Suppl* 33:1262, 1992.
38. Faubert J, vonGrünau M: Split-attention and attribute priming in motion induction, *Invest Ophthalmol Vis Sci Suppl* 33:1139, 1992.
39. Von Grünau M, Faubert J: Intra- and inter-attribute motion induction, *Perception* (In press).
40. Steinman SB, Steinman BA, Trick GL, Lehmkuhle S: A sensory explanation for visual attention deficits in the elderly, *Optom Vis Sci* 71:743-749, 1994.
41. Enroth-Cugell C, Robson DG: The contrast sensitivity of retinal ganglion cells of the cat, *J Physiol* 187:517-552, 1966.
42. Lennie P: Roles of M and P pathways. In Shapley R, Lam DK (eds): *Contrast sensitivity,* Cambridge, Mass, 1993, MIT Press.
43. Husain M: *Visuospatial and visuomotor functions of the posterior parietal lobe,* London, 1991, Macmillan Press.

44. Steinman BA, Steinman SB, Lehmkuhle S: Visual attention is dominated by the M stream, *Vision Res* (In press).
45. DeYoe EA, VanEssen DC: Concurrent processing streams in monkey visual cortex, *Trends Neurosci* 11:219-226, 1988.
46. Schiller PH, Logothetis NK, Charles ER: Role of color-opponent and broad-band channels in vision, *Vis Neurosci* 5:321-346, 1990.
47. Steinman BA, Garzia RP, Lehmkuhle S, Steinman SB: Transient visual attention deficit in a reading disabled adult, *Optom Vis Sci Suppl* 71:106, 1994.
48. Levi DM, Harwerth RS, Manny RE: Suprathreshold spatial frequency detection and binocular interaction in strabismic and anisometropic amblyopia, *Invest Ophthalmol Vis Sci* 18:714-735, 1979.
49. Geiger G, Lettvin JY: Peripheral vision in persons with dyslexia, *N Engl J Med* 316:1238-1243, 1987.
50. Shepard M, Findlay JM, Hockey RJ: The relationship between eye movements and spatial attention, *Q J Exp Psychol* 38(A):475-491, 1986.
51. Sereno AB: Programming saccades: the role of attention. In Rayner K (ed): *Eye movements and visual cognition,* New York, 1992, Springer-Verlag.
52. Burr DC, Morrone MC, Ross J: Selective suppression of the magnocellular visual pathway during saccadic eye movements, *Nature* 371:511-513, 1994.
53. Rayner K, Murphy LA, Henderson JM, Pollatsek A: Selective attentional dyslexia, *Cogn Neuropsychol* 6:357-378, 1989.

12

A Framework for Understanding Learning Difficulties and Disabilities*

Dale M. Willows

Key Terms

normal variation	language processing	visual processing
subtypes	spatial-numerical	deficits
symbol coding		

This chapter and the following are companion chapters: the first sets out a framework or working model for understanding learning difficulties and disabilities, and the second offers guidelines for assessment and programming for reading and writing difficulties based on that framework. The present chapter is directed to those who are interested in understanding the role that various types of processing deficits—including visual processing deficits—might play in reading, writing, and mathematics difficulties. The chapter can stand alone and is intended to be of interest to anyone reflecting on the potential causes of academic difficulties. Understanding of the next chapter, on assessment and programming for reading and writing difficulties, is,

*The author is grateful to Margie Golick and Sybil Schwartz for the inspiration to reflect on the nature of learning disabilities and to Karen Sumbler and Esther Geva for their construtive comments on an earlier draft on this chapter.

however, dependent on the framework presented here. The reference list at the end of this chapter includes the theory-based literature on which the framework is based, while the reference list and appendix at the end of the next chapter include books, articles, and materials relevant to the practical problems of assessment and programming.

A "Normal Variation" View of Learning Difficulties

Individuals who experience significant difficulties learning to read, write, or do mathematics—despite average general intelligence, normal educational opportunity, and a supportive social-emotional environment—have traditionally been referred to in the literature as "learning disabled." Much of the literature has conceptualized learning disabilities within a medical model, such that individuals with learning disabilities have been viewed as suffering from some type of neurological defect, and medical terminology such as *dyslexia, dysgraphia,* and *dyscalculia* has been coined to refer to difficulties in reading, writing, and mathematics, respectively. Although the use of medical terminology would suggest that there is a particular syndrome and etiology characteristic of individuals who are dyslexic, dysgraphic, or dyscalculic, there is, in fact, no generally accepted symptomatology associated with each of these terms other than a significant difficulty in the area implied by the term. The only widely accepted definition of any of these terms is an operational one: If an individual is substantially behind others of similar age in learning to read, write, or do mathematics (usually a delay of 2 or more years being the criterion)—despite average general intelligence, normal educational opportunity, and a supportive social-emotional environment—he or she may be said to qualify as learning disabled (in general) or as dyslexic, dysgraphic, or dyscalculic (in particular). On the basis of this type of operational definition, individuals whose test scores are ½ year or 1 year or even 1½ years below grade level in one or more of these domains do not "qualify" as learning disabled and are, by default, considered "normal." In fact, however, there is no demonstrable break in the distribution of scores on tests of reading, writing, or mathematics between so-called "learning disabled" and "normal" individuals; a full range of scores is represented in typical educational contexts.

CLINICAL PEARL

Individuals who experience significant difficulties learning to read, write, or do mathematics—despite average general intelligence, normal educational opportunity, and a supportive social-emotional environment—have traditionally been referred to in the literature as "learning disabled."

The framework developed in this chapter is based on the assumption that learning difficulties and disabilities—problems in learning to read, write, and do mathematics—are distributed along a continuum from mild difficulty to extreme disability.* Such an assumption seems warranted not only because an arbitrary distinction between individuals with learning difficulties and individuals with learning disabilities has not been justified in the literature but also because a variety of evidence is converging to support a "normal variation" view (in which difficulties and disabilities are conceptualized as reflecting quantitative rather than qualitative differences between individuals). This perspective is consistent with Levine's explanation of learning disorders[1] as an expression of developmental variation in basic cognitive and linguistic processes. It is also consistent with the recent findings of Shaywitz et al.[2] who have presented data showing that reading ability is normally distributed within the population, in contradistinction to the traditional medical model view that "reading disability" or "dyslexia" is a biologically based disorder distinct from less specific "garden variety" reading problems.† Finally, the position that the reading disabled are different in degree rather than in kind from poor readers and normally achieving readers is supported by evidence from the experimental literature comparing "less skilled" and "skilled" readers. An examination of this research demonstrates that the processing domains distinguishing these two groups, both "within the normal range," are the same ones that distinguish "disabled" from "normal" readers in other studies.[3]

Subtyping Versus an Individual-Differences Perspective on Learning Disabilities

Just as varying strengths in a number of domains may contribute to skillful learning, differing degrees of weakness in these areas may result in learning difficulties. To examine the possibility of differences among individuals in the types of processing deficits underlying

---

*This is not to say that there are no distinctive cases. Clearly some rare "hole-in-the-head" cases exist in which the symptoms of learning disability are idiosyncratic. For example, instances of mirror writing, in which a learning-disabled individual writes *entirely* in mirror orientation, have occasionally been documented in the literature. When such cases arise, however, it is usually assumed that the symptoms reflect some type of brain injury rather than a variation on the normal pattern. Although mirror image "reversal" is common in both the reading and the writing of learning-disabled individuals and of young children in the beginning stages of written language, such orientation confusions are very inconsistent in these situations.
†Although not all learning disabilities involve reading and writing problems, the vast majority do. Thus, much of the literature in the field of learning disabilities has focused on written language disabilities, especially reading disabilities, because these are the most frequent and most disabling school learning problems.

learning disabilities, clinicians and researchers have attempted to determine whether there might be relatively homogeneous "subtypes" among the learning disabled. A variety of approaches have been used to explore this possibility, ranging from subjective clinical judgments to more objective multivariate statistical techniques. There is now a large literature on this topic, including several large-scale subtyping studies.[4,5] Based on a clinical approach, Mattis[6,7] and Mattis et al.[8] reported subtypes of reading-disabled individuals with (1) articulatory and graphomotor dyscoordination, (2) language deficit, and (3) visual-spatial perceptual disorder. Based on a statistical subtyping approach involving cluster analysis, Watson and Willows[9] obtained the following three clusters of reading-disabled subjects: (1) a group with weak short-term auditory memory and sound-symbol knowledge, (2) a group with the same deficits as cluster 1 plus visual processing/memory deficiencies, and (3) a group with the same deficits as cluster 1 plus deficits in visual processing and rapid automatized naming. Also using the statistical technique of cluster analysis, but examining a relatively unselected sample of learning disabled children, Morris and Satz[10] and Satz and Morris[11] identified subtypes with impairments in (1) global language, (2) specific language—naming, (3) global language and perception, and (4) visual-perceptual motor processing. Satz and Morris[11] commented further that these four subtypes confirm the clinical finding that language problems, some type of visual problem, and mixed problems can all be associated with learning disability. Taken together, the subtyping literature has produced considerable evidence that a variety of factors must be involved in learning disabilities, but no set of subtypes has emerged consistently from the studies.

CLINICAL PEARL

Taken together, the subtyping literature has produced considerable evidence that a variety of factors must be involved in learning disabilities, but no set of subtypes has emerged consistently from the studies.

There are a number of possible explanations for the failure to find consistent patterns in the search for subtypes of learning disability, one of which is the diversity of methodologies and conceptual frameworks in the literature. Because the selection criteria for the learning-disabled samples, the test batteries used, and the approaches taken in determining subtypes have varied widely, the findings could not be expected to be comparable from study to study.[12] Another explanation that follows from the discussion of the normal-variation conceptualization in the preceding section is that the differences in learning abilities of those who have "disabilities," "difficulties," and "normal" functioning might be more parsimoniously described in terms of multifaceted individual variation along cognitive, linguistic, and other processing dimensions. Implicit in many of the subtyping studies is the all-or-none assumption that an individual either "fits" a subtype or does not. An alternative perspective is that all individuals vary on a range of processing dimensions and that their specific learning strengths and weaknesses on particular tasks such as reading, writing, and mathematics reflect a potentially unique product or interaction of their various processing abilities.

Given that each learning task involves certain information-processing demands, a rational approach to conceptualizing learning difficulties and disabilities is to consider how well an individual's particular pattern of information-processing strengths and weaknesses fits with the demands of learning tasks like reading, writing, or doing mathematics. Such processing demands undoubtedly vary depending on the learning stage and the particular facet of the task considered. For example, in reading and writing acquisition the processing demands change as skill develops.[13,14] In the early stages, recognizing and recalling the visual forms of letters and words is an attention-demanding component of the learning task, whereas later, when word recognition is automatized, more cognitive resources can be allocated to the processing of sentence and passage meanings. Similarly, in mathematics the ability to memorize number facts might be relatively important for success in simple arithmetic but be largely irrelevant to the manipulation of shapes in space required to excel in geometry.

CLINICAL PEARL

In reading and writing acquisition, the processing demands change as skill develops. In the early stages, recognizing and recalling the visual forms of letters and words is an attention-demanding component of the learning task, whereas later, when word recognition is automatized, more cognitive resources can be allocated to the processing of sentence and passage meanings.

A Framework for Understanding Reading, Writing, and Mathematics Difficulties

Based on a normal-variation assumption, difficulties and disabilities in reading, writing, and mathematics can thus be understood by analyzing each learning task into its particular set of demands and comparing an individual's processing abilities against the demands of that task. In areas where an individual is deficient in the type of processing involved in a learning task, that individual would be expected to have a corresponding deficit in learning or achievement.

When the general findings from the subtyping literature and the evidence from information-processing literature in the field of learning disabilities are viewed together, it is possible to generate constellations of processing weaknesses that seem to characterize the problems of most individuals with learning difficulties and disabilities. In the framework or working model developed here, three "areas of difficulty" are proposed as underlying the problems of individuals with reading, writing, and mathematics difficulties and disabilities—Area 1, symbol-coding difficulty; Area 2, language-processing difficulty; and Area 3, spatial-numerical difficulty. The first two are common sources of difficulty among individuals with school learning problems, while the third is a relatively less frequent source of difficulty. Individuals with reading, writing, or mathematics problems may have a weakness in one, two, or all three of these areas, but the nature of their difficulties will reflect their areas of processing weakness. In Figure 12-1 the processing difficulties associated with Areas 1, 2, and 3 are represented by three intersecting circles, with a gradient of shading ranging from very light to very dark representing degrees of processing difficulty (from mild to severe) in each of these areas.

CLINICAL PEARL

Three "areas of difficulty" are proposed as underlying the problems of individuals with reading, writing, and mathematics difficulties and disabilities—Area 1, symbol-coding difficulty; Area 2, language-processing difficulty; and Area 3, spatial-numerical difficulty.

The processing weaknesses of the vast majority of individuals with reading and writing difficulties can be represented in the combined area defined by the first two intersecting circles, Areas 1 and 2. The degree of difficulty in written language acquisition would be the product of an individual's symbol-coding and language-processing difficulties. Although some individuals' reading and writing problems may reflect only a symbol-coding or a language-processing difficulty, each of which can vary in severity, a significant portion of children with written language difficulties and disabilities have, to some degree, processing weaknesses of both types. The darker shading in the area of overlap between symbol-coding and language-processing difficulties represents the assumption that individuals who have processing weaknesses of both types, particularly if their processing

**Areas of Processing Difficulty
Contributing to
Written Language Difficulty**

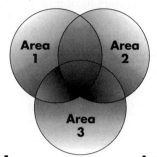

**Area 1:
Symbol-coding
difficulty**
Decoding and encoding of:

Letters
Orthographic patterns
Whole words

**Area 2:
Language-processing
difficulty**
Reception and expression of:

Phonology
Morphology
Semantics and syntax

**Area 3:
Spatial-numerical difficulty**
Processing of:

Visual-spatial information
Visual-motor integration
Numerical concepts

* Note: shading represents degree of difficulty,
ranging from mild (lightest) to severe (darkest).

FIGURE 12-1 A framework for understanding learning difficulties
and disabilities.

weaknesses are severe, would be less able to compensate by relying on
strengths in the other area.

In the context of this framework, the term *learning disabled* is a
relative one. Whether a particular degree of processing weakness is
considered disabling seems to depend on both its severity and the
demands of the learning task. Moreover, a range of affective factors
(e.g., self-efficacy, motivation, interest) undoubtedly modulates the
expression of these difficulties, rendering their effects more or less
disabling. In addition, the extent to which a teaching program accom-
modates to individuals' specific patterns of strengths and weaknesses
at various stages probably determines, in part, whether difficulties
become disabilities. The processing weaknesses themselves are assumed to represent **fairly stable individual differences,** but their

effects might range considerably.* The same combination of process-ing weaknesses may play a major role, a minor role, or an insignificant role in an individual's level of learning and achievement depending upon which component of a task is involved and the particular stage in development of skill.

CLINICAL PEARL

The term learning disabled *is a relative one. Whether a particular degree of processing weakness is considered disabling seems to depend on both its severity and the demands of the learning task.*

Area 1: Symbol-Coding Difficulties

Although the mechanisms are not yet well understood, evidence is converging from theory-based research on reading acquisition and reading disabilities that the primary problem of children with reading difficulties and disabilities is decoding and encoding the alphabetical symbols to oral language. A very large portion of children who experience some degree of difficulty in learning to read, spell, and write share the characteristic that they do not process letters, ortho-graphic (i.e., spelling) patterns (the building blocks of words), and whole words in context-free conditions as quickly and accurately as other children do.[15-19]

CLINICAL PEARL

Evidence is converging from theory-based research on reading acquisition and reading disabilities that the primary problem of children with reading difficulties is decoding and encoding the alphabetical symbols to oral language.

The characteristic processing weakness associated with symbol coding has been variously described[20-22] as a deficit in phonemic analysis, in phonemic awareness, and in phonological encoding. Whereas children who have real strengths in the symbol-coding area seem to extract the symbol-sound patterns of the written language

---

*In a sense, the distinction between the medical-model view and the present individual-differences view may be more semantic than real, because the individual-differences view does not deny a possible, indeed probable, neurological/genetic origin for many learning difficulties and disabilities. The key distinction is between the medical-model notion that an individual is either abnormal (i.e., dyslexic, dysgraphic, dyscalculic, etc.) or normal and the individual-differences view that all humans differ on a whole range of information-processing dimensions, many of which may be constitutional and most of which probably have some effect on their learning and functioning in the world.

with relatively little instruction, children with processing weaknesses in the same area have extreme difficulty learning the letter-sound associations required to decode and encode words, even when they have intensive direct instruction.[23] Such individuals are insensitive to the orthographic patterns of the written language so that even though there are common spelling patterns such as *ph, ght, ow, er* that carry information about the pronunciation of words, individuals with symbol-coding difficulties often fail to make use of these patterns to decode new words or pseudowords and to spell words.[23-25]

If we ask, "What is the underlying cause of these phonological coding difficulties?" again there are a number of potential "candidates" to explain them. Deficits in short-term or working memory, verbal efficiency, auditory temporal perception, naming automaticity, and basic visual processes might play some role; or, perhaps, some even more fundamental factor such as processing capacity, speed of processing, or attention might be involved.[26-30] Although it is clearly too early to draw firm conclusions concerning the underlying mechanisms, there is fairly general agreement that some type of weakness in symbol coding is central to written language difficulties and disabilities. Moreover, the more serious the weakness in symbol coding, the more severe is the difficulty in learning to read, spell, and write.

The concept of "specific" reading disability reflects the fact that there appears to be a discrepancy between the oral and written language-processing abilities of many individuals. In other words, some learning-disabled individuals appear to function quite normally in oral language and it is only in written language that their learning disabilities become apparent. Children who have been functioning in school at a normal or even above-normal level before the introduction of written language have sometimes been referred to as unexpected reading failures. They are *unexpected* because nothing obvious in their oral language development has suggested an area of weakness or disability. In fact, in many cases their oral language functioning will reflect superior language-processing ability, making their school failures all the more surprising. Such individuals seem to have primary processing problems in symbol coding and relative strengths in more general language processing.

Area 2: Language-Processing Difficulties

Not all children with reading and writing difficulties have well-developed oral language processes, however. Reading and writing are both written *language* processes—the former receptive, the latter expressive—so that, if an individual is deficient in receptive and/or expressive oral language functions he or she will almost inevitably experience difficulties in the written domain as well. The child who is not sensitive to the sound patterns of language, who does not know the meanings of as many words as other children the same age, and who is less mature in grammatical development will experience language-processing difficulty. Such difficulty can arise because the child has a developmental delay or deficit in linguistic functioning and/or comes from a linguistically impoverished or linguistically different environment.[31-33] Because the processing of written language, both receptive and expressive, is directly dependent on the phonology, morphology, semantics, and syntax of oral language,* the individual who is language deficient, for whatever reason, will not comprehend well in reading and will not express ideas well in writing. The amount and type of intervention required will, however, depend on the nature of the language-processing weakness.

Many learning-disabled individuals have very serious language-processing difficulties in both the oral and the written domain.[1,31,34] As early as 1937, Samuel Orton,[35] in his case studies of "word blind" children (the term then used for dyslexia or reading disability) observed that many of them appeared to have subtle oral language-processing difficulties. There is now considerable evidence[21,36,37] pointing to both subtle and not-so-subtle language-processing difficulties among the reading disabled. These are evident in disabled readers' phonological ability, morphological ability, semantic processing, and syntactic processing.[38-41] When compared with groups of normally achieving readers, the reading disabled (variously defined) consistently lag behind in one or more of these abilities. Similar patterns are also evident in comparisons of "skilled" and "less skilled" readers in the primary grades.[42-43]

CLINICAL PEARL

There is now considerable evidence pointing to both subtle and not-so-subtle language-processing difficulties among the reading disabled. These are evident in disabled readers' phonological ability, morphological ability, semantic processing, and syntactic processing.

Although, when compared as a group, the reading disabled usually differ from normal readers in the language processes mentioned previously, the evidence does not demonstrate that every individual in the group manifests the pattern reflected by the group mean. Indeed, it is a rare study in which the pattern of results is so "clean" that there is no overlap in the distribution of scores. In other words, it is very likely that whereas some individuals with symbol-coding weaknesses have language-processing weaknesses as well, others may actually have strengths in language processing. Although there is a

---

*Definitions: *semantics* is the system of meanings of the language, *morphology* refers to the rules of word formation, and *syntax* refers to the rules of sentence formation.

tendency in the literature to lump written language disabilities together and attribute them all to some general language-processing deficit, it may be premature to do so.[21] There is clearly considerable variation in the oral language-processing abilities of children with learning disabilities, and these variations account for only part of the variance in reading/spelling/writing abilities.[34] As discussed earlier, the subtyping literature[4,44] has repeatedly pointed to varying processing patterns among subgroups of the learning/reading disabled. The model adopted here allows for a great deal of overlap between the two areas of processing weakness—the amount of overlap in the figure is arbitrary and does not purport to represent the amount in the general population of learning difficulties and disabilities—but allows, as well, for the possibility that some individuals may have a processing weakness of one type or another alone that could affect their acquisition of written language at some stage.

There is also support in the theoretical and research literature for the importance of symbol-coding abilities and language-processing abilities in *combination* as a means of accounting for individual differences in the development of reading and writing. Areas 1 and 2 in the present framework roughly correspond to the two components in Gough and Tunmer's "simple view of reading,"[45] which suggests that reading ability reflects the product of two factors, decoding and comprehension. Decoding is the process involved in both the "sounding out" of words and the recognizing of whole words (context-free) because, in an alphabetical orthography, word recognition skill is dependent upon knowledge of letter-sound correspondence rules or the "orthographic cipher."[46] Comprehension in the "simple view" is the process of linguistic comprehension (not reading comprehension), by which words, sentences, and discourse are interpreted. Longitudinal research investigating the utility of the "simple view"[47] has found that the variance in decoding/encoding and comprehension ability largely accounts for differences in reading and writing development from first through fourth grades.

CLINICAL PEARL

There is also support in the theoretical and research literature for the importance of symbol-coding abilities and language-processing abilities in combination *as a means of accounting for individual differences in the development of reading and writing.*

Area 3: Spatial-Numerical Difficulties

The primary evidence for a significant area of weakness related to the processing of spatial and numerical information comes from the clinical and neuropsychological literature. Repeatedly in this literature[48-51] a fairly consistent pattern of difficulty has been described in which a relatively small portion of learning-disabled individuals— with learning difficulties and disabilities in handwriting and mathematics—have been found to be deficient in processing spatial orientation, visual-spatial-motor organization, number concepts, body image, and social problem-solving that requires observation, analysis, and synthesis. Individuals with this pattern of processing weaknesses are described[49,52] as having some or all of the following characteristics: clumsiness in gross motor tasks, awkwardness in fine motor tasks, right-left disorientation, weakness in visual-motor integration, and confusion about space, time, and number concepts.

It seems likely that all three areas of processing weakness in the framework could play some role in school difficulties and disabilities in mathematics. Although the primary focus of this and the next chapter is on reading and writing difficulties, it is probable that an examination of how an individual functions in mathematics could provide useful insights into the nature of processing weaknesses involved in reading and writing difficulties. Children with a weakness in any of the three areas in the framework would be expected to experience some type of difficulty in mathematics at some point, but the nature of the difficulties resulting from deficits in Areas 1, 2, and 3 would be substantially different. For example, given that numbers are symbols, a primary weakness in symbol-coding ability would be expected to result in difficulties processing the symbols involved in mathematics. Individuals with a weakness in Area 1 might make errors such as reversing and transposing numbers and confusing operational signs in the computation of addition, subtraction, multiplication, and division questions. On the other hand, individuals with a primary weakness in Area 2 would be expected to have difficulty with the language in mathematics, especially the vocabulary and grammar. They might not understand the meaning of terms such as *magnitude* or *divisor* and might have trouble comprehending word problems in which they had to read a short passage to "figure out" what was being asked. Finally, a primary weakness in Area 3—which seems to entail some fundamental deficiency in spatial and numerical processing—would be associated with basic conceptual problems in mathematics, reflecting a deficit in making the connections and comparisons between objects that is required to establish correspondence rules and to solve problems involving amount and quantity. Both the degree of processing weakness in any particular area and the number of areas of weakness involved (one, two, or all three) would obviously influence how much difficulty individuals experience in their learning and performance of mathematics. In turn, the types of difficulty demonstrated in mathematics might provide useful insights into the pattern of processing abilities underlying an individual's reading and writing skill.

The Role of Visual-Processing Deficits in the Framework

Although, as discussed earlier, there are theorists who argue fairly convincingly that phonological-coding and linguistic processing deficits account for virtually all reading and writing difficulties,[21,22] evidence in this and other books questions that contention.[53] In view of the fact that the evidence and arguments concerning the role of phonological and linguistic deficits[36,54,55] have been presented at length in several books already, I will not discuss them further here. Rather, because the present book is specifically concerned with vision and reading, the potential role of visual processing deficits in the three areas of difficulty within the framework are discussed following.

Both Area 1 (symbol-coding difficulties) and Area 3 (spatial-numerical difficulties) could involve significant visual processing components of some sort, but it is most unlikely that the same visual components are involved in these two areas of weakness. The typical visual processing difficulty associated with Area 1 is specific to associating symbols with language or, at least, to processing visual information with the visual (high–spatial frequency) characteristics of print.[56] Many individuals with a weakness in symbol coding apparently have no difficulty processing representational (low–spatial frequency) visual information in pictures.[57] As Aaron and Guillemard[58] have argued, it appears that Leonardo da Vinci had the type of specific reading/writing disability characteristic of a deficit in the symbol-coding area, but he obviously had no difficulty processing other kinds of visual information. Moreover, it is not uncommon in clinical settings to find very talented artists among those with severe symbol-coding difficulty. On the other hand, individuals with weakness in the type of spatial-numerical processing that is characteristic of Area 3 are deficient in visual-spatial integration and visual-motor processing, and artistic talent is inevitably lacking.

Area 1: Symbol-coding difficulties

If some disabled readers have delays or deficits in their basic visual processing abilities, such weaknesses could be a factor in their apparent difficulties in differentiating between similar-looking letters and words—especially in analyzing and remembering the orthographic patterns in words and in processing letters and words at a rapid rate in text.[30] Clinical observations and case reports, correlational evidence from studies using standardized psychometric instruments, and visual deficit subtypes from clinical and neuropsychological studies all point to some role of visual-processing deficits in reading disabilities. Evidence from basic research involving early visual processes[59-61] also suggests that there is some relation between visual processing deficits and reading disabilities. At this point, however, the potential role of visual processing weaknesses in symbol-coding problems is not well enough understood to draw confident conclusions.[53]

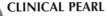

CLINICAL PEARL

If some disabled readers have delays or deficits in their basic visual processing abilities, such weaknesses could be a factor in their apparent difficulties in differentiating between similar-looking letters and words.

Clinicians and educators in the field of learning disabilities should certainly keep an open mind about the possibility that visual processing deficits contribute in some way to reading disabilities. Prudence would dictate that both assessment approaches and teaching techniques should be devised on the assumption that the reading-disabled child may have some difficulty in coping with the visual demands of a task. The findings indicating that younger disabled readers (6 to 8 years of age) may be more likely to have some sort of visual perceptual and/or visual memory deficits are worthy of special note. The visual demands of the beginning stages of reading acquisition are probably more significant than those at later stages of reading acquisition, when linguistic processes may play a greater role.[13,14,62]

Area 3: Spatial-numerical difficulties

Research investigating the type of nonverbal learning difficulties described in Area 3 of the framework[49,51] have often differentiated a nonverbal learning–disabled group on the basis of performance on some or all of the nonverbal subtests (including Picture Completion, Picture Arrangement, Block Design, Object Assembly, Coding, and Mazes) of the *Wechsler Intelligence Scale for Children* (the most recent edition being the *WISC-III*) in contrast with performance on the verbal subtests. In particular, three subtests in the nonverbal set—Block Design, Object Assembly, and Mazes—seem to tap processing abilities that are relatively distinct from those that might overlap the symbol-coding and language-processing areas. The Block Design subtest of the *WISC-III* is used to assess a child's ability to reproduce geometric designs from a model using colored blocks and is thought to measure nonverbal abstract problem-solving, visual-analytical, ability, and spatial relations–perceiving capabilities. The Object Assembly subtest involves assembling familiar objects from puzzlelike forms without a model and appears to measure visual-motor ability, visual integration ability, and the understanding of part-whole relationships. The Mazes subtest involves completing pencil mazes of increasing difficulty and is considered to measure visual-motor coordination and planning and anticipation. It is a very reasonable possibility that deficits in the visual-analytical, visual-spatial, and visual-motor abilities tapped by these subtests are implicated in the handwriting and mathematics deficits associated with Area 3 problems. Because extreme deficits in these processing areas are relatively rare and because mild difficulties in these areas have been little explored, conclusions with respect to the role of visual processes in spatial-numerical difficulties and disabilities (Area 3), within the individual-differences perspective offered here, are by necessity quite speculative.

Estimates in the literature of the proportion of learning-disabled or reading-disabled individuals who are thought to have visual processing deficits vary widely, and it may well be that these conflicting estimates are based on quite different types of visual processing demands. Careful research is needed to clarify the role that visual processing weaknesses of various types might play in reading, writing, and mathematics difficulties.

Other Contributing Factors

In addition to the three areas of processing weakness discussed in this chapter, there are other obvious modulating factors that often contribute to learning problems. Low levels of attention, self-esteem, motivation, background knowledge, educational opportunity, social-emotional support, and physical health can all have devastating consequences for an individual's success in school.* Any assessment should explore these and other potential contributing factors to determine the extent to which they may be involved. It also must be asked whether a factor is a cause or an effect, or both, of a learning problem. Individuals who have a history of failure often are not motivated or do not pay attention in school as a result of their learning problems.[64] Once appropriate intervention to ameliorate the learning difficulties has begun, the individual's self-esteem usually goes up and, along with it, his or her attention and motivational problems may "miraculously" disappear.

---

*A fairly large number of children with learning disabilities are described by their teachers as having "attention problems." Only a fraction of these, however, do in fact have *attention deficit disorder*.[63] Most children who have trouble reading and writing manifest some "attention problems" in school as a result of the fact that they are frustrated or bored. Observation of such children across various situations makes it evident that they are able to pay attention for extended periods in situations where they have the skills to be successful. Thus, it is important to distinguish true ADD from the situationally generated attention problems that *result from* other types of learning disabilities.

Using the Framework

The framework offered in this chapter is intended as a rough "working model" for understanding learning difficulties and disabilities. Its usefulness will be determined by the extent to which it contributes to theory and/or practice. Whether it can be useful to theoreticians in generating better research questions will be left to others to discover. The chapter following this one, however, is an attempt to put the framework into practice by using it as a basis for developing a practical guide to assessment and programming for reading and writing difficulties.

References

1. Levine MD: *Developmental variation and learning disorders,* Cambridge, Mass, 1987, Educators Publishing Service.
2. Shaywitz SE, Escobar MD, Shaywitz BA et al: Evidence that dyslexia may represent the lower tail of a normal distribution of reading ability, *N Engl J Med* 326:145-193, 1992.
3. Perfetti CA: Continuities in reading acquisition, reading skill, and reading disability, *Remed Spec Educ* 7:11-21, 1986.
4. Feagans L, Short E, Meltzer L (eds): *Subtypes of learning disabilities,* Hillsdale, NJ, 1991, Lawrence Erlbaum.
5. Hooper SR, Willis WG: *Learning disability subtyping,* New York, 1989, Springer-Verlag.
6. Mattis S: Dyslexia syndromes: a working hypothesis that works. In Benton AL, Pearl D (eds): *Dyslexia: an appraisal of current knowledge,* New York, 1978, Oxford University Press.
7. Mattis S: Dyslexia syndromes in children: toward the development of syndrome-specific treatment programs. In Pirozzolo FJ, Wittrock MC (eds): *Neuropsychological and cognitive processes in reading,* New York, 1981, Academic Press.
8. Mattis S, French J, Rapin I: Dyslexia in children and young adults: three independent neuropsychological syndromes, *Dev Med Child Neurol* 17:150-163, 1975.
9. Watson C, Willows DM: Information processing patterns in specific reading disability, *J Learn Disabil* 28(4):216-231, 1995.
10. Morris R, Satz P: Classification issues in subtype research: an application of some methods and concepts. In Malatesha RN, Whitaker HA (eds): *Dyslexia: a global issue,* The Hague, 1984, Martinus Nijhoff Publishers.
11. Satz P, Morris R: Learning disability subtypes: a review. In Pirozzolo FJ, Wittrock MC (eds): *Neuropsychological and cognitive processes in reading,* New York, 1981, Academic Press.
12. Feagans LV, McKinney JD: Subtypes of learning disabilities: a review. In Feagans LV, Short EJ, Meltzer LJ (eds): *Subtypes of learning disabilities: theoretical perspectives and research,* Hillsdale, NJ, 1991, Lawrence Erlbaum.
13. Chall JS: *Stages of reading development,* New York, 1983, McGraw-Hill.
14. Willows DM: A "normal variation" view of written language difficulties and disabilities: implications for whole language programs, *Except Educ Can* 1:73-103, 1991.
15. Biemiller AJ: Relationships between oral reading rates for letters, words, and simple text in the development of reading achievement, *Read Res Q* 13:223-253, 1977-78.

16. Corcos E, Willows DM: The role of visual processes in good and poor readers' utilization of orthographic information in letter strings. In Wright S, Groner R (eds): *Studies in visual information processing,* Amsterdam, 1992, North Holland Elsevier.
17. Corcos E, Willows DM: The processing of orthographic information in reading. In Willows DM, Kruk R, Corcos E (eds): *Visual processes in reading and reading disabilities,* Hillsdale, NJ, 1993, Lawrence Erlbaum.
18. Perfetti CA: *Reading ability,* New York, 1985, Oxford University Press.
19. Stanovich KE: The interactive-compensatory model of reading: a confluence of developmental, experimental, and educational psychology, *Remed Spec Educ* 5:11-19, 1984.
20. Williams JP: The role of phonemic analysis in reading. In Torgesen JK, Wong BYL (eds): *Psychological and educational perspectives on learning disabilities,* Orlando, Fla, 1986, Academic Press.
21. Mann V: Language problems: a key to early reading problems. In Wong BYL (ed): *Learning about learning disabilities,* New York, 1991, Academic Press.
22. Stanovich KE: Explaining the differences between the dyslexic and the garden-variety poor reader: the phonological-core variable-difference model, *J Learn Disabil* 21:590-604, 1988.
23. Lovett MW, Ransby MJ, Hardwick N et al: Can dyslexia be treated? Treatment-specific and generalized treatment effects in dyslexic children's response to remediation, *Brain Lang* 37:90-121, 1989.
24. Snowling M: The development of phoneme-grapheme correspondences in normal and dyslexic readers, *J Exp Child Psychol* 29:294-305, 1980.
25. Schwartz S: Spelling disability: a developmental linguistic analysis of pattern abstraction, *Appl Psycholinguist* 4:303-316, 1983.
26. Siegel LS, Ryan EB: The development of working memory in normally achieving and subtypes of learning disabled children, *Child Dev* 60:973-980, 1989.
27. Torgesen JK: Memory processes in reading disabled children, *J Learn Disabil* 18:350-357, 1985.
28. Tallal P: Auditory temporal perception, phonics, and reading disabilities in children, *Brain Lang* 9:182-198, 1980.
29. Bowers PG, Steffy R, Tate E: Comparison of the effects of IQ control methods on memory and naming speed predictors of reading ability, *Read Res Q* 23:304-319, 1988.
30. Willows DM: Visual processes in learning disabilities. In Wong BYL (ed): *Learning about learning disabilities,* New York, 1991, Academic Press.
31. Wiig EH, Semel EM: *Language assessment and intervention for the learning disabled,* ed 2, Columbus, Ohio, 1984, Charles E Merrill.
32. Entwisle DR: The child's social environment and learning to read. In Waller TG, MacKinnon GE (eds): *Reading research: advances in theory and practice,* New York, 1979, Academic Press.
33. Cummins J: Empowering minority students: a framework for intervention, *Harvard Educ Rev* 56:18-36, 1986.
34. Donahue M: Linguistic and communicative development in learning-disabled children. In Cici SJ (ed): *Handbook of cognitive, social, and neuropsychological aspects of learning disabilities,* Hillsdale, NJ, 1986, Lawrence Erlbaum.
35. Orton ST: *Reading, writing, and speech problems in children,* London, 1937, Chapman & Hall.
36. Vellutino FR: *Dyslexia: theory and research,* Cambridge, Mass, 1979, MIT Press.
37. Vellutino FR: Dyslexia, *Sci Am* 256:34-41, 1987.
38. Liberman IY, Shankweiler D: Phonology and beginning reading: a tutorial. In Rieben L, Perfetti CA (eds): *Learning to read: basic research and its implications,* Hillsdale, NJ, 1991, Lawrence Erlbaum.
39. Vogel SA: A qualitative analysis of morphological ability in learning disabled and achieving children, *J Learn Disabil* 16:416-420, 1983.

40. Wiig EH, Becker-Redding U, Semel EM: A cross-cultural, cross-linguistic comparison of language abilities of 7- to 8- and 12- to 13-year-old children with learning disabilities, *J Learn Disabil* 16:576-585, 1983.

41. Siegel LS, Ryan EB: Development of grammatical-sensitivity, phonological, and short-term memory skills in normally achieving and learning disabled children, *Dev Psychol* 24:28-37, 1984.

42. Ehri L: Sources of difficulty in learning to read and spell. In Wolraich MI, Routh D (eds): *Advances in developmental and behavioral pediatrics*, Greenwich, Conn, 1986, JAI Press.

43. Willows DM, Ryan EB: The development of grammatical sensitivity and its relationship to early reading achievement, *Read Res Q* 23:253-266, 1986.

44. Watson C, Willows DM: Evidence of a visual-processing-deficit subtype among disabled readers. In Willows DM, Kruk R, Corcos E (eds): *Visual processes in reading and reading disabilities*, Hillsdale, NJ, 1993, Lawrence Erlbaum.

45. Gough PB, Tunmer WE: Decoding, reading, and reading disability, *Remed Spec Educ* 7:6-10, 1986.

46. Gough PB, Hillinger, ML: Learning to read: an unnatural act, *Bull Orton Soc* 30:179-196, 1980.

47. Juel C: Learning to read and write: a longitudinal study of 54 children from first through fourth grade, *J Educ Psychol* 80:437-447, 1988.

48. Badian N: Dyscalculia and nonverbal disorders of learning. In Myklebust HR (ed): *Progress in learning disabilities*, New York, 1983, Grune & Stratton.

49. Johnson DJ: Nonverbal learning disabilities, *Pediatr Ann* 16:133-141, 1987.

50. Kinsbourne M, Warrington EK: Developmental factors in reading and writing backwardness. In Money J, Schiffman G (eds): *The disabled reader: education of the dyslexic child*, Baltimore, 1966, John Hopkins Press.

51. Myklebust HR: Nonverbal learning disabilities: assessment and intervention. In Myklebust HR (ed): *Progress in learning disabilities*, New York, 1975, Grune & Stratton.

52. Golick M: Learning disabilities and the school age child, *Learn Disabil Information Please:* 1-8, 1978.

53. Willows DM, Kruk R, Corcos E: Are there differences between disabled and normal readers in their processing of visual information? In Willows DM, Kruk R, Corcos E (eds): *Visual processes in reading and reading disabilities*, Hillsdale, NJ, 1993, Lawrence Erlbaum.

54. Gough PB, Ehri LC, Treiman R: *Reading acquisition*, Hillsdale, NJ, 1992, Lawrence Erlbaum.

55. Rieben L, Perfetti CA (eds): *Learning to read: basic research and its implications*, Hillsdale, NJ, 1991, Lawrence Erlbaum.

56. Lovegrove W, Martin F, Slaghuis W: A theoretical and experimental case for a visual deficit in specific reading disability, *Cogn Neuropsychol* 3:225-267, 1986.

57. Hinshelwood J: *Congenital word-blindness*, London, 1917, HK Lewis & Co.

58. Aaron PG, Guillemard JC: Artists as dyslexics. In Willows DM, Kruk R, Corcos E (eds): *Visual processes in reading and reading disabilities*, Hillsdale, NJ, 1993, Lawrence Erlbaum.

59. Breitmeyer B: Sustained (P) and transient (M) channels in vision: a review and implications for reading. In Willows DM, Kruk R, Corcos E. (eds): *Visual processes in reading and reading disabilities*, Hillsdale, NJ, 1993, Lawrence Erlbaum.

60. Kruk R, Willows DM: Toward an ecologically valid analysis of visual processes in dyslexic readers. In Wright S, Groner R (eds): *Studies in visual information processing*, Amsterdam, 1993, North Holland Elsevier.

61. Lovegrove WJ, Williams MC: Visual temporal processing deficits in specific reading disability. In Willows DM, Kruk R, Corcos E (eds): *Visual processes in reading and reading disabilities*, Hillsdale, NJ, 1993, Lawrence Erlbaum.

62. Vernon MD: Varieties of deficiency in reading processes, *Harvard Educ Rev* 47:396-410, 1977.
63. Douglas V: Attention and cognitive problems. In Rutter M (ed): *Developmental neuropsychiatry*, New York, 1983, Guilford Press .
64. Butkowsky IS, Willows DM: Cognitive-motivational characteristics of children varying in reading ability: evidence for learned helplessness in poor readers, *J Educ Psychol* 72:408-422, 1980.

13

Assessment and Programming for Reading and Writing Difficulties*

Dale M. Willows

Key Terms

symbol coding	spelling	visual processes
language processing	short-term/working	language
spatial-numerical	memory	development
assessment	long-term/rote	programming
writing difficulties	memory	

The ultimate goal of research on reading and writing processes is to improve the level of literacy in society, through better instruction and through detecting and correcting difficulties. As reflected in the framework described in Chapter 12, significant advances have been made over the last 25 years in our theoretical understanding of reading and writing processes, and, to some extent, these gains have filtered down into practice. With respect to reading instruction, basic research has now led to some well-grounded frameworks for under-standing reading and writing acquisition that have direct implications for teaching practices.[1,2] Moreover, theory-based models on which to

* The author wishes to thank Margie Golick and Sybil Schwartz for sharing their wealth of clinical wisdom and Karen Sumbler and Esther Geva for their helpful comments on an earlier version of this chapter.

develop clinical approaches for the assessment and remediation of difficulties and disabilities are beginning to emerge.[3,4] Despite these advances, however, there is a considerable way to go before we can prescribe with certainty the best approach to the assessment and remediation of reading and writing problems—because there is still much to learn about the processes involved in acquisition and disabilities, and because translating theory into practice is far from a precise science.

Practitioners whose role it is to assess the nature of students' reading and writing difficulties and to plan and/or implement programs to alleviate them do not have the luxury of waiting until the theoreticians all agree on which direction to take. Thus, it is incumbent on those who have a familiarity with current theories and models of reading processes and reading disabilities to attempt to translate theory into practice. It was with this responsibility in mind that 12 years ago, after having spent over 10 years as a basic researcher in the field of reading, I took a sabbatical leave and "apprenticed" at a highly respected university hospital learning center with an outstanding team of clinicians whose credentials included master's and doctor's degrees in such fields as psychology, education, linguistics, and communication disorders. For over a quarter of a century this team had been assessing students' learning disabilities and developing and implementing programs for them. By working with these experts, I hoped to determine whether the theories and models emanating from basic research had validity and utility in the real world of practice. Although my knowledge of research literature and theories of reading prepared me in some ways to profit from that clinical experience, what I learned from those clinicians and their clients contributed more to my understanding of reading and writing processes than did my previous 10 years of "laboratory" study. During the years since that clinical internship, I have maintained an active involvement in basic research and theories of reading processes and reading disabilities.[5] At the same time, I have remained deeply involved in clinical/educational practice in the fields of reading acquisition and learning difficulties and disabilities.[6,7] In both schools and clinics I now deal with the problems that face educators and clinicians on a regular basis, doing my best to make recommendations and use approaches that are consistent with the latest "theory-based wisdom"; but at the same time, when the latest theories and models do not suggest clear answers, I rely a great deal on the "clinical wisdom" that I have gained from my mentors and from my own years of clinical experience.

My goal in this chapter is to share with clinicians and educators some practical guidelines for the assessment and remediation of reading and writing difficulties and disabilities. Based on the framework presented in the preceding chapter, the present chapter applies a synthesis of theory-based wisdom with clinical wisdom to generate specific recommendations. The remainder of the chapter is organized into three main sections. The first presents an abbreviated version of the framework advanced in Chapter 12 for understanding variations in patterns of reading and writing difficulties. Following from that framework, the second section presents a practical guide to the assessment of reading and writing difficulties. And the third offers programming recommendations consistent with assessment findings. As mentioned in Chapter 12, the reference list and appendix at the end of this chapter include books, articles, and materials relevant to the practical problems of assessment and programming.

I. Framework for Assessment and Programming

As described in the framework developed in the previous chapter, there are three main areas of processing weakness that seem to underlie the problems of individuals with learning difficulties and disabilities—Area 1, symbol-coding difficulty; Area 2, language-processing difficulty; and Area 3, spatial-numerical difficulty. The first two areas are common sources of difficulty among individuals with school learning problems, whereas the third much less so. Individuals with reading/writing difficulties may have problems in one, two, or all three of these areas. However, because the third area of difficulty is far less clearly understood and articulated than the other two, and because difficulties in Areas 1 and 2 account for the vast majority of reading and writing problems, Area 3 will not be discussed in this chapter. Rather, an abbreviated version of the framework, including only Areas 1 and 2, will be used as an organizer. The processing difficulties associated with these areas are represented by the two intersecting circles in Figure 13-1, with a gradient of shading from very light to very dark representing degrees of processing difficulty from mild to severe.

CLINICAL PEARL

There are three main areas of processing weakness that seem to underlie the problems of individuals with learning difficulties and disabilities—Area 1, symbol-coding difficulty; Area 2, language-processing difficulty; and Area 3, spatial-numerical difficulty.

Throughout the sections on assessment and programming, it is important to remember that both Area 1 and Area 2 may be components

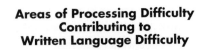

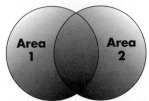

Area 1:
Symbol-coding
difficulty
Decoding and encoding of:

Area 2:
Language-processing
difficulty
Reception and expression of:

Letters
Orthographic patterns
Whole words

Phonology
Morphology
Semantics and syntax

* Note: shading represents degree of difficulty,
  ranging from mild (lightest) to severe (darkest).

FIGURE 13-1   Framework for understanding reading and writing
difficulties.

of an individual's learning difficulties and it is essential that they both
be explored to ensure that the major potential sources of difficulty have
been examined. An individual who is having reading/writing difficulties may have a weakness only in Area 1, or may have weakness in Area
2 as well. Other potential contributing factors (e.g., attention deficit,
poverty of background knowledge, lack of motivation) should, of
course, also be investigated. To design an appropriate program for
intervention, it is important to ascertain the areas of processing weakness involved. The following sections, in which assessment and programming are discussed, are both organized around the two areas of
weakness described in the framework in Figure 13-1.

II. Assessing Reading and Writing Difficulties

What to Look for in Assessment

Any good clinician knows that testing and assessment are not one
and the same. A person might be a competent "tester," in the sense of
being well versed in the technical requirements involved in administering and scoring standardized test instruments, but know little
about assessing learning problems. There is no adequate test or even

battery of tests that, when administered, will provide a clear explanation for an individual's reading and writing difficulties and disabilities. Although it is simple enough to demonstrate that a child is having reading difficulties by administering one of the many "quick-and-dirty" tests of word recognition (as is often done in research) and showing that the child is performing below some arbitrary level, such a demonstration is trivial and rarely tells the tester anything that the classroom teacher or parents could not have told the clinician without formal testing—that the child is indeed having difficulty reading. To be of real value to clinicians, a test must point to the potential cause(s) of an individual's difficulties so a special program can be developed to ameliorate the situation. However, reading/writing difficulties and disabilities reflect such a complex interaction of processing weaknesses that it is unlikely this interaction will ever be adequately captured in one test, or even a battery of tests. There are dozens of tests available that could be used in some aspect of the assessment of reading/writing difficulties, but it is very telling that no particular one has emerged as the "test of choice" among clinicians (other than the standard, the *Wechsler Intelligence Scale for Children–III*). In fact, it is typical for good clinicians to make use of a combination of informal and formal assessment techniques and, in their formal testing, to select sub-tests (rather than whole tests) from the variety of test batteries available. Thus assessment of reading/writing difficulties is a rather individualized matter in which each clinician chooses the set of "tools" with which he or she feels most comfortable. How successful clinicians are in accurately assessing the nature of reading/writing difficulties is a reflection more of how well they understand what they are looking for than of which particular formal tests they choose to use. Despite numerous attempts to come up with an early screening battery to select in advance those children who are likely to have difficulty learning to read and write, or, for that matter, to specify which individuals are already "genuinely" disabled in their reading/writing processes, there is no general agreement in the clinical literature as to what tests should be included. If there were an ideal test or test battery for the assessment of reading/writing difficulties, then surely clinicians in the field would have discovered it.

CLINICAL PEARL

There is no adequate test or even battery of tests that, when administered, will provide a clear explanation for an individual's reading and writing difficulties and disabilities.

CLINICAL PEARL

To be of real value to clinicians, a test must point to the potential cause(s) of an individual's difficulties so a special program can be developed to ameliorate the situation.

As discussed in Chapter 12, there is considerable evidence in the literature that certain types of processing weakness underlie difficulties in reading and writing. The key to effective assessment is knowing what to look for. Thus, in this chapter, the focus is not on tests per se but on providing a clear description of the *symptoms* of the processing weaknesses that underlie reading/writing difficulties. These symptoms—the characteristic patterns of difficulty—are organized around the two areas of processing weakness presented in the framework in Figure 13-1. Equipped with a knowledge of these symptoms, clinicians can undertake informal assessment techniques (if they have extensive experience and good "internal norms") or choose from among a range of potential testing instruments (a few of which are mentioned specifically in this chapter). Although some might dispute that the symptoms pointing to the causes of reading and writing disabilities are as clear cut as those for physical illnesses, I would argue that they are usually fairly obvious if the clinician "looks for clues" by exploring the extent to which the individual manifests "symptoms" of Area 1 and/or Area 2 difficulties.

Throughout this section specific examples and suggested tests are mentioned, to make the guidelines as explicit as possible. (See Table 13-1 for a list of the tests mentioned and their abbreviations.) It is not the intent to imply, however, that the specific tests given as examples are the only, or even the best, ones available to assess the processing area under consideration They are simply intended as models to demonstrate the types of "data" that should be useful in determining the areas of processing weakness underlying an individual's reading and writing problems. It would have been much easier to be vague and general in these recommendations in order to avoid controversy, but the intent of this chapter is to provide practical information. Although some of the suggestions in this section (on assessment) and in the next (on programming) cannot be corroborated with "hard evidence" from theory-based research, they are well grounded in clinical wisdom.

Assessing Area 1: Characteristics Associated with Symbol-Coding Weakness

The box on p. 256 summarizes the characteristic learning difficulties associated with a symbol-coding weakness. These difficulties become evident when the child first encounters print, and they continue to be manifested in various forms as the child progresses through school. The remainder of this section expands on the characteristic difficulties summarized in the table, with the intent of preparing clinicians and teachers to recognize the learning patterns of individuals who have a processing weakness in the symbol-coding area. These characteristic difficulties are elaborated under four main headings—*Reading* (with subheadings of Letter recognition, Word recognition, Reading fluency, and Reading comprehension), *Writing* (with subheadings of Letter formation, Spelling, and Written composition), *Memory* (with sub-headings of Short-term/working memory and Long-term/rote memory), and *Visual Processes.*

Reading

Letter recognition. From the very beginning, children with a weakness in symbol coding often have problems learning to identify letters and numbers, so they are slower than other children at learning to recognize visual symbols when they see them. This is true both for print and cursive writing and for the uppercase and lowercase forms of print. When shown an array of letters and asked to "show me the [letter]," for example, they may not be able to recognize some of the letters of the alphabet quickly and accurately at an age when others can do so without effort. Letters that are visually similar seem to

TABLE 13-1
Standardized Assessment Instruments

Test name	Abbreviation
Boston Naming Test	BNT
Clinical Evaluation of Language Fundamentals–Revised	CELF-R
Detroit Test of Learning Aptitude–2	DTLA-2
Developmental Test of Visual-Motor Integration	VMI
Durrell Analysis of Reading Difficulty–Revised	DARD-R
Goldman-Fristoe-Woodcock Auditory Skills Test Battery	G-F-W
Lindamood Auditory Conceptualization Test	LAC
Peabody Picture Vocabulary Test–Revised	PPVT-R
Screening Tests for Identifying Children with Specific Language Disability	Slingerland, Malcomesius
Test of Auditory Perceptual Skills	TAPS
Test of Visual-Perceptual Skills	TVPS
Test of Written Language–2	TOWL-2
Wechsler Intelligence Scale for Children–III	WISC-III
Wide Range Achievement Test–Revised	WRAT-R
Woodcock Reading Mastery Tests–Revised	WRMT-R

Assessing Area 1: Learning Difficulties Associated with Symbol-Coding Weakness

Reading

Letter recognition

Difficulty recognizing letters
Visually similar letters confused
Mirror-image letters confused

Word recognition

Poor word recognition "by sight"
Word analysis skills weak
Recognition based on first letter and overall word shape

Reading fluency

Slow and inaccurate reading
Overreliance on context for word recognition
Words and parts of words omitted
Familiar stories recited instead of read

Reading comprehension

Comprehension limited as a result of poor word recognition
Listening comprehension superior to reading comprehension
Comprehension poor on first reading, rereading required

Writing

Letter formation

Slow at copying and writing
Poorly formed letters
Letter orientation "reversals"
Uppercase and lowercase letters intermixed
Printing used after others begin writing

Spelling

Spelling an area of persistent difficulty
Insensitivity to orthographic patterns of the language
Words spelled better in lists than in compositions
Spelling phonetic, based on sounds in words
Letters reversed and letter-order transposed
Difficulty checking own spelling "by sight"

Written composition

Content of written composition well below level of oral expression
Words omitted and repeated
Word endings or parts of words omitted
Punctuation and details omitted
Inappropriate spacing between words
"Sloppy" written work

Memory

Weak short-term/working memory
Weak long-term/rote memory

represent a particular source of confusion. For example, letter pairs with some visual similarity, such as *h-n, E-F,* and *v-y,* and especially letters that can be transformed to other letters by a change of orientation—*b-d, u-n, f-t,* and *M-W*—are especially problematical. While most children experience some difficulty with these types of discriminations in the beginning stages of reading acquisition, such visual confusions often persist into the later grades and sometimes even into adulthood (especially the classic "reversal error" involving a *b-d* confusion) for individuals with symbol-coding weakness.

CLINICAL PEARL

From the very beginning, children with a weakness in symbol coding often have problems learning to identify letters and numbers, so they are slower than other children at learning to recognize visual symbols when they see them.

Word recognition. Although children with weak symbol-coding abilities may not have difficulty recognizing single letters and numbers (only a few of which are confusable on a visual basis, and there are only 10 numbers and 26 letters to learn), they inevitably have difficulty recognizing whole words, because these "strings of letters" have many visual features in common (e.g., "spot," "spat," "stop," "step") and there are thousands of them to learn. Thus children with a symbol-coding weakness are slow learning to recognize words out of context (e.g., as determined by the Reading subtest of the *WRAT-R*) and, in context, have to "sound them out" or guess at them based on pictures and semantic/syntactic cues. It is characteristic that children with symbol-coding weakness cannot read nearly as many words "by sight," quickly and effortlessly, as others their age and may even have difficulty recognizing very high-frequency words they have seen hundreds of times. As they progress through school, word recognition continues to be a source of difficulty. Their word analysis skills are also poor, so they fail to analyze the internal structure of words (e.g., as measured by the Word Attack subtest of the *WRMT-R*). Even when they recognize quite a few words apparently by sight, their misidentifications or word substitutions show that they often rely on partial cues such as initial letters, final letters, and/or overall word shapes to identify words (e.g., "hose" is read as "house," "either" as "enter"). Sometimes, too, the child appears not to know where to start or in which direction to go when decoding a word and will begin at the end of a word, reading "saw" for "was" and "stop" for "pots." Across the grades, the development of a *sight vocabulary* by children with symbol-coding weakness is much slower than that of other children, taking considerably longer to automatize the recognition of words.

CLINICAL PEARL

Children with a symbol-coding weakness are slow learning to recognize words out of context and, in context, have to "sound them out" or guess at them based on pictures and semantic/syntactic cues.

Reading fluency. A salient characteristic of the oral reading of individuals with a symbol-coding weakness is that it lacks fluency (e.g., as measured by the Oral Reading subtest of the *DARD-R*). Such individuals read in a word-by-word manner, slowly and inaccurately. They often approach words that they have seen numerous times before by trying to "sound them out" as though they do not realize that the words should be familiar. As is the case for all children, word recognition is easier in context than out. However, children with a symbol-coding weakness overrely on context, compensating for inadequate word-recognition skills. As mentioned previously, they often misread words on the basis of partial cues, with word endings being missed or added. Figure 13-2 presents a transcript of contextual reading that demonstrates poor word analysis and the overuse of context by a reading disabled student.

CLINICAL PEARL

A salient characteristic of the oral reading of individuals with a symbol-coding weakness is that it lacks fluency. Such individuals read in a word-by-word manner, slowly and inaccurately.

Reading comprehension. Although children with a processing weakness in Area 1 may have excellent oral language (if they have strength in Area 2) and their oral language comprehension may be outstanding, they often have serious comprehension difficulties in reading (e.g., as reflected in a discrepancy between performance on the Listening Comprehension and Silent Reading Comprehension subtests of the *DARD-R*). The reading-comprehension difficulties arise not as a result of language comprehension problems per se but

JOE AND MOE AT THE GOLF COURSE

hurts

Joe and Moe are toads. Joe likes Moe. Moe hates Joe.

gets   hop   in   gets   hop   in

Moe goes to hole nine. Joe goes to hole nine.

hops   leap in trip for

Moe hides in the hole. Will Joe land on top of Moe?

leaps   net   must   snore

Joe lands on Moe's nose. He makes Moe's nose sore.

might and

My! Moe is mad at Joe.

FIGURE 13-2 Transcript of contextual reading by a 9-year-old student with symbol-coding difficulty.

because of a lack of automaticity of word recognition. This deficit in automaticity hinders their ability to process the meaning of what they read. Their limited cognitive and attentional resources are taken up in decoding the individual words in text, so they have limited resources available to process larger units of meaning. On first reading a text, the individual with a symbol-coding weakness may comprehend little of what has been read; but on rereading, when more attentional resources are freed from the demands of decoding, comprehension may be much improved.

Writing

Letter formation. In addition to the difficulty with recognition that affects their reading, children with symbol-coding difficulty have trouble recalling how letters look in order to write them. This is reflected in their being slow to learn the formation of letters (both in print and in cursive writing, in uppercase and lowercase). When a child with this weakness is attempting to write the alphabet, he or she may say "What does a [any letter] look like?" Thus, unless copying from a model, such children's letter formation is usually poor. As in the case of recognition, children with symbol-coding weakness confuse visually similar letters and have particular difficulty with letters that are mirror images (e.g., *b-d, u-n, M-W, f-t*). Moreover, in their written work they sometimes reverse the orientation of nonreversible letters and numbers (ịọ, ꓘ, Ɛ, and ꜀). Thus they demonstrate that their problem with orientation is not just the result of a problem of mislabelling (which could explain the *b-d* confusions), as some theorists have argued. In the case of nonreversible letters children with symbol-coding weakness demonstrate that they know what letters they wish to make, they just cannot remember which way they go. Figure 13-3 presents examples of letter-orientation errors in the printing of students with symbol-coding weakness.

Jared   8 years

Nick   9 years

David   10 years

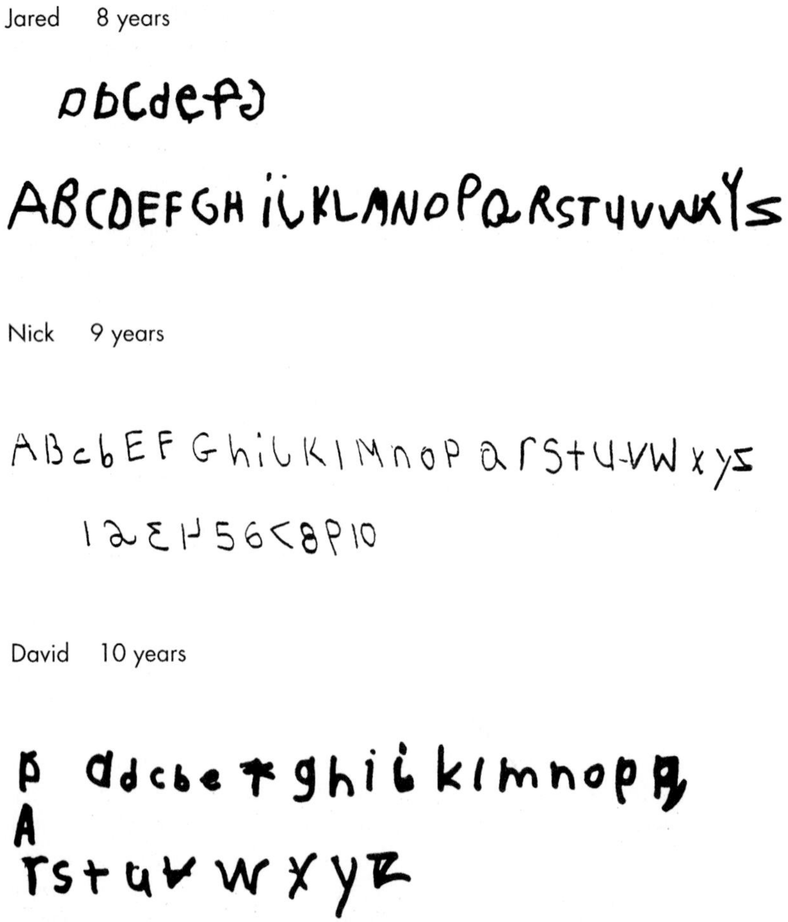

FIGURE 13-3 Examples of letter-orientation errors by students with Area 1 weakness.

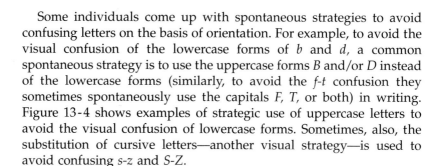

CLINICAL PEARL

In addition to the difficulty with recognition that affects their reading, children with symbol-coding difficulty have trouble recalling how letters look in order to write them. This is reflected in their being slow to learn the formation of letters.

Some individuals come up with spontaneous strategies to avoid confusing letters on the basis of orientation. For example, to avoid the visual confusion of the lowercase forms of *b* and *d*, a common spontaneous strategy is to use the uppercase forms *B* and/or *D* instead of the lowercase forms (similarly, to avoid the *f-t* confusion they sometimes spontaneously use the capitals *F, T,* or both) in writing. Figure 13-4 shows examples of strategic use of uppercase letters to avoid the visual confusion of lowercase forms. Sometimes, also, the substitution of cursive letters—another visual strategy—is used to avoid confusing *s-z* and *S-Z*.

Spelling. Recalling how words look is even more difficult. So spelling is an area of extreme and persistent difficulty. In describing the spelling of children with symbol-coding weakness, it is common for clinicians to observe that "it doesn't look like English." This observation reflects the fact that such children have great difficulty learning the orthographic (i.e., spelling) patterns of the language. Long after other children have learned that *t* always precedes *h* in the *th* digraph, children with symbol-coding weakness show an insensitivity to the pattern. Thus, even in a copying task they sometimes transpose *th* to *ht* and fail to notice that a very high-frequency word (e.g., "hte" for "the" or "wiht" for "with") does not look right. If the difficulty were only at the level of phonological encoding, then after misspelling a common orthographic pattern children with symbol-coding weakness should recognize "by sight" that it doesn't look right. But the inability of most such individuals to check their own spelling by sight is very well known to clinicians.

From the beginning of writing, the child with symbol-coding weakness is slow learning to spell. As in reading, even the commonest words present a problem. So, for example, by the end of first grade children with this problem may not be able to spell "the," "are," "come," or even their own names. Children who have been taught sound-symbol correspondences may be able to spell regular words (e.g., and, but, stop) much more easily than words that do not follow a direct sound-letter relationship. In fact, such children may spell very high-frequency words that they have seen many times in print the way they sound rather than the way they look (e.g., *"ov"* for "of," *"wun"* for "one," *"laf"* for "laugh"). Even when they are able to read quite well, their spelling errors still reflect a difficulty in remembering

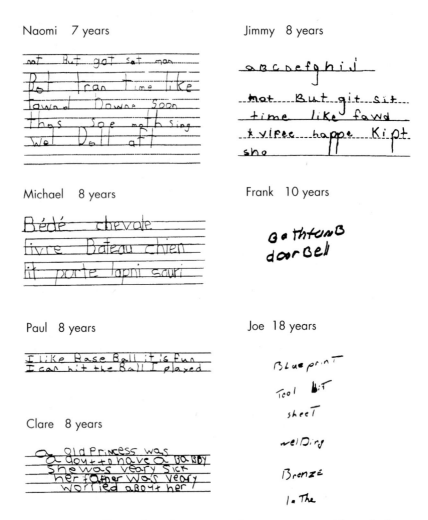

FIGURE 13-4 Examples of uppercase letter use to avoid confusions of lowercase forms.

how words look. Figure 13-5 shows a spelling sample from a student who has difficulty in the symbol-coding area. It can be seen that the student spells some very common words on the basis of how they sound rather than how they look. Spelling is often better out of context than in context. When children with symbol-coding problems have to learn a spelling list for school, they may study hard at home (reciting the spellings over and over) and get a high level of accuracy on the test the next day. Despite such good performance on spelling lists, they may make errors on the same words (even on the same day) in written compositions where their attentional resources are taken up expressing ideas.

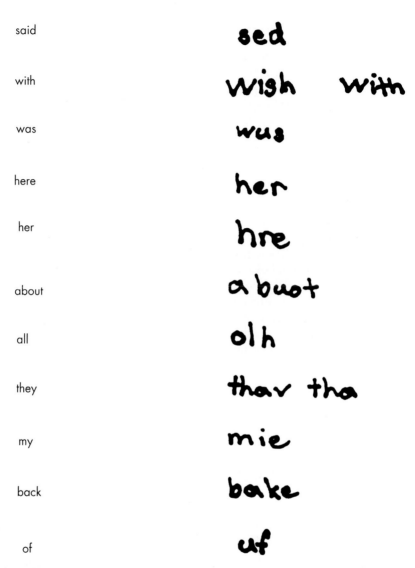

said	sed	
with	wish	with
was	wus	
here	her	
her	hre	
about	a buot	
all	ol h	
they	thav	tha
my	mie	
back	bake	
of	uf	

FIGURE 13-5 Spelling sample from a 12-year-old student with symbol-coding difficulty.

Written composition. The task of expressing ideas on paper is a daunting one for individuals with a weakness in symbol coding. The demands of remembering how to form letters and how to spell words already represent an enormous processing load. Thus, the content of the written compositions of individuals who are weak in Area 1 but who have average-or-above Area 2 abilities is usually far below their level of oral expression (e.g., a comparison of their oral and written production to the same stimulus picture, such as those used in the

TOWL-2, provides a graphic demonstration of the contrast between the oral and written language of an individual with weakness in symbol coding and strength in language processing/production). Their handwriting often deteriorates (compared with their performance on a copying task) and the quality of their vocabulary and grammar may suggest that of a child considerably younger. Although the underlying ideas expressed may be quite interesting, and even sophisticated, their presentation may be disjointed and "messy"— word endings or whole words omitted or repeated, punctuation and technical details overlooked, spacing between letters and words uneven—leaving an overall impression of "sloppy work."

Memory

Short-term/working memory. There is a great deal of evidence in the literature to suggest that individuals with what is here called a weakness in symbol coding have a deficit in short-term and/or working memory. Short-term memory is reflected by the ability to hold newly acquired "nonmeaningful"* information briefly in memory, as in holding a telephone number in mind after looking it up in the phone book, and working memory is the ability to hold information in mind while working on it, as in counting backwards from 100 by 7s. Transpositions of numbers (e.g., 12 becomes "21," 743 becomes "734") and letters ("left" becomes "felt," "about" becomes "abuot") that sometimes characterize the writing of individuals with Area 1 problems may also be a reflection of short-term and/or working-memory difficulties. Evidence of both types of memory weakness is readily obtained on digit span tests (e.g., the *WISC-III* Digit Span subtest), in which strings of numbers are presented and the task is to repeat them either in the same order (short-term memory) or in the reverse order (working memory). Individuals with a weakness in symbol coding usually perform below age expectations on such tasks.

CLINICAL PEARL

There is a great deal of evidence in the literature to suggest that individuals with a weakness in symbol coding have a deficit in short-term and/or working memory.

Long-term/rote memory. Perhaps as a result of their short-term/working-memory problems, individuals with symbol-coding weakness often also have auditory rote-memory problems. They are weak

---

*The term *nonmeaningful* is used to refer to types of information not meaningfully related in a semantic and/or syntactic sense, such as lists of random numbers or words.

in their ability to commit nonmeaningful rote facts to long-term memory. So, for example, such individuals may have considerable trouble commiting number facts to memory in mathematics and may persist in using their fingers to compute answers to simple addition, subtraction, multiplication, and division questions (e.g., "7 − 5 = ?," "6 × 4 = ?") at an age when others are able to remember such basic number facts "in their heads." Individuals with these difficulties, however, often become quite adept at using their fingers to do rapid calculations to come up with correct answers, so measures that assess only products and do not observe the process by which the product was obtained are not useful.*

Other evidence of their rote-memory weakness is demonstrated by the fact that, long after others their age are able to retain such information, they may not remember the days of the week or months of the year and may have difficulty remembering their own birth date, address, and home phone number. Having trouble remembering how to spell irregularly spelled words whose spellings must be committed to rote memory (e.g., *"people," "laugh," "ocean"*) is probably also a reflection of this rote-memory difficulty for nonmeaningful information. In contrast to poor memory for nonmeaningful information, individuals with symbol-coding weakness may—if they have strength in Area 2—be very capable of remembering meaningful information (i.e., information that can be readily associated with their semantic and syntactic network of background knowledge).

Visual processes

Given the possibility that symbol-coding weakness may well reflect some type of basic visual processing deficit, assessment should include measures explicitly designed to measure various aspects of visual processes. Obviously, a basic eye examination should precede any reading/writing assessment to ensure that vision is normal. In addition to the informal and more formal assessment measures outlined in the preceding sections on reading and writing (which have only an implicit visual processing component), measures that assess visual processes more directly should be utilized. Many clinicians find that the informal use (observing the child's strategies) of several subtests of the *Slingerland*—Far-Point Copying, Near-Point Copying, Visual-Perceptual Memory, Visual Discrimination, and Visual-Kinesthetic (Motor) Memory—can be particularly helpful in determining the locus of symbol-coding difficulties (although the norms of the test have been, justifiably, criticized in the literature). The usefulness

---

*Despite pervasive "technical problems" in their work—such as number reversals and transpositions, misreading of operational signs, and difficulty memorizing basic number facts—if they have strengths in Area 2, individuals with symbol-coding weakness may function amazingly well conceptually in math (as long as they are allowed to use aids such as number lines, number fact matrices, and calculators).

of the *Slingerland* comes from the fact that it involves assessing children's processing of both familiar symbols (letters, numbers, and words) and unfamiliar geometric forms under conditions that vary in the extent to which visual processing demands are combined with memory and motor requirements. It can be used with students from grades 1 to 6, and a more advanced version (the *Malcomesius*) is suitable for students in grades 6 to 8.

Other more generic measures of visual processes may also be of value when the previously mentioned measures indicate a visual-processing problem. The Coding subtest of the *WISC-III* (for children over the age of 8.0), for example, is useful as a standardized measure of symbol-coding difficulties. It assesses children's ability to form grapheme-to-grapheme associations as well as psychomotor speed. In addition, a range of other measures can be useful in determining whether deficits in visual perception, visual memory, and visual motor abilities might be implicated in a symbol-coding weakness. Various aspects of visual perception can be assessed with the Visual Discrimination, Visual Memory, Visual Spatial Relations, and Visual Form Constancy subtests from the *TVPS;* and visual-motor abilities can be assessed with the *VMI.*

Assessing Area 2: Characteristics of Language Processing/Production Weakness

Many, though not all, individuals with symbol-coding difficulties have a weakness in the language-processing area as well. This is reflected in difficulties understanding and/or producing language in both oral and written modalities. The box on p. 267 summarizes the characteristic learning difficulties associated with a language-processing weakness. These difficulties, unless very subtle, usually first become evident when the child begins to acquire aural/oral language, and they are manifested in various forms as the individual progresses through school and beyond.

Language development

Although a child whose only serious processing weakness is in the symbol-coding area may not show any apparent signs of learning difficulty before school, the individual with a language-processing/production weakness usually manifests problems long before school, even from the beginning of aural/oral language development. In some cases the difficulty may be fairly subtle and evident only to the speech and language professional; but in other cases, when the language-processing problem is more severe, it may be obvious to the parents from the earliest stages of language acquisition. Language-processing/production difficulties are reflected directly in phonological, semantic, and syntactic development and indirectly in reading, writing, and memory processes.

Assessing Area 2: Difficulties Associated with Language Processing/Production Weakness

Language development
Phonological development
Speech unclear
Misperception and/or mispronunciation of words

Semantic and syntactic development
Late in learning to talk
Vocabulary growth slow
Word-finding difficulties
"Immature" syntax

Reading
Decoding/word recognition
Weak grapheme-phoneme knowledge
Mispronunciation of words
Weak knowledge of word meanings
Word retrieval problems

Reading fluency
Slow dysfluent reading
Insensitivity to contextual cues

Reading comprehension
Weak comprehension, both in aural language and in reading

Writing
Spelling
Words misspelled on the basis of phonological confusions
Voiced-unvoiced confusions
Similar sounds confused
Hard-to-hear sounds omitted
Vowels with similar place of articulation confused
Weak analysis of sounds in longer words
Memory for spellings of nonphonetic words weak

Written composition
Expression weak, both in oral language and writing
Inappropriate word usage
Limited vocabulary
Immature grammatical structures
Confusion about abstract concepts
Repetitive language patterns
Limited productivity

Memory
Pervasive memory problems
Weak short-term/working memory
Weak long-term/rote memory
Weak long-term semantic memory

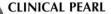

CLINICAL PEARL

Although a child whose only serious processing weakness is in the symbol-coding area may not show any apparent signs of learning difficulty before school, the individual with a language-processing/production weakness usually manifests problems long before school, even from the beginning of aural/oral language development.

Phonological development. In addition to difficulties with the content and form of language (i.e., semantics, syntax, and morphology),* some individuals with a language-processing problem have trouble with the sounds of language—the phonology. They have difficulty differentiating the sound units in the spoken language. This becomes apparent in the early stages of language acquisition in that the child's oral language is unclear and hard to understand. Such a difficulty may be the result of either receptive or expressive weakness, or both. The child may not perceive clearly the fine differences between similar sounds (e.g., as assessed by the Auditory Word Discrimination subtest of the *TAPS*) and/or, although able to perceive differences, may not be able to articulate them. The former, the receptive problem, may be indicative of fundamental and deep-seated difficulties in processing the sounds in language; the latter may merely reflect an immature or defective speech apparatus that mechanically interferes with the child's ability to correctly articulate speech sounds. If the phonological problem is only an expressive one, reflecting an articulatory deficit, then time and/or speech therapy may completely eliminate it. If either receptive deficits alone or receptive and expressive deficits together are involved, unclear speech may be a precursor of further confusion about the sounds of speech. Receptive and expressive phonological difficulties may be manifested in the misperception and mispronunciation of words over the long run. The analysis of sounds in auditory sequences presents a particular problem for individuals with phonological processing deficits (these problems can be assessed using the *LAC* test). Such difficulties cause problems in analyzing sequences of sounds in words (e.g., a child might say "aminal" for "animal" at an age when most other children no longer make this type of error) and in recognizing the constituent sounds in words (the child might think the second month of the year is called "Vemberry"). Phonological processing weaknesses have direct academic consequences for decoding (in reading) and encoding (in spelling) the sounds in words.

---

*Definitions: *semantics* is the system of meanings of the language, *morphology* refers to the rules of word formation, and *syntax* refers to the rules of sentence formation.

Semantic and syntactic development. The first sign of language-processing/production difficulty may come in the form of timing of a child's first words. Children who later manifest full-blown language disorders generally lag behind developmental norms in all aspects of their speech and language acquisition. They are late in learning to talk, and often their speech is unclear. Their weakness is also apparent in limited vocabulary growth in that they do not know the meanings of as many words as others their age do. This problem may be reflected in receptive or expressive vocabulary, or both. If individuals have difficulty in receptive vocabulary, not understanding the meanings of words said to them (e.g., as measured by the *PPVT-R*), then they will almost certainly not be able to express word meanings in spoken language at a level commensurate with their ages (e.g., as measured by the *WISC-III* Vocabulary subtest). The converse is not necessarily true, however: Individuals with expressive vocabulary weakness may not demonstrate any evidence of receptive language difficulties; they may understand perfectly well what is said to them, but still have great difficulty expressing themselves clearly.

Another characteristic of some but not all individuals with a language-processing weakness is retrieval or word-finding difficulties (sometimes referred to as dysnomia). For example, children with word-finding problems overuse empty words such as "the thing" or "whatever" to refer to objects or activities. Such difficulties may be masked in informal observations of natural speech by the child's facility at circumlocutions (e.g., the child may say "the thing that cuts the grass" to refer to a lawnmower). Moreover, given enough time, the child may be able to retrieve the precise word, sometimes through semantic or phonological associations. In assessment, word-finding difficulties can be evaluated with confrontation-naming tasks in which the child is shown a series of pictures depicting common nouns and is expected to respond immediately with a single appropriate word or words to identify each (e.g., as reflected by the *BNT*). Such tasks make it readily apparent when the child is resorting to circumlocution or hesitating until the word becomes available.

"Immature" grammar is another characteristic of weakness in processing language. Individuals with this difficulty tend to use grammatical structures typical of younger children. Although grammatical development occurs as they advance in age, a lag between their age and the maturity of their grammar usually persists. Assessment of grammatical development normally requires the assistance of a knowledgeable speech and language professional or at least the use of a well-established formal test of language processing (e.g., the *CELF-R*). As in vocabulary development, comprehension (receptive language) normally surpasses production (expressive language), such that people understand more than they are able to express adequately in words.

A particular conundrum for speech and language clinicians is distinguishing between "delays" and "deficits" in the semantic and syntactic development of children in the early school grades. Given that normal variation has a fairly broad range, especially up to the age of 7 or 8, what may appear as a basic language-processing weakness may simply be the expression of developmental variation and, a year later, all evidence of the "problem area" may have vanished. In many cases, however, what originally appeared to reflect a delay in development may turn out to be indicative of a genuine area of deficit. Because such distinctions are fine ones, they should clearly be left to specialists.

Another potential confounding factor in assessments of grammatical development is the cultural/linguistic models that served as the basis for the particular grammatical forms adopted. Because there are dialectical and regional variations in what are considered "standard" grammatical structures, it is essential that judgments of the appropriateness of children's grammar be made in the context of their personal linguistic environment. Simply comparing an individual's grammatical usage with "standard English" can result in very inappropriate conclusions, so assessment should be done at least in part by someone who is conversant with the child's linguistic environment.

Reading

Aural/oral language functions are fundamental to the development of skill in reading. If children's phonological, semantic, and syntactic development is weak, they will have difficulties in all aspects of reading acquisition, including decoding/word recognition, reading fluency, and comprehension.

CLINICAL PEARL

Aural/oral language functions are fundamental to the development of skill in reading. If children's phonological, semantic, and syntactic development is weak, they will have difficulties in all aspects of reading acquisition, including decoding/word recognition, reading fluency, and comprehension.

Decoding/word recognition. If children are deficient in their ability to process the sounds of the aural/oral language with speed and accuracy, they will be weak in phonemic awareness and will find phonemic analysis—a key element in decoding words—to be problematical. In attempting to decode the graphemes (letters) in a printed word to the associated phonemes (sounds), the individual with language-processing weakness may not know the sounds that are associated with the letters in a printed word and may not be able to synthesize (blend) them into the correct word (e.g., as assessed by the Sound-Symbol Battery of the *G-F-W* and the Word Attack subtest of the *WRMT-R*). Moreover, even if the letter-sound decoding is achieved, the individual may not be able to match the phonological representation to a known word because of deficits in vocabulary and word finding (i.e., although they may "decode" the letters in a word to phonemes, they may not be able to retrieve the appropriate word meaning to make sense of what they have decoded and pronounce it properly).

Reading fluency. To recognize words in text, children need to know the meanings of the words in their aural/oral language (i.e., have a representation of them in their lexicon or internal dictionary). In addition, if they have not yet learned the printed form of the words they must make use not only of phonological information but of contextual information to "figure them out" (i.e., the psycholinguistic guessing game). For children with weak semantic and syntactic processing, their ability to make use of context to supplement the visual information on the page is limited because they are insensitive to semantic and syntactic cues in the text (e.g., as reflected in the semantic and syntactic appropriateness of their word substitutions in oral reading).

Reading comprehension. Even if individuals are able to recognize the printed words on the page, their weak language-processing ability will interfere with their comprehension of the meaning of the text. Children with language-processing weakness should not be expected to understand something in print that they would not understand in aural/oral language. Tests that compare Listening Comprehension with Silent Reading Comprehension (e.g., as in the *DARD-R*) will indicate that comprehension in both modes is below age/grade expectations.

Writing

Spelling. When attempting to encode phonemes to graphemes in writing, children with Area 2 problems are at a great disadvantage. Weak phonological processing causes them to confuse phonemes that differ only by minor articulatory features, failing to clearly differentiate the voiced and voiceless pairs /b-p/, /d-t/, /v-f/, and /g-k/ (e.g., misspelling "mapy" for "maybe," "trop" for "drop"), mixing up similar sounds such as /m-n/ and /sh-ch/, omitting hard-to-hear sounds (e.g., spelling *"simig"* for *"swimming,"* "thik" for "think," "wet" for "went"), and confusing vowel sounds have a similar place of articulation in the mouth, as in the short sounds of *e-i-a* (e.g., spelling "wit" for "what," "want" for "went"). There is also difficulty analyzing all of the sounds in longer words so the child with a language-processing problem may drop or add whole syllables (e.g., as reflected in the Phonic Spelling subtest of the *DARD-R*).

Written language. Given that the oral language production of individuals with an Area 2 weakness is generally substandard, it is self-evident that written production will be as well. In view of the multiple simultaneous linguistic demands in written language, it is not surprising that this area is seriously impoverished. The written production of those with language-processing/production weakness is characterized by inappropriate word usage, limited vocabulary, immature grammatical structures, confusion about abstract concepts, repetitive language patterns, and limited productivity. These types of difficulties are reflected in their writing of stories in response to picture prompts (e.g., as in the Spontaneous Writing component of the *TOWL-2*).

Memory

Whereas individuals who have a primary weakness in Area 1 and no apparent difficulty in Area 2 usually have some memory difficulties in the form of short-term/working memory and long-term/rote memory, those who have weakness in Area 2 (with or without Area 1 problems) have much more pervasive memory problems, affecting immediate memory (both short-term and working memory) and long-term memory (for both nonmeaningful and meaningful information). These memory weaknesses are often reflected in low scores on the *WISC-III* subtests that make up the Memory Factor (also known as the Freedom-From-Distractibility Factor) score—Arithmetic, Coding, Information, and Digit Span (i.e., the "ACID pattern"). Such extensive memory problems invariably have serious consequences for school learning.

Short-term/working memory. Difficulties in short-term/working memory are characteristic of the vast majority of individuals with reading/writing problems. Individuals with Area 2 weakness have a hard time holding newly acquired information in mind, be it non-meaningful (e.g., lists of unrelated words or of number sequences, as assessed in the Word Sequences subtest of the *DTLA-2* and the Digit Span subtest of the *WISC-III*) or meaningful (as in the Sentence Imitation subtest of the *DTLA-2*). This weakness is strikingly demonstrated when instructions or explanations are given verbally in class at school. Under these circumstances children with Area 2 problems may ask about something just explained seemingly as though they were not paying attention, but in fact they have forgotten (and, possibly, not understood) some or all of the instructions just heard.

Long-term/rote memory. As is the case with individuals who have Area 1 problems, memory for nonmeaningful information, which must be retained through rote repetition (e.g., number facts, spellings of irregular words, days of the week and months of the year), is weak.

Long-term semantic memory. In contrast with individuals who have a primary weakness in symbol-coding (Area 1) and strength in language processing/production (Area 2), individuals who have a weakness in Area 2 (irrespective of their strength or weakness in Area 1) have difficulty retaining meaningful information in long-term semantic memory. After seeing a favorite TV program, or after hearing a story read to them (e.g., as in the Listening Comprehension subtest of the *DARD-R*), children with weakness in Area 2 may not be able to respond correctly to questions about the program or story. Not surprisingly, this problem may be compounded in situations where they must retain information they have read themselves.

III. Programming for Reading and Writing Difficulties

The goal of this section is to offer recommendations for teaching students who have processing difficulties in one or both of the areas in the framework used in this chapter. The suggestions are intended as guidelines for those who are expected to offer practical recommendations following from assessment findings and those who are charged with implementing special programs. Both generic and specific suggestions are included.

The term *remediation* is specifically avoided in this section because—within the context of a chapter in which reading and writing difficulties are conceptualized as a reflection of normal variation in basic information-processing abilities—it is felt to convey the impression of a disease or defect that requires a remedy rather than individual differences that call for individualized programming.

Programming for Area 1: Symbol-Coding Weakness

Visual deficits and programming. As was discussed in the previous sections on assessment, a very large number of individuals with reading/writing difficulties have a weakness in the symbol-coding area. This is reflected in difficulties with processing and remembering visual symbols in both reading and writing. As discussed in the previous chapter, whether what appears to involve some type of visual processing deficit will ultimately turn out to reflect visual processes per se or other basic processing deficits (e.g., processing speed and/or memory) is, I believe, uncertain. The evidence that individuals who manifest symbol-coding difficulties perform below normal readers on a range of tasks apparently assessing visual processes is very compelling, but so too is the extensive evidence implicating other types of processing deficits, especially phonological-coding deficits. What seems essentially indisputable on the basis of the evidence to date is that associating visual symbols with language is a source of enormous difficulty for the vast majority of individuals who have trouble learning to read. From a clinical point of view, the distinction between whether the problem in coding symbols is in the visual domain or the phonological domain, or at the interface between the two, may be largely immaterial with respect to intervention. Both research evidence and clinical experience show that approaches that assist in the symbol-coding process—involving both visual and phonological components—appear to be an effective route toward ameliorating reading and writing difficulties.

CLINICAL PEARL

Associating visual symbols with language is a source of enormous difficulty for the vast majority of individuals who have trouble learning to read. From a clinical point of view, the distinction between whether the problem in coding symbols is in the visual domain or the phonological domain, or at the interface between the two, may be largely immaterial with respect to intervention.

Although there is a considerable amount of research indicating that disabled readers exhibit a variety of types of visual processing deficits, evidence that interventions designed to overcome such deficits result in improved reading and writing is still limited and highly controversial.[5] At this point, the only approach to intervention that I can recommend with any degree of confidence is specialized educational programming. Both research and clinical evidence demonstrate that appropriate teaching can be of great benefit to the reading/writing disabled.

Reading

Word recognition. For children with a weakness in symbol coding, word recognition is clearly the fundamental problem underlying difficulties in reading fluency and comprehension. Because such children seem to have difficulty remembering what words look like, the teaching program must be designed to reduce the memory demands involved in word recognition and to facilitate discrimination between similar-looking words. The former can be achieved by using reading material with a carefully controlled vocabulary of high-frequency sight words (see examples of *High Interest/Controlled Vocabulary Material* suitable for students of different ages in the Appendix at the end of this chapter), and the latter can be achieved by providing children with the word analysis skills to decode words they cannot recognize by sight (through programs such as *Phonics They Use: Words for Reading and Writing, The Phonics Handbook, Recipe for Reading,* and *The Benchmark School Word Identification/Vocabulary Development Pro-*

gram). Two books that provide an excellent foundation for developing appropriate word recognition programs are *Beginning to Read* and *Stages of Reading Development*.[1,2]

Because students with reading/writing difficulties and disabilities have serious problems remembering visual symbols, they require much more repetition of letters and words before they can retain them. Such repetition could become "dull drill," especially in the early stages of the program before they have a sufficiently large repertoire of words that can be recognized "by sight" or "sounding out" (i.e., phonics). There are few books at the beginning stages using either controlled sight vocabulary or decodable words that are sufficiently stimulating to motivate students over an extended period. Well-chosen games are useful in providing the repetition needed to reinforce the word recognition and decoding developed in the instructional program. Games provide motivation to practice skills long after the student would have become bored reading controlled-vocabulary books. Card games, board games, and computer games can be used to supplement the reading texts (examples are presented in the Appendix).

Writing

Spelling. Because students with symbol-coding difficulties and disabilities seem to have serious problems remembering what the letters, orthographic (spelling) patterns within words (e.g., *ght, ing, oi*), and whole words look like, their spelling program must be very systematic in introducing the orthographic patterns of the language, beginning with the least complex. The most common spelling patterns of English should be introduced with "phonics" and "word families" approaches (e.g., *Phonics They Use: Words for Reading and Writing*). To reduce the memory load, the spelling program should be closely coordinated with the reading program, following similar principles. Some students can learn to spell irregular words (i.e., words that are not spelled the way they sound, such as "laugh," "people") by repeating them many times in games. If spelling of irregular words is taught this way, it is important to have the students practice spelling the words in sentence context, as well. Many students with specific reading/writing difficulties and disabilities have weak rote memory for nonmeaningful sequences, however. These students may find it very difficult to remember how to spell irregular words by repetition, and they can benefit from a focus on the patterns in words through learning a simple set of rules (e.g., *The Spell of Words*) and/or being taught the morphological patterns in words (e.g., *Morphographic Spelling*). Also, because it is easier to recognize (read) words than to recall (spell) them, students with poor memory for the spellings of irregular words need to use a special alphabetized word list (e.g., *Spelling Reference Book*) to look up the spellings of words they can read but cannot spell. It is usually very difficult for students with Area 1 problems to check over their work for spelling errors, so for some (especially older) students a computer spell checker can be useful.

Written composition. The task of written composition is extremely taxing for students with a symbol-coding weakness because it involves the processing demands of handwriting, spelling, and creative writing (composition) simultaneously. To reduce this load and promote the creative expression of ideas, students should be allowed to do written composition without concerns about neatness of handwriting or correctness of spelling. Students should be encouraged to spell words the way they sound (inventive spelling) in their rough drafts and to consult a *Spelling Reference Book* or use a computer spell checker to correct their spelling in work they want to share with others. In the early stages, an assisted-composition approach (e.g., *Composition Guided-Free* or *Writing About Pictures*) can facilitate the coordination of handwriting, spelling, and composition processes. To develop letter formation and handwriting skills, specific instruction will facilitate the student's development of legibility.

Programming for Area 2: Language-Processing/Production Difficulties

Oral Language

As discussed in the section on assessment, weakness in receptive/ expressive oral language often, though not always, accompanies symbol-coding weakness. If it does, then the recommendations presented in this section must be combined with those in the previous section dealing with symbol-coding weakness. It must be recognized, however, that, because oral language processes are the substrate upon which written language processes are built, intervention must begin by establishing a good oral language foundation. Unless the oral language weakness is a mild one, intervention in this area will require the assistance of a qualified speech and language clinician. General information about programming for oral language disorders is available in such texts as Wiig and Semel's *Language Assessment and Intervention for the Learning Disabled,*[8] and very useful intervention techniques are outlined in the *Handbooks of Exercises for Language Processing (H.E.L.P.)*, Books 1 to 4, and *H.E.L.P. Language Games,* and in *Language Remediation and Expansion.* The recommendations in this section will focus only on programming for written language processes—reading and writing.

Reading

Reading comprehension. The reading comprehension of students with Area 2 difficulties will virtually always lag behind their oral language comprehension, because those who have problems with oral language processing/production will not understand in reading what they do not understand in oral language. In addition to building up their phonological, grammatical, morphological, and pragmatic knowledge through oral language intervention, it is important to provide instruction explicitly designed to foster reading comprehension. There are now excellent practical theory-based guidelines for developing semantic and syntactic processing in reading through improving reading vocabulary (e.g., *Teaching Reading Vocabulary*) and promoting reading comprehension (*Reading Comprehension: New Directions for Classroom Practice*). Explicit development of vocabulary and background knowledge is essential to the formation of schemas, which in turn provide semantic and syntactic networks that allow for the assimilation and accommodation of new ideas.

Writing

Spelling. To improve the spelling of individuals with Area 2 problems, it is important to employ a systematic phonics program in which the student is sensitized to the articulatory differences between similar sounds. Unless students with weak phonological processing skills are able to discriminate between the articulatory movements involved in similar phonemes, they will have great difficulty spelling accurately. Comprehensive phonological processing intervention such as Lindamood's *Auditory Discrimination in Depth* program are needed to sensitize the child to the articulatory and phonological distinctions between phonemes. Suitable approaches for spelling instruction are presented in the previous section on reading/writing difficulties and disabilities (Area 1). Students who persist in making "phonological confusions" (e.g., *p-b, m-n, ch-sh*) should be taught to use a *Spelling Reference Book* so they can rely on visual processes to verify their spelling efforts based on unreliable auditory cues.

Written composition. Just as the student who is weak in symbol-coding abilities is extremely handicapped in written language, so also is the student who is weak in oral language-processing/production abilities, but for different reasons. For students with Area 1 weakness, written language is challenging because of the processing demands of encoding speech sounds to visual symbols. Students with Area 2 weakness have trouble not only because of their phonological-coding difficulties but also because of their pervasive language difficulties. In written language tasks, students who are weak in terms of vocabulary and grammatical knowledge are under enormous stress because they must call upon their deficient oral language abilities and at the same time cope with the demands of spelling and handwriting. As in the case of Area 1 problems, it is important to teach composition, spelling, and handwriting separately. However, development of oral language is a prerequisite to written tasks for the language-disabled student.

Moreover, for students with weakness in both areas, intensive and lengthy intervention is required for improvement in the written domain.

Present Practice and Future Frameworks

In presenting the practical guidelines offered in this chapter, I have been painfully aware of the "risks" involved in attempting to take the leap from theory to practice. However, as someone who teaches graduate courses on reading and writing processes and disabilities to classroom teachers, special educators, school psychology students, and speech and language clinicians, I have learned from my students that the application to assessment and remedial interventions of the framework presented here is considered by those in the field as being of great practical utility. The present working model will undoubtedly require revision in future, to keep up with advances in our theoretical understanding of reading and writing processes, but given the rich foundation of clinical wisdom underlying the recommendations, it seems likely that future changes will be minor rather than major.

References

1. Chall JS: *Stages of reading development,* New York, 1983, McGraw-Hill.
2. Adams MJ: *Beginning to read: thinking and learning about print,* Cambridge, Mass, 1990, MIT Press.
3. Levine MD: *Developmental variation and learning disorders,* Cambridge, Mass, 1987, Educators Publishing Service.
4. Lipson MJ, Wixon KK: *Assessment and instruction of reading disability: an interactive approach,* New York, 1991, Harper Collins.
5. Willows DM, Kruk R, Corcos E (eds): *Visual processes in reading and reading disabilities,* Hillsdale, NJ, 1993, Lawrence Erlbaum.
6. Willows DM: A "normal variation" view of written language difficulties and disabilities: implications for whole language programs, *Except Educ Can* 1:73-103, 1991.
7. Willows DM: Visual processes in learning disabilities. In Wong BYL (ed): *Learning about learning disabilities,* New York, 1991, Academic Press.
8. Wiig EH, Semel EM: *Language assessment and intervention for the learning disabled,* ed 2, Columbus, Ohio, 1984, Charles E Merrill.

Appendix: Assessment and Programming Resources

Assessment Instruments

Boston Naming Test (BNT)
Philadelphia, 1983, Lea & Febiger

Clinical Evaluation of Language Fundamentals–Revised (CELF-R)
San Antonio, 1987, The Psychological Corporation

Detroit Test of Learning Aptitude–2 (DTLA-2)
Austin, 1985, Pro-Ed

Developmental Test of Visual-Motor Integration (VMI)
Cleveland, 1989, Modern Curriculum Press

Durrell Analysis of Reading Difficulty–Revised (DARD-R)
San Antonio, 1980, The Psychological Corporation

Goldman-Fristoe-Woodcock Auditory Skills Test Battery (G-F-W)
Circle Pines, Minn, 1974, American Guidance Service

Lindamood Auditory Conceptualization Test (LAC)
Allen, Texas, 1979, DLM Teaching Resources

Peabody Picture Vocabulary Test–Revised (PPVT-R)
Circle Pines, Minn, 1981, American Guidance Service

Screening Tests for Identifying Children with Specific Language Disability
(Slingerland, grades 1 to 6; *Malcomesius,* grades 6 to 8)*
Cambridge, Mass, 1974, Educators Publishing Service

Test of Auditory-Perceptual Skills (TAPS)
Seattle, 1982, Psychological Assessment Resources

Test of Visual-Perceptual Skills (TVPS)
Seattle, 1982, Psychological Assessment Resources

Test of Written Language–2 (TOWL-2)
Austin, 1988, Pro-Ed

Wechsler Intelligence Scale for Children–III (WISC-III)
San Antonio, 1991, The Psychological Corporation

Wide Range Achievement Test–Revised (WRAT-R)
San Antonio, 1984, The Psychological Corporation

Woodcock Reading Mastery Tests–Revised (WRMT-R)
Circle Pines, Minn, 1987, American Guidance Service

Programming Resources

Decoding/Encoding Programs

Benchmark Word Identification Program
Media PA, 1986, Benchmark Press
Gaskins RW, Gaskins JC, Gaskins IW: A decoding program for poor readers—and the rest of the class, too! *Lang Arts* 68:213-225, 1991

Making Words
Making Big Words
Cunningham PM, Hall DP: Columbus, Ohio, Good Apple

Phonics They Use: Words for Reading and Writing
Cunningham PM: New York, 1991, Harper Collins

Recipe for Reading: A Structured Approach to Linguistics
Traub N: Cambridge, Mass, 1990, Educators Publishing Service

The Phonics Handbook
Lloyd S: Chigwell, Essex, UK, 1994, Jolly Learning Ltd.

High-Interest/Controlled-Vocabulary "Sight" Reading Material

Dolch Read and Comprehend Series
Allen, Texas, DLM Teaching Resources

Giant First-Start Readers
First-Start Easy Reader
Mahwah, NJ, Troll Associates

Heinemann Guided Readers
London, Heinemann Educational Books

New PM Story Books
New York, Scholastic Inc.

Sprint Gold Medal Collection
New York, Scholastic Inc.

Stars Magazine and other high-interest/low-vocabulary reading
Seattle, Turman Publishing

STEP into Reading
STEP-UP Classic Chillers
New York, Random House

Resources for Reading Comprehension

Reading Comprehension: New Directions for Classroom Practice (ed 3)
McNeil JD: New York, 1992, Harper-Collins

Teaching Reading Vocabulary (ed 2)
Johnson DD, Pearson PD: New York, 1984, Holt, Rinehart & Winston

Resources for Spelling

Phonics They Use: Words for Reading and Writing.
   Cummingham PM: New York, 1991, Harper Collins

Morphographic Spelling
   Engelmann-Becker SRA

The Spell of Words
Spellbound
Spellbinding
   Cambridge, Mass, Educators Publishing Service

Spelling Reference Book
   Allen, Texas, DLM Teaching Resources

Spelling: Sharing the Secrets
   Scott R: Toronto, Gage Publishing

Spellex Word Finder
Spellex Thesaurus
   North Billerica, Mass, Curriculum Associates

Resources for Written Composition

Composition: Guided-Free
Writing About Pictures
   New York, Teachers College Press

Recipes for Writing
   Menlo Park, Calif, Addison-Wesley

Resources for Language Development

H.E.L.P. (Handbooks of Exercises for Language Processing)
   East Moline, Ill, LinguiSystems

Language Remediation and Expansion: 150 Skill Building Reference Lists
   Tucson, Communication Skill Builders

Games

Dolch Puzzle Books
   Allen, Texas, DLM Teaching Resources

H.E.L.P. Language Games
   East Moline, Ill, LinguiSystems

Magic Squares
   Cambridge, Mass, Educators Publishing Service

Road Race (reading, spelling, vocabulary)
   North Billerica, Mass, Curriculum Associates

Short Vowel and Long Vowel Gameboards and Reproducible Worksheets
   Palos Verdes Estates, Calif, Frank Schaffer Publications

14

A Wavelength-Specific Intervention for Reading Disability

Mary C. Williams
Katie LeCluyse
Richard Littell

Key Terms

transient system	metacontrast	scotopic sensitivity
sustained system	wavelength	syndrome
perceptual deficits	visual discomfort	
visual masking	syndrome	

Visual Factors in Specific Reading Disability

Specific reading disability is a broad term that encompasses reading disabilities arising from a number of sources. A specific-reading-disabled child (SRD) is defined here as one of normal or better intelligence with no known organic or behavioral disorders who, despite normal schooling and average progress in other subjects, has a reading disability of at least 2.5 years.[1-6] Because reading involves a dynamic visual processing task that requires the analysis and integration of visual pattern information across fixation-saccade sequences, studies in the area of reading disability have explored the possibility that visual processing abnormalities contribute to reading difficulties. A number of studies have provided evidence for basic visual processing differences between normal and disabled readers, especially at early stages of visual processing. Differences have been reported in visual information store duration,[6-8] in the rate of transfer of information from visual information store to short-term memory,[7, 8] and in the characteristics of visual short-term memory itself.[9] These results indicate that some disabled readers process information more slowly and have a more limited processing capacity than normal readers do. However, studies that have used tasks relying less on dynamic visual processing and temporal resolution, and more on pattern-formation processes and long-term memory,[10-17] have failed to show visual processing differences between normal and disabled readers, although the validity of these studies has been called into question.[18, 19] Thus the long-standing debate as to whether visual factors play a significant role in reading difficulties has been complicated by the differences in methodologies and the failure to distinguish between measurements of temporal versus pattern-formation processes.

CLINICAL PEARL

Some disabled readers process information more slowly and have a more limited processing capacity than normal readers do.

Transient-Sustained Theory of Visual Processing

It has been suggested[20-24] that the processing of temporal and pattern information is accomplished by two separate but interactive subsystems in vision with different spatial-temporal response characteristics. A short-latency transient system is most sensitive to low spatial frequencies, has a high temporal resolution and short response persistence, and is thought to be involved in the perception of motion, the control of eye movements, and the localization of targets in space. A longer-latency sustained system is most sensitive to high spatial frequencies and stationary or slowly moving targets, has a long response persistence or integration time and low temporal resolution, and is thought to be involved in the identification of patterns and resolution of fine detail. According to this theory, the transient system is a fast-operating early warning system that extracts large amounts of global information. The sustained system, on the other hand, responds more slowly and subsequent to the transient response and is dependent to an extent upon output of the transient system.

CLINICAL PEARL

It has been suggested that the processing of temporal and pattern information is accomplished by two separate but interactive subsystems in vision with different spatial-temporal response characteristics.

This transient-sustained processing distinction has recently been reconceptualized[25-28] in light of evidence for separate parvocellular (P) and magnocellular (M) pathways in primates, which have been found to have largely sustained and transient response properties respectively. The sustained P pathway appears to be additionally involved in the perception of color, texture, and fine stereopsis, while the transient M pathway is involved in the perception of flicker and motion.

Transient-Sustained Processing and Reading Disability

There is evidence that this transient-sustained relationship is different in normal and disabled readers. Lovegrove et al.[29,30] and Martin and Lovegrove[31] have shown that visual processing differences between normal and disabled readers are evident when transient system processing is involved but fail to surface under sustained processing conditions. For example, disabled readers are less sensitive than normal readers to low spatial frequencies, but equally or more sensitive to high spatial frequencies. Additionally, disabled readers show lower overall temporal sensitivity[31] and a different pattern of temporal processing across spatial frequencies,[1,5,29] but these temporal processing differences between normal and disabled readers are eliminated when transient system activity is reduced. These findings indicate that disabled readers have a deficient transient system. Measures of sustained channel processing, such as orientation band width, spatial frequency band width, and the oblique effect, have not provided evidence of differences between normal and disabled readers,[3,4] suggesting that the integrity of the sustained system is intact.

CLINICAL PEARL

Visual processing differences between normal and disabled readers are evident when transient system processing is involved but fail to surface under sustained processing conditions.

Williams and co-workers (Brannan and Williams,[32-34] Williams and Bologna,[35] Williams and LeCluyse,[36] and Williams et al.[37-40]) have expanded on Lovegrove's work by studying the perceptual consequences of a transient deficit in disabled readers. These studies demonstrate the existence of a number of perceptual deficits in disabled readers that would be predicted by a transient deficit (i.e., the perceptual skills affected are those most likely mediated by the transient system). The evidence suggests that the nature of the transient deficit is a slowed or sluggish response from the transient system, such that it does not clearly precede and provide output to the sustained system.

CLINICAL PEARL

Studies have demonstrated the existence of a number of perceptual deficits in disabled readers that would be predicted by a transient deficit (i.e., the perceptual skills affected are those most likely mediated by the transient system).

Visual Masking Studies

More direct measures of the temporal aspects of visual processing in normal and disabled readers have been obtained in recent visual masking studies.[38,39]

Williams et al.[38] used a metacontrast masking paradigm to index the processing rate in both foveal and peripheral vision. In metacontrast, a target is briefly presented and is followed at various delays by a spatially adjacent masking stimulus. Accuracy of detecting the target is measured as a function of the delay between the target and the mask. The time course of the accuracy function is thought to represent the time course of processing the target and mask. The accuracy functions typically obtained in metacontrast experiments are U-shaped, much like the schematic in Figure 14-1, *B*. Accuracy first decreases, reaches a low point at an intermediate delay, and then increases again to the baseline level. Two-component metacontrast theories[23,24,41-43] attribute U-shaped metacontrast functions to the interaction of transient and sustained components of visual response. These models posit metacontrast masking as the result of the faster transient response to the later-occurring mask's catching up with, and inhibiting, the slower sustained response to the target. For this to occur, the mask must be delayed relative to the target. Figure 14-1, *A*, illustrates these timing assumptions. The dip, or lowest accuracy point in the function is the point of maximum inhibition. As the dip shifts rightward toward longer delays, it can be assumed that some

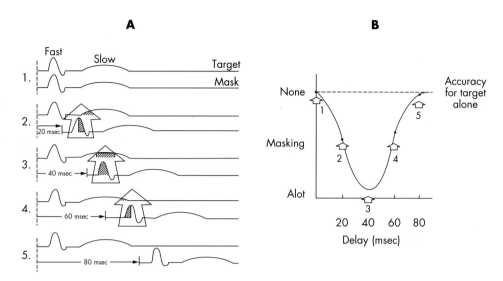

FIGURE 14-1 U-shaped metacontrast function together with hypothetical visual responses to a target and a mask. **A,** The responses. *(1)* Simultaneous onset of the target and mask. Transient response does not overlap sustained response, and there is no masking (*arrow* labeled *1* on right). *(2)* Target leading the mask by 20 msec. Transient response to the mask slightly overlaps the beginning of the sustained response to the target and some interference occurs. There is a small amount of masking (*arrow 2*). *(3)* Difference in onsets of the target and mask produce maximum overlap of transient and sustained components and thus the greatest amount of interference (*arrow 3*). *(4)* Target leading the mask by 60 msec, with the transient response to the mask again only slightly overlapping the sustained response to the target and the amount of interference, again, small. Masking begins to decrease (*arrow 4*). *(5)* Target leading the mask by a long delay. No interference occurs, and from this point on there is no masking. **B,** The metacontrast function. Accuracy is plotted against delay. (From Williams M, Weisstein N: The effects of perceived depth or metacontrast functions, *Vision Res* 24:1279-1288, 1984.)

aspect of the transient (inhibitory) response to the mask is traveling faster, simply because a response that is activated later has to travel faster to catch up. Thus, according to these models, dips at long delays between the target and mask imply faster transient processing, and dips at short delays imply slower transient processing.

Using diagonal line segments as targets and a surrounding outlined square as a masking stimulus, Williams et al.[38] obtained the metacontrast functions shown in Figure 14-2. The different dip locations in the functions obtained from adults, normal readers, and disabled readers indicate that the foveal transient response is fastest in normal adults, slowest in reading-disabled children, and intermediate in

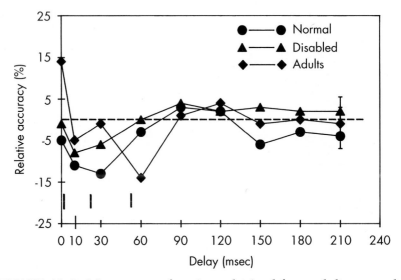

FIGURE 14-2 Metacontrast functions obtained from adults, normal readers, and disabled readers. The accuracy (measured as percent correct) for detecting target lines followed by the masking stimulus at various delays is plotted against the accuracy (*dashed line*) for target lines alone, which was set at a level between 70% and 80% before each session. (From Williams M, Molinet K, LeCluyse K: Visual masking as a measure of temporal processing in normal and disabled readers, *Clin Vis Sci* 4:137-144, 1989.)

normal-reading children. These findings are consistent with the findings from previous reports of increased temporal resolution with age[33,34] and, additionally, suggest that temporal processing in disabled readers is sluggish compared with that in normal readers.

The magnitude of metacontrast masking increased in the peripheral retina of adults and normal readers (Figure 14-3, *A* and *B*), which is consistent with previous reports of increased masking effects in the periphery.[44-46] There was, however, an absence of metacontrast masking in disabled readers with peripheral presentations (Figure 14-3, *C*), a finding compatible with that of Geiger and Lettvin's,[47] in which dyslexic subjects show a smaller magnitude of simultaneous lateral masking in the periphery. Geiger and Lettvin attribute the reduced masking effect to an attentional strategy of dyslexic subjects to allocate more processing capacity to peripheral than to foveal areas of the visual field. An alternate explanation can be derived from the two-component masking theories described previously, which attribute metacontrast masking to the inhibition of slow sustained channels by fast transient channels. These theories would predict that a transient channel deficit leads to an attenuation or elimination of metacontrast masking.

This masking study[38] suggests that the nature of transient system deficits in disabled readers is a slowed or sluggish response from the

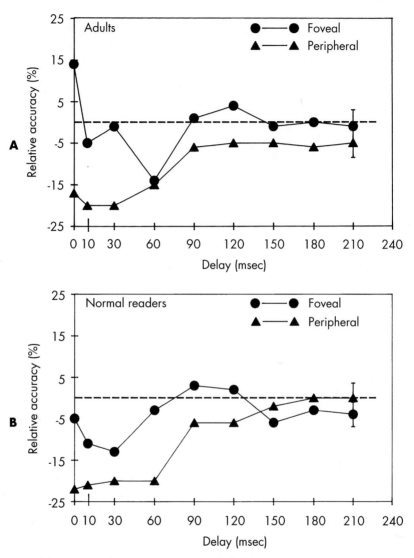

FIGURE 14-3 Metacontrast functions obtained from adults (*A*) normal readers (*B*) and disabled readers (*C*) with foveal viewing (*circles*) and peripheral viewing (*triangles*). The accuracy (measured as percent correct) for detecting target lines followed by a masking stimulus at various delays is plotted against the accuracy (*dashed line*) for the target lines alone, which was set at a level between 70% and 80% before each session. (From Williams M, Molinet K, LeCluyse K: Visual masking as a measure of temporal processing in normal and disabled readers, *Clin Vis Sci* 4:137-144, 1989.)   *Continued*

transient system. Additional evidence for temporal processing differences between normal and disabled readers is provided by studies of the effect of wavelength on temporal aspects of visual processing.

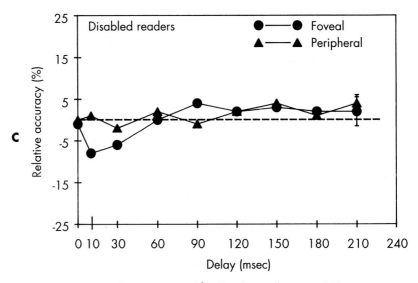

FIGURE 14-3, cont'd. For legend see p. 289.

Recent psychophysical and physiological data indicate that the wavelength of a stimulus differentially affects the response characteristics of transient and sustained processing channels. Physiological investigations of the primate visual system indicate that there are differences in the color selectivity of these systems[27] and that a steady red background light attenuates the response of transient channels.[48-50] A recent investigation by Breitmeyer and Williams[51] provides evidence that variations in wavelength produce similar effects in the human visual system. These authors found that the magnitude of both metacontrast and stroboscopic motion decreased when red, as compared with the use of equiluminant green or white backgrounds. According to transient-sustained theories of metacontrast and stroboscopic motion, the activity of transient channels is attenuated by red backgrounds. Using a metacontrast paradigm, Williams, Breitmeyer, Lovegrove, and Gutierrez[39] additionally found that the rate of processing in transient channels increases as wavelength decreases and that red light enhances the activity of sustained channels.

CLINICAL PEARL

The wavelength of a stimulus differentially affects the response characteristics of transient and sustained processing channels. The activity of transient channels is attenuated by red backgrounds.

In the context of these findings, Williams and colleagues used a metacontrast paradigm to obtain direct measures of the effects of wavelength on temporal visual processing in normal and disabled readers. Using white diagonal lines as targets, and a white, red, or blue 12 c/deg flanking grating as a mask, they obtained the metacontrast functions shown in Figures 14-4 and 14-5. Normal readers showed differences in both enhancement and dip location with the different colored masks (see Figure 14-4). The fact that the delay of maximum masking was shorter for the red than for the other masks suggests that the processing rate in transient channels is slowest with the red masks. This finding may be related to previous findings[48,51] that red light inhibits the activity of transient channels. Along the same lines, the fact that the delay in maximum masking occurred at a longer delay for the blue than for the other masks suggests that blue light may enhance the processing rate in transient channels.

CLINICAL PEARL

Blue light may enhance the processing rate in transient channels.

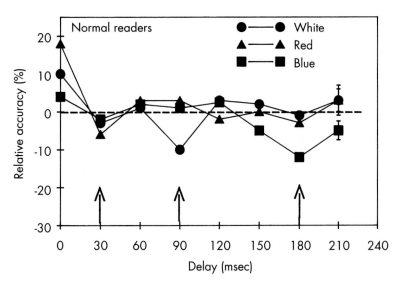

FIGURE 14-4 Metacontrast functions collected on normal readers with masks varying in wavelength. The accuracy for target lines followed by a flanking grating mask is plotted against the accuracy for target lines alone *(dashed line)*. A positive accuracy indicates that the mask enhanced the visability of the target, a negative accuracy impaired the visability.

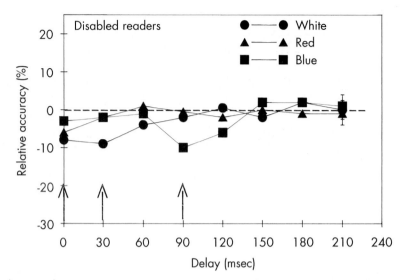

FIGURE 14-5 Metacontrast functions collected on disabled readers with masks varying in wavelength. The accuracy for target lines followed by a flanking grating mask is plotted against the accuracy for target lines alone *(dashed line).* A positive accuracy indicates that the mask enhanced the visability of the target, a negative accuracy impaired the visability.

Next, consider the differences found in the magnitude of masking at the dips in functions. Again, this is the point in the metacontrast function where the transient response to the mask maximally overlaps with, and inhibits, the sustained response to the target. Because the target is always the same, differences in the magnitude of masking at the dip can be attributed to differences in the response magnitude of transient channel activity generated by the mask. The fact that there was a smaller magnitude of masking with the red than with the shorter wavelength masks suggests that transient channels respond less vigorously to long-wavelength stimuli.

At simultaneous presentation of the target and mask, accuracy for detecting the target was enhanced over the accuracy level when the targets were presented alone. This finding is consistent with previous reports of contextual information enhancing the detectability of briefly presented targets.[46,52,53] According to masking models based on transient-sustained theory, this is the part of the function wherein figural information carried by the sustained components of response to the target and mask can interact. Because the enhancement effect varied with the wavelength of the mask, it appears that the sustained component of visual response is sensitive to variations in wavelength. The results indicate that sustained channels respond with greater sensitivity to red light than to blue or white light.

Disabled readers also showed differences in dip location and magnitude of masking with the wavelength of the mask (see Figure 14-5). Overall, dip locations occurred at shorter delays for disabled than for normal readers, suggesting that the processing rate in transient channels is slower in disabled readers. As with the normal readers, however, the processing rate in transient channels appeared to be slowest with the red mask and fastest with the blue mask. Disabled readers generally showed a smaller magnitude of masking than normal readers did, again suggesting that, overall, transient channels respond less vigorously in disabled readers. As with the normal readers, there was a smaller magnitude of masking with the red than with the shorter-wavelength masks, suggesting that transient channels respond less vigorously to long-wavelength stimuli. Finally, it is interesting to note that the function produced by the blue mask in disabled readers was similar in time course to the function produced by the white mask in normal readers, again suggesting that blue light may produce a normal time course of processing in disabled readers. This is consistent with the contention that blue light may enhance the processing rate in transient channels.

CLINICAL PEARL

Blue light may produce a normal time course of processing in disabled readers. This would be consistent with the contention that it may enhance the processing rate in transient channels.

The Use of Color as an Intervention for Reading Disability

Given the systematic effects of wavelength on the visual processing of reading-disabled children, combined with the fact that blue light can render their performance comparable to that of normal readers, Williams, LeCluyse, and Rock-Faucheux[40] investigated the effects of wavelength on actual reading performance. In this study, passages from graded reading books were covered with blue, green, red, gray, and clear plastic overlays and presented to normal and reading-disabled children. The grade level of the passages was determined by each subject's performance on a standardized reading test. The children read passages at their current measured reading levels, whether normal or delayed, and were instructed to read each passage at a rate that was comfortable for them. They also were to pay close attention to what they were reading, because they would be asked to answer questions at the end of each passage. Multiple-choice questions of literal comprehension were presented after the passages to check reading comprehension. An experimenter read each question to the children to ensure that they understood. A group of 36 children (18 normal readers and 18 disabled readers) participated in the study. They all read one story in each color condition, with the presentation order of the conditions counterbalanced among the readers. Percent correct on the reading comprehension questions and reading rate were the dependent measures.

Figure 14-6 shows the percent correct on reading comprehension questions obtained with the different colored overlays and the different groups of children. As can be seen, the blue and gray overlays produced significant improvement in the reading comprehension of

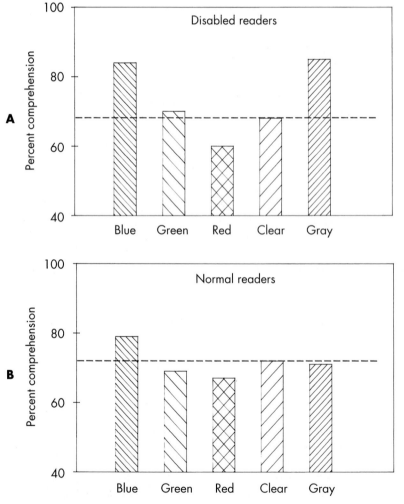

FIGURE 14-6 Reading comprehension (as measured by questions of literal recall) for passages covered with various colored overlays. **A,** Disabled readers. **B,** Normal readers.

disabled readers compared with clear overlays, whereas red overlays produced a significant decrement in performance. The performance with green overlays did not differ significantly from that with clear overlays. Among the disabled readers tested, 75% showed this pattern of results. Normal readers, likewise, showed significant improvement with the blue overlays only and a significant decrement in performance with red overlays. Reading rate increased with blue overlays compared with clear overlays in both normal and disabled readers. Disabled readers also showed an increase in reading rate with gray overlays and a significant decrease in reading rate with red overlays. Normal readers showed a decrease in reading rate with red overlays compared with the clear overlays, but this effect did not reach significance.

CLINICAL PEARL

Blue and gray overlays produced significant improvement in the reading comprehension of disabled readers compared with clear overlays, whereas red overlays produced a significant decrement in performance.

In disabled readers blue and gray overlays had equivalent effects on reading performance. It is likely, however, that these were due to effects on different visual processing mechanisms produced by these two overlays. Although the use of short-wavelength backgrounds has been found to increase the response magnitude and speed in transient channels,[39] gray filters, by reducing stimulus luminance or contrast, may instead slow the response of sustained channels more than those of transient channels.[54,55] Thus, although the mechanisms may be different, the effects on reading performance of using blue and gray overlays in reading-disabled children are the same—a temporal separation between transient and sustained responses may be created, which apparently compensates for the visual deficit of disabled readers. Normal readers, on the other hand, show reading gains only with the blue overlay, which may be due mainly to the increased magnitude of the transient response observed in visual processing of short-wavelength stimuli[39] in normal readers, resulting in greater efficiency of visual processing. Reducing contrast, however, may not be expected to benefit normal readers, because the creation of a temporal separation is not necessary in this group, and delaying sustained processing is not likely to result in greater efficiency of visual processing.

The use of a red overlay produced significant decreases in the reading performances of both normal and disabled readers. This finding may be related to the previous finding[39,51] that the use of red stimuli weaken and slow transient processing. This would serve to exacerbate the visual deficit of disabled readers and simulate a transient processing deficit in normal readers.

CLINICAL PEARL

The use of a red overlay produced significant decreases in the reading performances of both normal and disabled readers. This finding may be related to the previous finding that the use of red stimuli weaken and slow transient processing.

It should be noted that there are some individual differences that are obscured by the averaged data. For example, approximately 80% of disabled readers demonstrated an effect of color, the remaining 20% performing best with clear overlays. Furthermore, not all disabled readers showed best performance with the blue overlay; a small subgroup (approximately 5%) showed beneficial effects of red overlays. It is believed that this subgroup is representative of another type of visual syndrome called visual discomfort, which is discussed in the section that follows.

Visual Discomfort Syndrome

It is possible that a sluggish transient system represents one end of a continuum of transient system contributions to reading disability. At the other end of this hypothesized continuum lies an overactive transient system that may also result in visual perceptual impairment. As with a sluggish transient system, faster than normal transient processing may interfere with synchronization of the transient and sustained systems. Such a relationship can only be hypothesized at this point, but recent evidence suggests a neurological basis for such a phenomenon.

Williams et al.[40] found that there was also a small subgroup of children with reading disabilities who performed better with the use of red backgrounds and overlays. It is unlikely that this small subgroup of disabled readers experienced sluggish transient activity, because red filtering would attenuate transient functioning and exacerbate the transient deficit, resulting in greater reading difficulties. Rather, it is possible that this subgroup may represent a group of individuals whose transient systems are excessively fast, resulting in a visual-perceptual disorder that has been labeled *visual discomfort.*

Visual discomfort is a syndrome characterized by illusions of shape, color, and motion.[56-59] Impaired reading is only one consequence associated with this syndrome. Other impairments are frequently associated with physical symptoms of discomfort that include eye strain, headache, nausea, dizziness, and (rarely) seizures. The stimuli used to experimentally induce visual discomfort consist of square wave gratings of black and white stripes. The properties of these provocative stimuli have been identified as falling into a critical range of contrast and spatial frequency. Critical contrast is in the range of 5% to 30% Michelson; critical spatial frequency range is 1 to 8 c/deg. It has been observed[56] that many forms of text share similar spatial features with the experimental gratings and may therefore be expected to produce similar symptoms and illusions associated with visual discomfort in susceptible readers.

CLINICAL PEARL

Visual discomfort is a syndrome characterized by illusions of shape, color, and motion. Impaired reading is only one consequence. Other impairments are eye strain, headache, nausea, dizziness, and (rarely) seizures.

The mechanism by which visual discomfort is triggered is not known at this time, nor has the syndrome been investigated within a theoretical framework, as has been done for specific reading disability. There is, however, some evidence that such a syndrome may exist. Anecdotal evidence for visual anomalies in disabled readers was provided by Meares.[60] Several of the children with whom she worked described various illusions while reading, such as the encroachment of the white background on the black text, as well as shimmering, moving, and jumping of the text itself. In addition, there were complaints of physical discomfort, such as headaches and eyestrain, while trying to read. Some of these children noticed that reading was improved if they read from blackboards through colored report covers or by shading the page from the light source. All of these strategies have in common the act of contrast reduction. Unrelated studies[57,61] have found that contrast reduction is beneficial to disabled readers.

Indirect physiological evidence for visual discomfort has been provided through a series of comparisons made between photosensitive epileptogenic patients and nonepileptogenic volunteers. Wilkins et al.[58] found the same stimuli that evoked epileptiform activity in patients with photosensitive epilepsy induced self-reported symptoms of visual discomfort in nonepileptic individuals. A strong relationship was, likewise, found between the number and type of headaches and other symptoms suffered and the spatial and temporal characteristics of the test stimuli. This has not yet been tested with nonepileptogenic disabled readers to determine if they experience similar patterns of cortical activity when viewing striped patterns. Recent investigations,[62,63] however, have found abnormal EEG patterns associated with reading disability.

In an effort to empiricize visual discomfort, a pilot study[64] was recently undertaken using normal and reading-disabled children.

First, ratings of visual discomfort were collected based on a self-report questionnaire in which the children were questioned about perceptual or physical difficulties they experienced while reading.[65] Then a direct measure of visual distortion was taken that involved the children's viewing high-contrast black and white gratings composed of either square waves or typed letters. After they had viewed each stimulus for 30 seconds, they were asked to indicate if various distortions or physical symptoms of discomfort occurred. Based on their answers, an index of perceptual experience was derived. The children then viewed each stimulus through transparent colored overlays of red, blue, gray, and clear and were asked to judge whether or not the filters improved viewing of the grating. In this manner a score was obtained for each color condition.

The results provided a basis for future study of the association between visual discomfort and colored overlays. Blue and clear overlays were negatively correlated with both measures of visual discomfort, indicating that children who exhibited a high degree of visual discomfort symptoms did not benefit from viewing the stimuli through blue or clear overlays. There was also a trend, although not significant, toward a positive relationship between the self-report score and the red overlay, suggesting that, given a larger sample, red overlays might be beneficial for children reporting a large number of symptoms of visual discomfort. The data indicate that the filter color that produced greatest reading improvement for each child is associated more closely with the direct measure of visual discomfort than with the self-report measure. This particular result has implications for diagnosis and intervention, arguing for the importance of carefully researched and objective performance measures.

Wilkins has speculated that visual discomfort arises from hypersensitive transient system activity. Preliminary research with subjects experiencing a high degree of visual discomfort has indicated that their transient systems may be hypersensitive rather than deficient.[65] Thus the use of red overlays, which would function to inhibit the transient response, might be expected to reduce visual discomfort and improve reading performance. Given evidence that red stimuli attenuate transient activity and reduce visual discomfort, it is logical to assume that visual discomfort may involve, at least partially, a hypersensitive transient system that is adjusted by the application of red stimuli.

CLINICAL PEARL

Preliminary research with subjects experiencing a high degree of visual discomfort has indicated that their transient systems may be hypersensitive rather than deficient.

Comparison of SRD and Visual Discomfort

Although there are some parallels to be drawn between specific reading disability (SRD) and visual discomfort, there are many important differences that must be addressed as well. The two appear to be confused as synonymous, which also seems to be the case with *scotopic sensitivity syndrome*.[66,67] Scotopic sensitivity syndrome is defined as "a perceptual dysfunction which is related to difficulties with light source, luminance, intensity, wavelength and color contrast."[67] To date, however, there has been no documented scientific evidence to support the notion of scotopic sensitivity syndrome.[68]

The method devised by Irlen involves the use of colored glasses while reading and is based on the assumption that dyslexic individuals experience visual perceptual deficiencies. The subjects are diagnosed as reading disabled based on self-report (or, in the case of children, teacher/parent report) rather than on an objective standardized measure of reading performance. It appears that no effort is made to determine whether the subjects meet standardized criteria for dyslexia. The candidates look at various nontext stimuli through colored overlays and report if an overlay helps them read faster and more comprehensively while increasing attention and reducing fatigue. Again, objective standardized measures are not taken to determine the accuracy of the candidates' reports. Based on a positive self-report, candidates are then prescribed glasses with colored lenses.

The entire concept of scotopic sensitivity syndrome, therefore, represents a nonvalidated intervention. This ultimately leads to an invalid diagnostic and clinical picture. It is not surprising that the results of the various studies designed to investigate Irlen lenses are equivocal (for review, see Evans and Drasdo[69]).

Unfortunately, Wilkin's work in the area of visual discomfort and reading disability has involved only subjects diagnosed through the Irlen method, thus making the results difficult to interpret within a theoretical framework. In fact, the symptoms reported by Irlen as forming the basis for her clients' reading disabilities are similar in many respects to the symptoms of visual discomfort. Yet to label this syndrome "reading disability" may be inaccurate.

Visual discomfort is not a disability specific to the reading process because it appears to be potentially disruptive of many processes that may be affected by glare. Clinically, visual discomfort has not been reliably linked to standardized measures of reading disability. From a diagnostic standpoint, objective measures do not yet exist for the identification of visual discomfort.

It is possible that the conflicting findings regarding visual perceptual etiologies of reading disability are related to confusion between visual discomfort and SRD. The disorders are similar insofar as they are both visual perceptual disorders. Individuals suffering them likely share similar clinical profiles in terms of impaired reading in the absence of problems with visual acuity. Both likely involve deficits in the way the transient system processes information. Therefore, neither would necessarily show up in tasks that rely upon sustained system processing. A sole reliance upon sustained system measures might lead to the impression that a visual perceptual disorder does not exist. Visual discomfort and SRD can be further confused because of their similar effects on the reading process; that is, both affect the reading process. Finally, clinical manifestations are likely to differ between the two. SRD would appear to be the more challenging deficit to diagnose, because physical symptoms are apparently not associated with it.

These individual differences stress the need for individualized and accurate diagnostic assessment procedures, using standardized, objective instruments to distinguish different disorders. Such instruments could include psychometric measures (e.g., IQ, achievement measures), psychophysical measures (e.g., flicker photometry, masking, equiluminance studies), physiological studies (electroencephalography), and inferences drawn from intervention results as well as subjective data collected from surveys.

Summary

SRDs occur in a relatively large population of individuals afflicted with subtle visual deficits. The families of children with SRDs usually suffer years of frustration and an inordinate financial burden as they attempt to remedy the disorder. Children with SRD often endure repeated evaluations, undergo expensive treatment programs, and continue to experience frustration and disappointment as each new attempt fails. Because the deficit underlying the reading disability has not been well understood, past attempts at intervention have been ill focused and often expensive. We have found that simply reducing the contrast of text materials, or using color overlays in books, at practically no expense to the client, produces definite and measurable results. We encourage caution because there are individual differences in the effects of different colors. An objective measure of the reading performance of each individual must be obtained with various colored and gray overlays before an assignment is made. Additionally, a thorough evaluation and appropriate diagnosis of reading disability must be established before any intervention is employed. The protocol we use for colored overlay testing and assignment is presented in the Appendix.

References

1. Badcock D, Lovegrove W: The effects of contrast, stimulus duration, and spatial frequency on visible persistence in normal and specifically disabled reader, *J Expl Psychol Hum Percept Perform*, 7:495-505, 1981.
2. Critchley M: *Developmental dyslexia*, London, 1964, Heinemann.
3. Lovegrove W, Billings G, Slaghuis W: Processing of visual contour orientation information in normal and disabled reading children, *Cortex* 14:268-278, 1978.
4. Lovegrove W, Martin F, Slaghuis W: A theoretical and experimental case for a visual deficit in specific reading disability, *Cogn Neuropsychol* 3:225-267, 1986.
5. Slaghuis W, Lovegrove W: Flicker masking of spatial frequency dependent visible persistence and specific reading disability, *Perception* 13:527-534, 1984.
6. Stanley G: Visual memory process in dyslexia. In Deutsch D, Deutsch J (eds): *Short-term memory*, New York, 1975, Academic Press.
7. Lovegrove W, Brown C: Development of information processing in normal and disabled readers, *Percept Mot Skills* 46:1047-1054, 1978.
8. Stanley G, Hall R: A comparison of dyslexics and normals in recalling letter arrays after brief presentations, *Br J Educ Psychol* 43:301-304, 1973.
9. Stanley G, Hall R: Short-term visual processing information in dyslexia, *Child Dev* 44:841-844, 1973.
10. Benton A: Dyslexia in relation to form perception and directional sense. In Money J (ed): *Reading disability: progress and research needs in dyslexia*, Baltimore, 1962, Johns Hopkins Press.
11. Benton A: Developmental dyslexia: neurological aspects. In Freidman WJ: *Advances in neurology*. Vol 1, *Current reviews of higher order nervous system dysfunction*, New York, 1975, Raven Press.
12. Vellutino F: Alternative conceptualizations of dyslexia: evidence in support of verbal-deficit hypothesis, *Harvard Educ Rev* 47:334-354, 1977.
13. Vellutino F: The validity of perceptual deficit explanations of reading disability: a reply to Fletcher and Satz, *J Learn Disabil* 1:160-167, 1979.
14. Vellutino F: *Dyslexia: theory and research*, Cambridge, Mass, 1979, MIT Press.
15. Vellutino F: Dyslexia, *Sci Am* 256:34-41, 1987.
16. Vellutino F, Steger J, DeSetto L, Phillips F: Immediate and delayed recognition of visual stimuli in poor and normal readers, *J Exp Child Psychol* 19:223-232, 1975.
17. Vellutino F, Steger J, Kaman M, DeSetto L: Visual form perception in deficient and normal readers as a function of age and orthographic-linguistic familiarity, *Cortex* 11:22-30, 1975.
18. Fletcher J, Satz P: Unitary deficits hypothesis of reading disability: has Vellutino led us astray? *J Learn Disabil* 12:155-159, 1979.
19. Fletcher J, Satz P: Has Vellutino led us astray? A rejoinder to a reply, *J Learn Disabil* 12:168-171, 1979.
20. Breitmeyer B: Unmasking visual masking: a look at the "why" behind the veil of the "how," *Psychol Rev* 87:52-69, 1980.
21. Breitmeyer B: Sensory masking, persistence, and enhancement in visual exploration and reading. In Raynor K (ed): *Eye movements in reading: perceptual and language processes*, New York, 1983, Academic Press.
22. Breitmeyer B: *Visual masking: an integrated approach*, New York, 1985, Oxford University Press.
23. Breitmeyer B, Ganz L: Implications of sustained and transient channels for theories of visual pattern masking, saccadic suppression, and information processing, *Psychol Rev* 83:1-36, 1976.

24. Weisstein N, Ozog G, Szoc R: A comparison and elaboration of two models of metacontrast, *Psychol Rev* 82:325-342, 1975.
25. Cavanagh P: The contribution of color to motion. In Valberg A, Lee BB (eds): *From pigment to perception*, New York, 1991, Plenum Press.
26. Livingstone MS, Hubel DH: Psychophysical evidence for separate channels for the perception of form, color, movement and depth, *J Neurosci* 7:3416-3468, 1987.
27. Livingstone MS, Hubel DH: Segregation of form, color, movement, and depth: anatomy, physiology, and perception, *Science* 240:740-749, 1988.
28. Maunsell JHR: Physiological evidence for two visual subsystems. In Vaina L (ed): *Matters of intelligence*, Amsterdam, 1987, Reidel.
29. Lovegrove W, Heddle M, Slaghuis W: Reading disability: spatial frequency specific deficits in visual information store, *Neuropsychologica* 18:111-115, 1980.
30. Lovegrove W, Martin F, Bowling A et al: Contrast sensitivity functions and specific reading disability, *Neuropsychologia* 20:309-315, 1982.
31. Martin F, Lovegrove W: Flicker contrast sensitivity in normal and specifically disabled readers, *Perception* 16:215-221, 1987.
32. Brannan J, Williams M: Allocation of visual attention in good and poor readers, *Percept Psychophys* 41:23-28, 1987.
33. Brannan J, Williams M: The effects of age and reading ability on flicker thresholds, *Clin Vis Sci* 3:137-142, 1988.
34. Brannan J, Williams M: Developmental versus sensory deficit effects on perceptual processing in the reading disabled, *Percept Psychophys,* 44:437-444, 1988.
35. Williams M, Bologna N: Perceptual grouping in good and poor readers, *Percept Psychophys* 38:367-374, 1985.
36. Williams M, LeCluyse K: Perceptual consequences of a temporal deficit in disabled reading children, *J Am Optom Assoc* 61:111-121, 1990.
37. Williams M, Brannan J, Lartigue E: Visual search in good and poor readers, *Clin Vis Sci* 1:367-371, 1987.
38. Williams M, Molinet K, LeCluyse K: Visual masking as a measure of temporal processing in normal and disabled readers, *Clin Vis Sci* 4:137-144, 1989.
39. Williams M, Breitmeyer B, Lovegrove W, Gutierrez C: Metacontrast with masks varying in spatial frequency and wavelength, *Vision Res* 31:2017-2033, 1991.
40. Williams M, LeCluyse K, Rock-Faucheux A: Effective interventions for reading disability, *J Am Optom Assoc* 63:411-417, 1992.
41. Matin E: The two-transient (masking) paradigm, *Psychol Rev* 82:451-461, 1975.
42. Weisstein N: A Rashevsky-Landahl neural net: simulation of metacontrast, *Psychol Rev* 75:494-521, 1968.
43. Weisstein N: Metacontrast. In Jameson D, Hurvich LM (eds): *Handbook of sensory physiology*, New York, 1972, Springer-Verlag.
44. Kolers P, Rosner B: On visual masking (metacontrast): dichoptic observations, *Am J Psychol* 73:2-21, 1960.
45. Stewart A, Purcell D: U-shaped masking functions in visual backward masking: effects of target configuration and retinal position, *Percept Psychophys* 7:253-256, 1970.
46. Williams M, Weisstein N: Spatial frequency response and perceived depth in the time-course of object-superiority, *Vision Res* 21:631-645, 1981.
47. Geiger G, Lettvin J: Peripheral vision in persons with dyslexia, *N Engl J Med* 316:1238-1243, 1987.
48. Dreher B, Fukuda Y, Rodieck R: Identification, classification, and anatomical segregation of cells with X-like and Y-like properties in the lateral geniculate nucleus of old-world primates, *J Physiol* 258:433-452, 1976.
49. Kruger J: Stimulus-dependent color specificity of monkey lateral geniculate neurones, *Exp Brain Res* 30:297-311, 1977.
50. Schiller P, Malpeli J: Functional specificity of lateral geniculate nucleus laminae of the rhesus monkey, *J Neurophysiol* 41:788-797, 1978.

51. Breitmeyer B, Williams M: Background color affects the magnitude of lateral masking and stroboscopic motion, *Vision Res* 30:1069-1075, 1990.
52. Weisstein N, Harris C: Visual detection of line segments: and object-superiority effect, *Science* 186:752-755, 1974.
53. Williams M, Weisstein N: The effects of perceived depth on metacontrast functions, *Vision Res* 24:1279-1288, 1984.
54. Breitmeyer B, Clark CD, Hogben JH, DiLollo V: The metacontrast masking in relation to stimulus size and intensity, *Rev Suisse Psychol* 50:87-96, 1990.
55. Harwerth R, Levi D: Reaction time as a measure of suprathreshold grating detection, *Vision Res* 18:1579-1586, 1978.
56. Wilkins A: Visual discomfort and reading. In Stein J (ed): *Reading and reading disabilities,* London, 1991, Macmillan.
57. Wilkins A, Nimmo-Smith I: On the reduction of eye-strain when reading, *Ophthalmic Physiol Opt* 4:53-59, 1984.
58. Wilkins A, Nimmo-Smith I, Tait A et al: A neurological basis for visual discomfort, *Brain* 107:989-1017, 1984.
59. Wilkins AJ, Neary C: Some visual, optometric, and perceptual effects of colored glasses, *Ophthalmic Physiol Opt* 11:163-171, 1991.
60. Meares O: Figure/ground, brightness contrast, and reading disabilities, *Vis Lang* 14:13-29, 1980.
61. Giddings EH, Carmean SL: Reduced brightness contrast as a reading aid, *Percept Mot Skills* 69:383-386, 1989.
62. Hughes JR: Evaluation of electrophysiological studies on dyslexia. In Gray DB, Kavanagh JF (eds): *Biobehavioral measures of dyslexia,* Parkton, Md, 1985, York Press.
63. Shucard DW, Cummins KR, Gay E et al: Electrophysiological studies of reading-disabled children: in search of subtypes. In Gray DB, Kavanagh JF (eds): *Biobehavioral measures of dyslexia,* Parkton, Md, 1985, York Press.
64. LeCluyse K, Williams M: Visual discomfort and reading disability. (In preparation, 1995.)
65. Lovegrove W: Personal communication, 1990.
66. Irlen H: Successful treatment of learning disabilities. Presented at the 91st Annual Convention of the American Psychological Association, Anaheim, Calif, 1983.
67. Irlen H, Lass MJ: Improving reading problems due to symptoms of Scotopic Sensitivity Syndrome using Irlen lenses and overlays, *Education* 109:413-417, 1989.
68. Solan HA: An appraisal of the Irlen technique of correcting reading disorders using tinted overlays and tinted lenses, *J Learn Disabil* 23:621-623.
69. Evans BJW, Drasdo N: Tinted lenses and related therapies for learning disabilities: a review, *Ophthalmic Physiol Opt* 11:206-217, 1991.
70. LeCluyse K, Williams M, Rock-Faucheux A: Towards an effective intervention for specific reading disabilities, *J Learn Disabil* (submitted).

Appendix Protocol For Colored Overlay Evaluation

To screen children for a specific reading disability, we recommend, in addition to a complete visual examination, an IQ measure, an individually administered standardized reading test, an auditory processing screen, language assessment, attentional measures, and a social/emotional measure.

Because poor reading skills can be the result of a variety of disabling factors, a child may be diagnosed as specifically reading disabled only if his or her IQ is average or above, the score on a standardized test of reading shows a 2-year delay, there is no behavioral or organic disorder, and normal sensory functioning is exhibited. Children meeting these criteria can be tested with the overlays.

A quiet room free of distractions, with a good light source, is required for the evaluation. The testing is conducted with a set of eight standardized reading passages that include multiple-choice comprehension questions.[70] The passages should be at the child's current reading grade level, whether normal or delayed, as determined by a standardized reading test. A set of four clean transparencies (red, blue, gray, clear) is also needed, along with an answer form on which to record the responses. The examiner should have a stopwatch and a separate form on which to record the passage number, overlay color, reading time, and comprehension score.

Testing Protocol

1. Choose the appropriate set of passages at the child's present reading level. Assign a passage to each overlay.
2. Present the following instructions:
   I am going to give you some stories to read. Read at a pace that is comfortable for you. Pay attention to what you read, because you will need to answer questions about the story at the end. While you are reading, keep the page completely covered with the plastic overlay that I give you. You may tilt the book so there is no glare on the page while you are reading. When you reach the end of the first page, continue on the next page until you reach the end of the story. Raise your hand when you are finished reading the story. Do you have any questions about the instructions?
3. Lay the overlay flat in the book. Help the child position the book so there is no glare coming from the overlay.
4. Tell the child to begin. Start timing immediately.
5. When the child is finished, stop the watch and record the time (minutes and seconds).
6. Immediately read the questions out loud as the child reads silently. Have the child use the same color overlay to read the questions. Have the child record answers on the answer sheet.

7. Repeat the procedure using all of the overlays twice, for a total of eight stories. Randomize the order of overlay presentation for each trial.

Calculate an efficiency ratio for each color of overlay by the following method: First, take the average comprehension score and reading rate for trial 1 and trial 2 of each color condition. Next, convert the rate into a proportion by dividing the number of seconds by 60 and adding that value to the number of minutes. Finally, divide the number of correct answers by the rate. Compare each efficiency ratio to the efficiency ratio for the clear overlay. If a colored overlay increases the efficiency ratio relative to the clear overlay, the child should be assigned overlays of that color. Assign the color overlay that produces the largest efficiency gain relative to the clear overlay. If the highest efficiency ratio is associated with the clear overlay, it should be assumed that there is no color overlay effect for that child.

If there is a demonstrated color overlay effect, present the child with the overlays (we provide two), instructing him or her to use the overlays at home and at school for any work that involves reading. To increase compliance, explain the benefits of the overlays (e.g., more comfort and ease of reading, better grades). It is important to explain to the parents that the use of overlays will enhance the reading process and have immediate effects on reading comprehension. Overlays do not, however, remedy poorly developed decoding abilities. Therefore, tutoring is often recommended to assist the child in catching up to grade level when the child's basic skills are significantly delayed. If there is no demonstrated color effect, it is important to explain to both the parents and the child that, while many children are helped with the overlays, there are many children who do not read better using colored overlays. Possible directions for remediation can then be appropriately addressed.

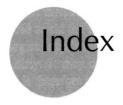

Index

Page numbers in *italic type* refer to figures. Tables are indicated by *t* following the page number.